Skull and Spine Imaging

An Atlas of
Differential Diagnosis

Skull and Spine Imaging

An Atlas of Differential Diagnosis

Ronald L. Eisenberg, M.D.
Chairman of Radiology
Highland General Hospital
Oakland, California
and
Clinical Professor of Radiology
University of California at San Francisco and Davis

Raven Press 🐾 New York

Raven Press Ltd., 1185 Avenue of the Americas, New York, New York 10036

Library of Congress Cataloging-in-Publication Data

Eisenberg, Ronald L.
    Skull and spine imaging : an atlas of differential diagnosis / Ronald Eisenberg.
        p.   cm.
    Includes bibliographical references and index.
    ISBN 0-7817-0047-7
    1. Skull—Imaging—Atlases.   2. Spine—Imaging—Atlases.   3. Diagnosis,
Differential.   I. Title.
    [DNLM: 1. Diagnosis, Differential—atlases.   2. Diagnostic Imaging—
atlases.   3. Skull—pathology—atlases.   4. Spine—pathology—
atlases.   WE 17 E36s]
    RC936.E47   1993
    617.5'140754'0222—dc20
    DNLM/DLC
    for Library of Congress   92—49419
                                                                                        CIP

9 8 7 6 5 4 3 2 1

To Zina, Avlana, and Cherina

Contents

SPINE PATTERNS

Preface

Pattern recognition leading to the development of differential diagnoses is the essence of imaging. When faced with a specific finding on a plain radiograph, CT scan, MR image, or myelogram, residents and practitioners in radiology, neurology, and neurosurgery are often unaware of the underlying disease and must suggest a differential diagnosis and a rational diagnostic approach. This book offers differential diagnoses for a broad spectrum of radiologic patterns involving the skull and spine. Added to these lists are descriptions of the specific imaging findings to be expected for each diagnostic entity as well as differential points to aid the reader in arriving at a precise diagnosis. This book includes numerous illustrations to point out the often subtle differences in appearance among conditions that can produce a similar overall radiographic pattern. Extensive cross-referencing is also included to limit duplication and to permit the reader to find various radiographic manifestations of the same condition.

For convenient use, this book is divided into two parts: *Skull Patterns*, with 45 diagnostic chapters, and *Spine Patterns*, with 26 diagnostic chapters. This approach will make the book easier to use by the busy practitioner and also will provide a logical basis for any general review of imaging of diseases of the skull and spine.

Ronald L. Eisenberg, M.D.

Skull Patterns
1

DIFFUSE DEMINERALIZATION OR DESTRUCTION
OF THE SKULL

Condition	Imaging Findings	Comments
Osteoporosis	Generalized demineralization of the skull.	Most commonly a condition of aging (senile or postmenopausal osteoporosis). Also a manifestation of deficiency states, endocrine disorders, and steroid therapy.
Hyperparathyroidism (Fig SK1-1)	Diffuse granular pattern of skull demineralization.	Irregular demineralization produces the characteristic salt-and-pepper skull. Individual brown tumors and hemorrhagic cysts may occur (best seen after the removal of a parathyroid adenoma because of remineralization of the surrounding bone).
Paget's disease (osteoporosis circumscripta) (Fig SK1-2)	Sharply defined lucent zone that is usually large and may involve more than half the calvarium. Primarily involves the outer table, sparing the inner table.	Represents the destructive phase of the disease that usually begins in the frontal or occipital area. The development of irregular islands of sclerosis during the reparative process results in a mottled, cotton-wool appearance.
Osteogenesis imperfecta (see Fig SK12-2)	Diffusely thin and lucent bones with abnormally wide sutures simulating increased intracranial pressure.	As calvarial ossification proceeds, a number of wormian bones may develop in the sutural gaps. Multiple fractures may occur in the paper-thin skull.
Hypophosphatasia (Fig SK1-3)	Large unossified areas in the skull simulate severe widening of the sutures.	If the infant survives and calvarial recalcification occurs, there may be premature closure of the sutures.
Rickets	Thin, lucent skull in infants with severe disease.	Fine lucent lines traversing the calvarium may mimic multiple fractures.

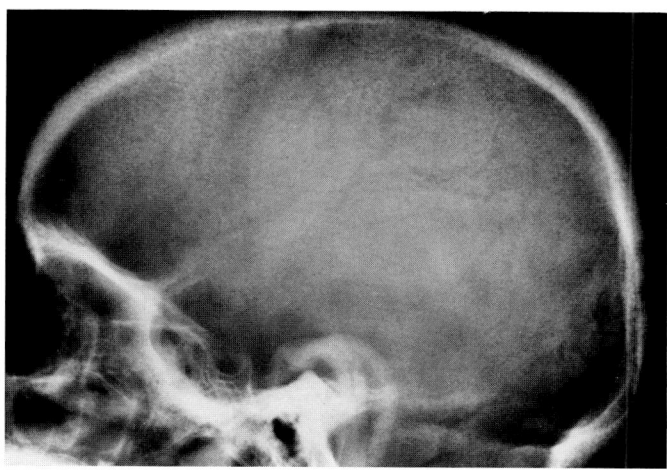

Fɪɢ SK1-1. **Hyperparathyroidism.** Characteristic salt-and-pepper skull.

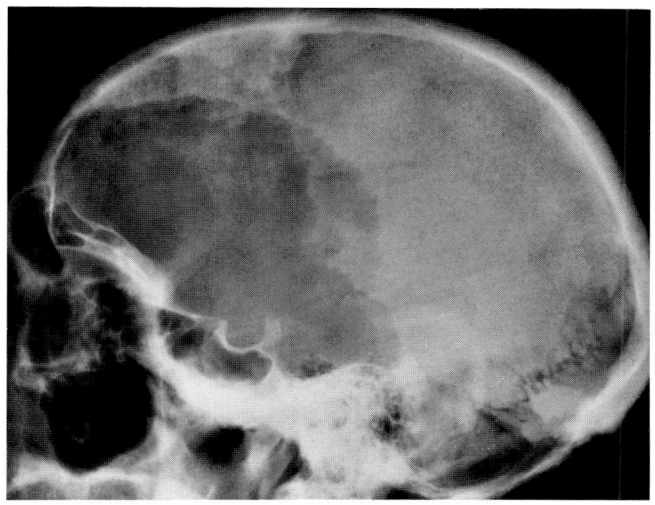

Fɪɢ SK1-2. **Paget's disease** (osteoporosis circumscripta).

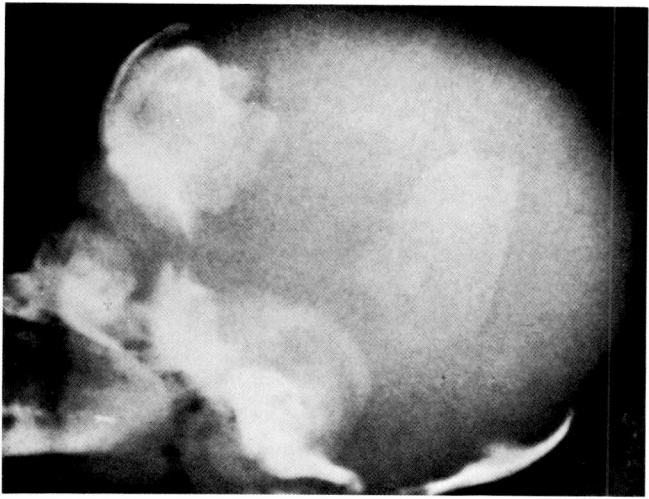

Fɪɢ SK1-3. **Hypophosphatasia.** Large areas of uncalcified osteoid in the membranous bones in the region adjoining the sutures and, to a lesser extent, at the base.[1]

LYTIC DEFECTS (SINGLE OR MULTIPLE) IN THE SKULL

Condition	Imaging Findings	Comments
Neoplasm **Metastases**	Multiple irregular, ill-defined lucent areas of various sizes. A solitary metastasis may occasionally present as a larger area of bone destruction.	Lytic metastases may arise from a wide spectrum of malignant neoplasms, most commonly carcinomas of the breast and lung. Solitary metastases are most likely to arise from carcinomas of the thyroid and kidney.
Multiple myeloma **(Fig SK2-1)**	Multiple sharply circumscribed ("punched-out") osteolytic lesions that are scattered throughout the skull and are relatively uniform in size.	Although often indistinguishable from metastatic carcinoma, the lytic defects in multiple myeloma tend to be more discrete and uniform in size. A solitary lytic defect (plasmacytoma) may occasionally exist for years and be the only osseous manifestation of a plasma-cell dyscrasia.
Lymphoma/leukemia	Multiple poorly defined lytic areas that may become confluent.	Most common in childhood leukemia. Spreading of cranial sutures indicates increased intracranial pressure secondary to central nervous system involvement.
Neuroblastoma	Widespread punctate areas of destruction.	Elevation of the periosteum causes radial bone spiculation extending into the soft tissues. A similar process occurring between the inner table and the dura with invasion of the sutures results in marked sutural spreading.
Primary sarcoma **of bone**	Large lytic area with poorly defined margins.	Rare site of osteosarcoma, chondrosarcoma, or fibrosarcoma. There may occasionally be radiating bony spicules in osteosarcoma or stippled calcifications in chondrosarcoma.
Meningioma	Purely lytic lesion with irregular margins and a faint reticular or spiculated internal architecture (on tangential view).	Unusual manifestation that occurs when a tumor infiltrating the bone causes erosion rather than the much more common hyperostosis. The association of enlarged dural arterial grooves or tumor calcification aids in making the diagnosis.
Hemangioma **(see Fig SK4-7)**	Expansile lytic lesion that arises in the diploic space.	Usually contains characteristic osseous spicules that radiate from the center to produce a sunburst pattern.
Direct extension **of tumor**	Destructive process involving the base of the skull.	Contiguous spread into adjacent areas of the skull from carcinoma of the paranasal sinuses or nasopharynx.
Erosion by other **intracranial tumors**	Indistinct, patchy area of lucency.	Rare manifestation of carcinoma metastatic to the brain and meninges. The underlying intracranial tumor dominates the clinical picture.
Neurofibromatosis **(Fig SK2-2)**	Irregular lytic defects in the occipital and temporal bones.	Rare manifestation. Neurofibromatosis more commonly produces orbital dysplasia, in which unilateral absence of a large part of the greater wing of the sphenoid and hypoplasia and elevation of the lesser wing result in a markedly widened superior orbital fissure.
Skin malignancy **(Fig SK2-3)**	Ill-defined lucent defect that initially affects the outer table.	Rare manifestation of extension of a malignant skin tumor to destroy the underlying skull.

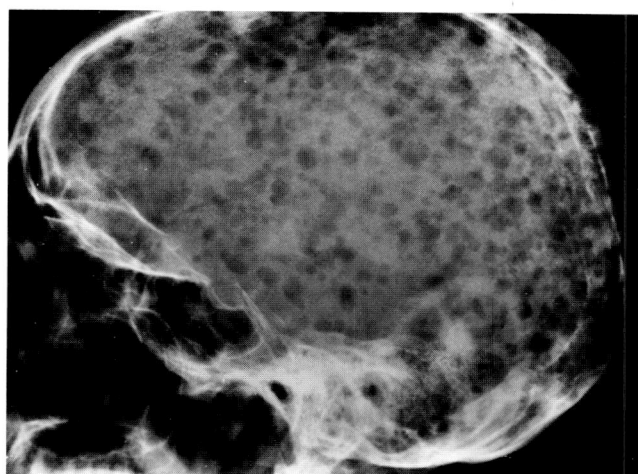

FIG SK2-1. Multiple myeloma. Diffuse punched-out osteolytic lesions scattered throughout the skull.

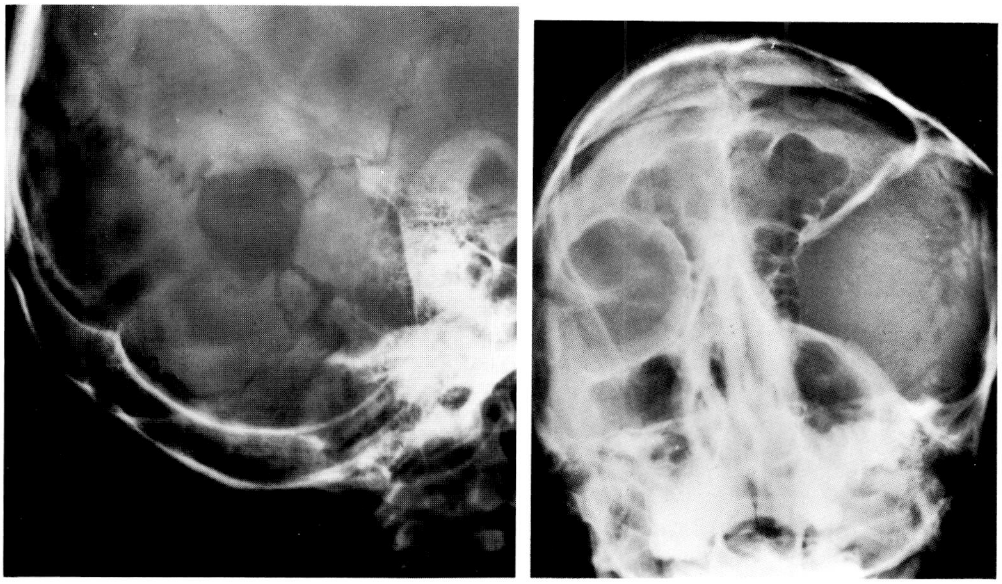

FIG SK2-2. Neurofibromatosis. (A) Mesenchymal defect in the lambdoid suture. (B) Severe orbital dysplasia with virtual absence of the posterolateral walls of the orbit.

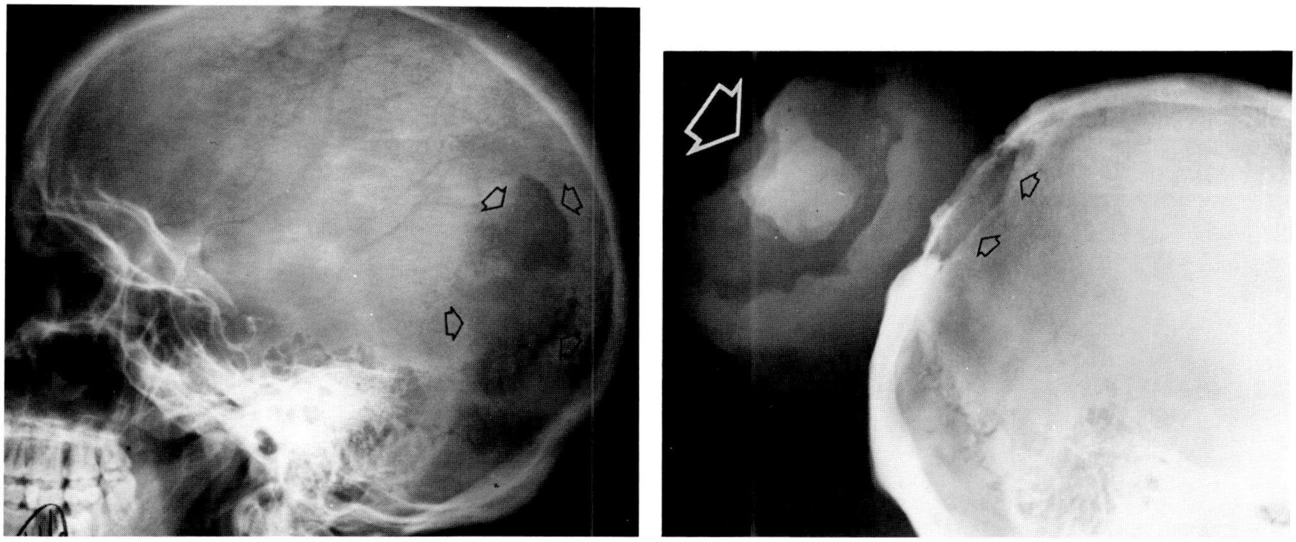

FIG SK2-3. Scalp malignancy. (A) Ill-defined lucency (arrows) representing erosion of the underlying skull. (B) Huge soft-tissue mass (white arrow) eroding the skull (black arrows).

Condition	Imaging Findings	Comments
Congenital or developmental defect		
Lacunar skull (Fig SK2-4)	Large radiolucent areas of calvarial thinning in newborns and infants, producing a pattern simulating exaggerated convolutional impressions.	Usually an underlying meningocele of the skull or spine or hydrocephalus due to aqueductal stenosis or an Arnold-Chiari malformation. There may even be a complete calvarial defect (fenestra).
Parietal foramina (Fig SK2-5)	Small, symmetric, smoothly marginated openings situated posteriorly on both sides of the sagittal suture and through which emissary veins pass.	Normal finding with no pathologic significance. Although these foramina are usually small, they may be as large as 2 to 3 cm in diameter.
Parietal thinning	Crescentic lucencies over the middle and upper parts of the parietal bones.	Normal variant consisting of marked thinning of the superior portion of the parietal bones.
Pacchionian depressions (Fig SK2-6)	Multiple smooth erosions of the inner table representing underlying dural venous pools. Usually located parasagittally within 3 cm of the midline.	Arachnoid granulations (pacchionian bodies) for the absorption of cerebrospinal fluid fill the parasagittal venous lakes, which receive blood laterally from hemispheric veins and communicate medially with the superior sagittal sinus.
Epidermoid (primary cholesteatoma) (Fig SK2-7)	Generally round, frequently lobulated, lytic lesion with a thin, well-defined sclerotic border.	Benign lesion caused by the congenital inclusion of ectoderm in the diploic space. The keratinizing epithelium proliferates and desquamates, resulting in slow expansion of the tumor with erosion of diploic bone and displacement of the inner and outer tables. Erosion of the tumor through the inner table occasionally results in a large intracranial component.
Arachnoid cyst (Fig SK2-8)	Smooth lucency, often with a thin sclerotic rim.	Localized pressure causes outward bowing of the inner table and thinning of the diploic space. Although usually congenital, may be due to trauma or inflammation.
Dermoid cyst	Small round lucency without surrounding sclerosis. Usually occurs near the midline.	Benign lesion arising in the diploic space as a result of the congenital inclusion of ectoderm and mesoderm.
Meningocele/ encephalocele	Midline bone defect that is generally round with smooth, well-defined, slightly sclerotic margins.	Herniation of brain, meninges, or both through a variably sized skull defect. Most commonly involves the occipital bone, followed by the frontal bone and the base of the skull.
Arteriovenous malformation	Localized area of skull thinning.	Infrequent manifestation overlying a superficial intracranial angioma.
Fibrous dysplasia (Fig SK2-9)	Blister-like expansion of bone with relative lucency in the center. There usually are areas of formless sclerosis lying in the lucent region and abnormally dense bone about the periphery of the lesion.	Radiolucency of the fibrous "cysts" is only relative because they are always surrounded by disorganized, densely woven bone. A mixed lytic and sclerotic pattern is the major calvarial manifestation.

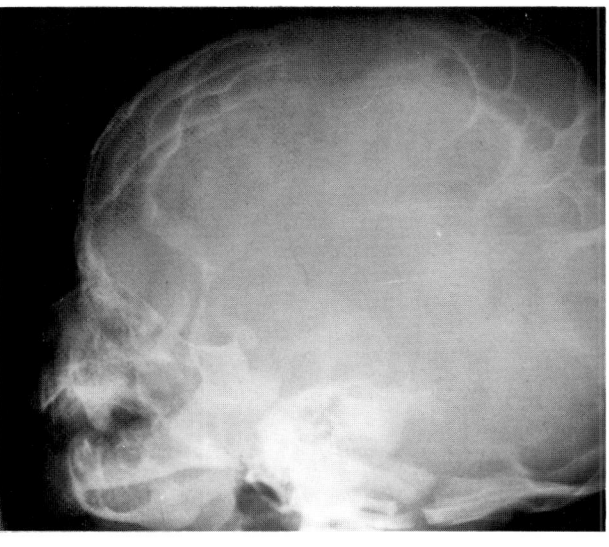

FIG SK2-4. Lacunar skull. Pattern resembling pronounced convolutional impressions.

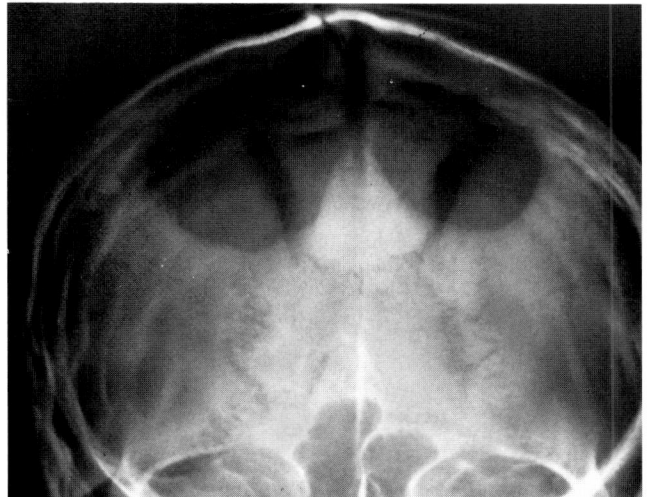

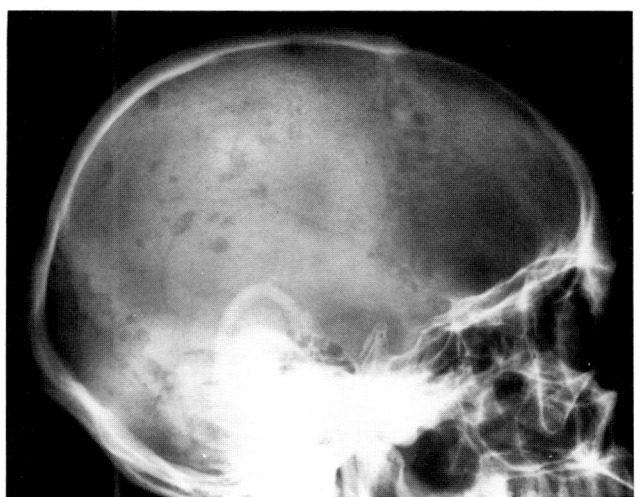

FIG SK2-5. Parietal foramina. (A) Plain skull radiograph. (B) Scan.

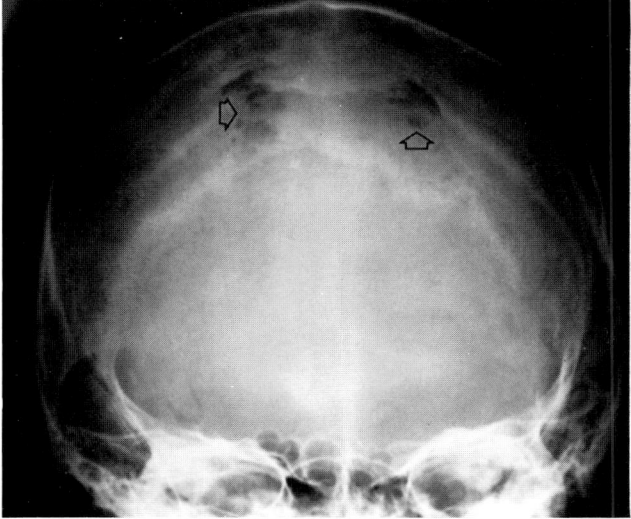

FIG SK2-6. Pacchionian depressions. (A) Frontal and (B) lateral views of the skull show multiple lucent venous lakes (arrows).

Condition	Imaging Findings	Comments
Trauma		
Burr hole/ craniotomy	Lytic defect of variable size.	Margins are initially beveled and smooth, but may become irregular with new bone formation.
Skull fracture (Figs SK2-10 and SK2-11)	Sharp lucent line that is often irregular or jagged and occasionally branches.	Must be distinguished from suture lines (which generally have serrated edges and tend to be bilateral and symmetric) and vascular grooves (which usually have a smooth curving course and are not as sharp or distinct as a fracture line). Fractures involving the sinuses or mastoid air cells may result in posttraumatic pneumocephalus. Fractures intersecting a suture and coursing along it (diastatic fractures) cause sutural separation.
Leptomeningeal cyst (growing fracture) (Fig SK2-12)	Enlarging bone defect that typically has smooth, scalloped, well-defined margins.	Complication of skull fracture in infants and children. Soft tissue or a pouch of arachnoid membrane interposed between the fracture edges prevents healing and leads to widening of the fracture line.
Inflammation		
Osteomyelitis (Fig SK2-13)	Multiple irregular, poorly defined lytic areas that may enlarge and coalesce centrally with an expanding perimeter of small satellite foci. As elsewhere in the skeleton, the radiographic changes often lag 1 to 2 weeks behind the clinical symptoms and signs.	Most commonly due to direct extension of a suppurative process from the paranasal sinuses, mastoids, or scalp. May also develop after direct contaminating trauma. Pyogenic calvarial osteomyelitis may remain a predominantly lytic process until treated and may closely resemble a malignant lesion. The appearance of a host response (poorly defined reactive sclerosis superimposed on the initial lytic changes) is characteristic of chronic osteomyelitis caused by syphilis, tuberculosis, or fungal infection.
Hydatid (echinococcal) cyst	Large expanding lesion causing thinning and destruction of bone.	Multilocular cysts usually break through the bone, resulting in erosion and destruction of bone and invasion of the cranial cavity. A unilocular cyst may become an enormous expanding lesion with walls covered by impressions as in convolutional atrophy.
Cholesteatoma	Well-circumscribed lytic defect centered on the attic and often extending into the mastoid antrum.	Complication of chronic otomastoiditis that usually arises in the presence of sclerotic, poorly pneumatized mastoid air cells. Typically causes displacement or erosion of the ossicles, blunting of the scutum, and erosion of Korner's septum.
Sarcoidosis	Smooth lytic defect without marginal sclerosis.	Infrequent and nonspecific manifestation of this granulomatous disease of unknown etiology.
Miscellaneous		
Parietal thinning of aging	Symmetric thinning of the middle and upper parts of the parietal bones.	Although occurring as a normal variant in younger individuals, there is evidence that parietal thinning may increase, become more obvious, or turn into true defects with advancing age.
Histiocytosis X (Fig SK2-14)	Solitary or multiple small punched-out areas that originate in the diploic space and expand to perforate the inner and outer tables.	Margins of an eosinophilic granuloma are usually well defined and often beveled. The calvarial defect may have a bony density in its center (button sequestrum). The more malignant forms of the disease can produce multiple larger and more irregular skull defects in young children.

(continued page 10)

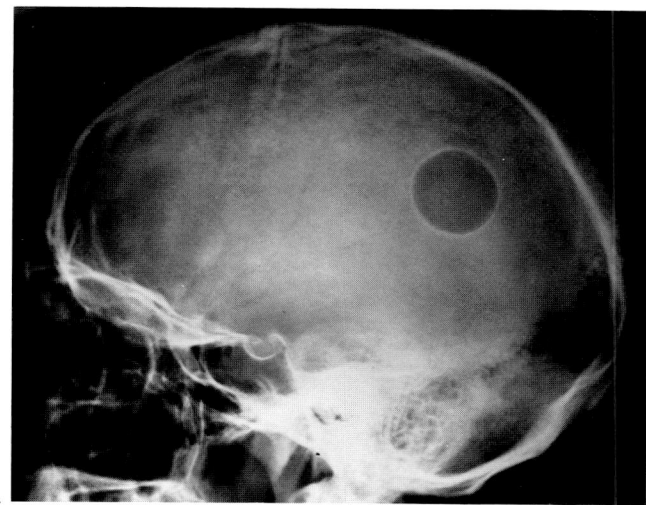 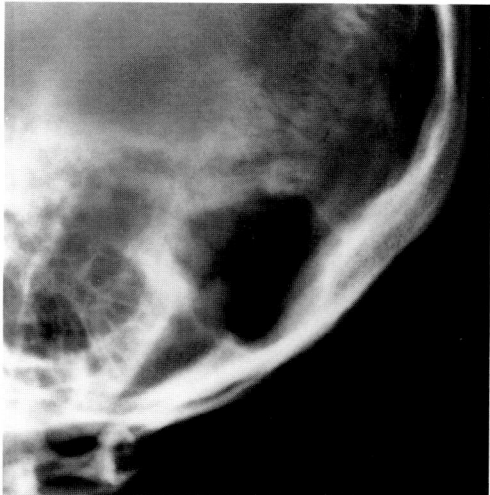

FIG SK2-7. Epidermoid. (A) Round lucent lesions with a smooth dense peripheral ring of sclerosis at the margin. (B) In another patient, there is erosion of the inner table of the posterior fossa.

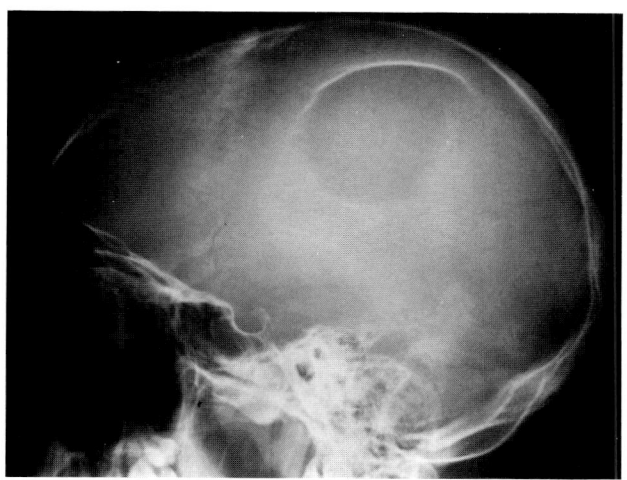

FIG SK2-8. Arachnoid cyst. Large parietal lucency with a thin sclerotic rim along its superior border.

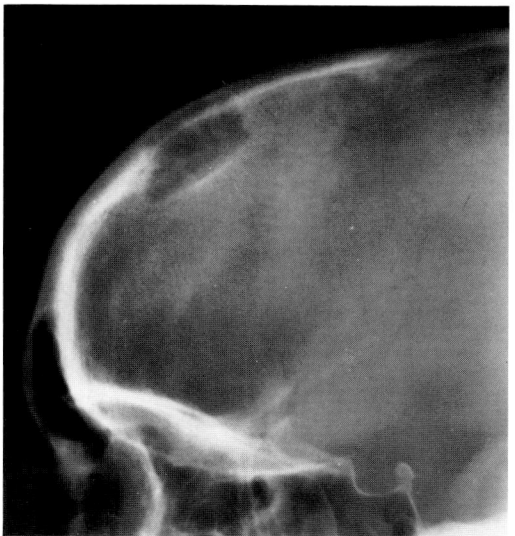 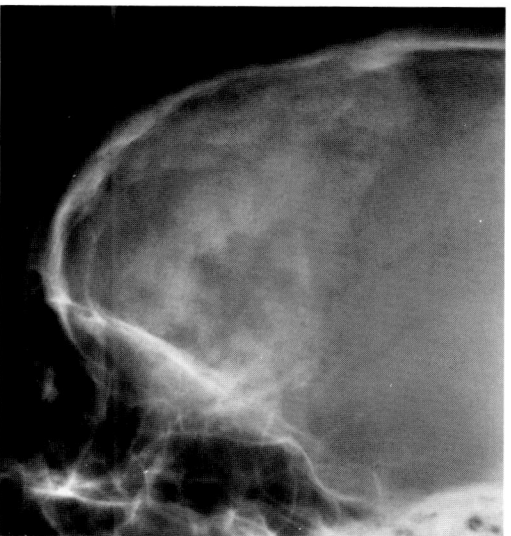

FIG SK2-9. Fibrous dysplasia. (A) Isolated lytic process. (B) In another patient, the lucent region is surrounded by abnormally dense bone.

Condition	Imaging Findings	Comments
Hyperparathyroidism (see Fig SK1-1)	Poorly defined lesions (solitary or multiple) surrounded by granular demineralization (salt-and-pepper skull).	Individual brown tumors and hemorrhagic cysts may be better seen after the removal of a parathyroid adenoma because of remineralization of the surrounding bone. After treatment, brown tumors heal by filling in with bone and may persist as sclerotic foci.
Radiation necrosis	Multiple lytic foci that coalesce. No evidence of sclerosis or periosteal new bone formation.	Aseptic necrosis of the skull, particularly a bone flap, may occur after the irradiation of an intracranial tumor. The appearance often mimics that of osteomyelitis, though it develops very slowly. The skull may return to an almost normal appearance after healing.
Paget's disease (osteoporosis circumscripta) (see Fig SK1-2)	Sharply circumscribed area of lucency representing the destructive phase of the disease. Primarily involves the outer table, sparing the inner table.	Deossification begins in the frontal or occipital area and spreads slowly to encompass the major portion of the calvarium. During the reparative process, the development of irregular islands of sclerosis in the inner table combined with thickening of the diploë and later the outer table results in the characteristic mottled, cotton-wool appearance.

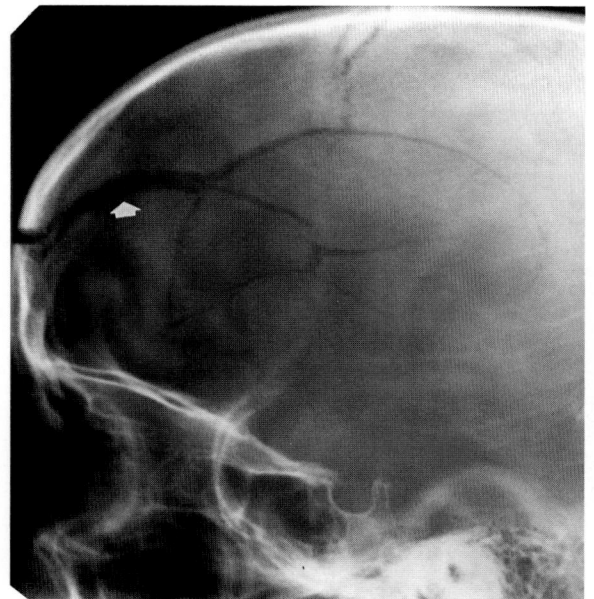

FIG SK2-10. **Skull fracture.** Widely diastatic fracture (arrow) extending to a stellate array of linear fractures.

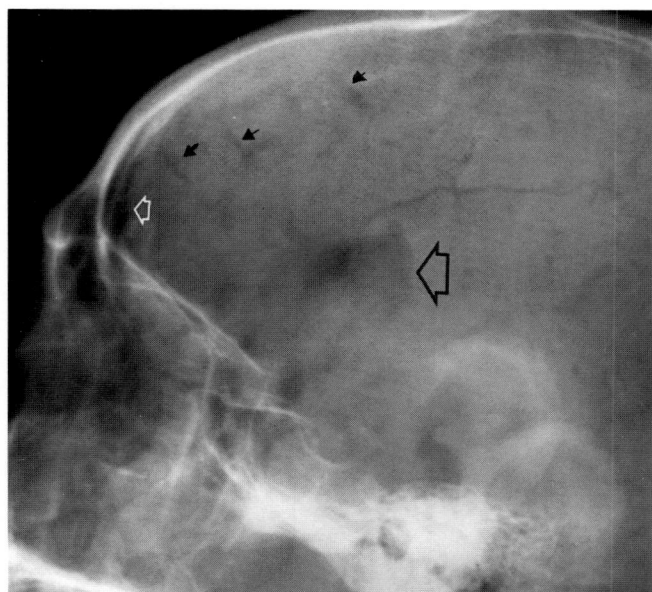

FIG SK2-11. **Posttraumatic pneumocephalus.** Lateral view of the skull made with a horizontal beam and the patient supine demonstrates air in the anterior recesses of the lateral ventricle (open black arrow), anterior to the frontal lobe (open white arrow), and in the subarachnoid space outlining the sulci (closed black arrows). The patient had sustained multiple facial fractures, some of which involved the walls of the sinuses.

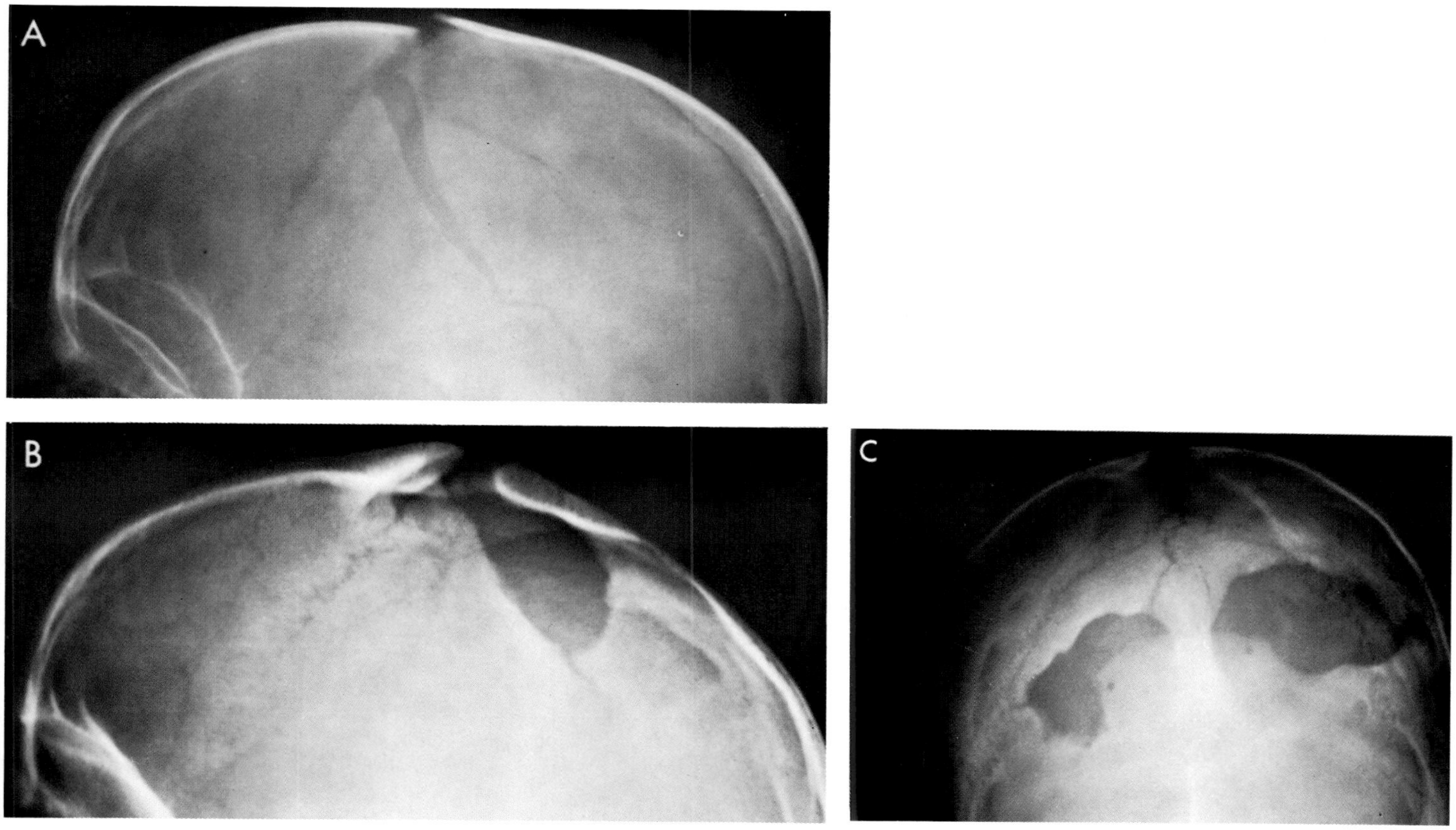

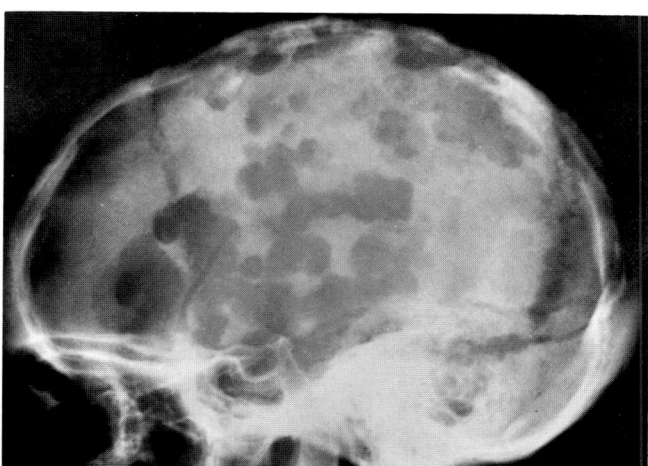

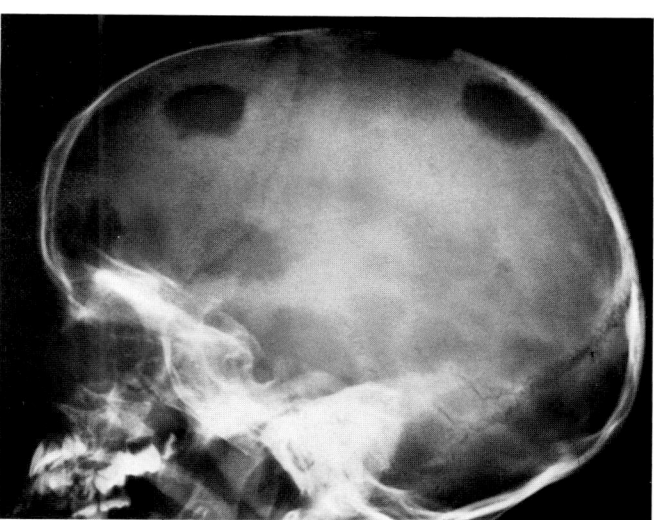

FIG SK2-12. Pulsating leptomeningeal cyst with residual bilateral large defects in the calvarium. (A) An initial lateral view shows diastatic bilateral comminuted parietal fractures after head injury during infancy. (B) Lateral and (C) frontal views 5 years later show large bilateral defects at the sites of the earlier parietal fractures. At surgery, the dura beneath the fractures was found to be torn. The bone on the margins of the defect is sclerotic and thickened.[2]

FIG SK2-13. Blastomycosis osteomyelitis. Diffuse areas of osteolytic destruction affect most of the calvarium.

FIG SK2-14. Histiocytosis X. Multiple punched-out lytic lesions in the skull. Note the beveled appearance of the inner margins.

BUTTON SEQUESTRUM*

Condition	Comments
Eosinophilic granuloma **(Fig SK3-1)**	Most common cause and usually associated with pain or tenderness over the area. The lesion originates in the diploic space and expands to perforate both the inner and outer tables. The margins are usually well defined and often beveled.
Neoplasm **(Fig SK3-2)**	Meningioma; metastases; dermoid cyst; epidermoid; hemangioma.
Infection **(Fig SK3-3)**	Tuberculous osteitis; staphylococcal abscess of the scalp.
Radiation necrosis	More commonly produces purely lytic areas of destruction in the skull that do not develop until at least 5 years after therapy.
Iatrogenic	Appearance mimicking that of a button sequestrum due to a superficially placed polyethylene shunt reservoir within a burr hole.
Calvarial "doughnut" **(Fig SK3-4)**	Lucent region containing densities of various sizes that is an incidental finding on routine skull radiographs. This entity invariably has a sclerotic outer border and is benign and asymptomatic, unlike button sequestra, which are frequently associated with localized pain or soft-tissue abnormalities in the region of the bony lesion.

*Pattern: Round, lucent calvarial defect with a bony density or sequestrum in its center.

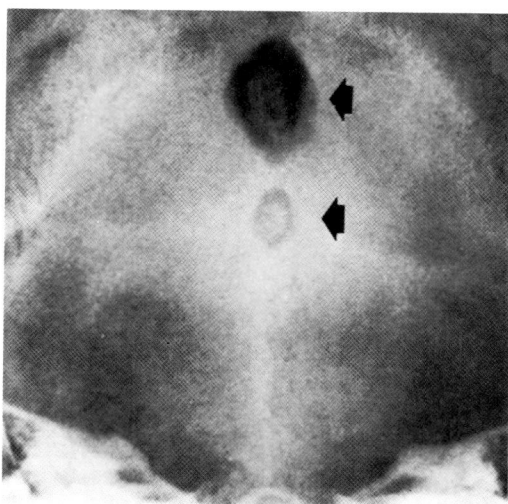

FIG SK3-1. **Eosinophilic granuloma.** Central retained bone is seen in each of two midline parietal lesions (arrows).[3]

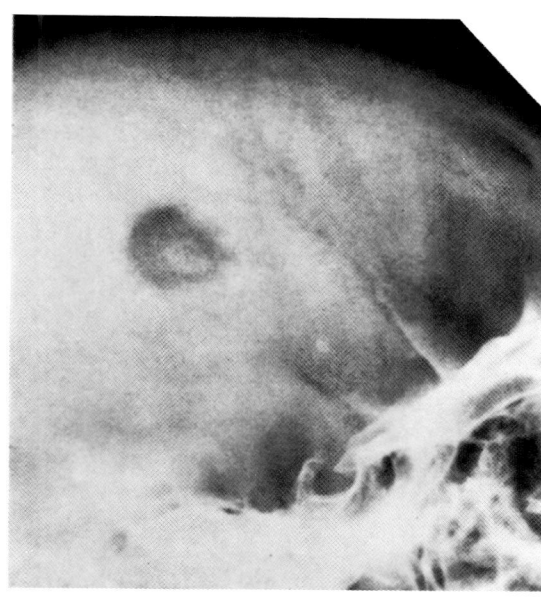

FIG SK3-2. **Meningioma.** The lucent lesion is irregularly marginated and residual bone remains in the center.[3]

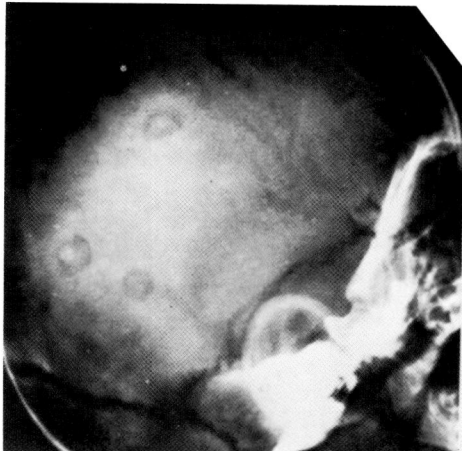

FIG SK3-3. **Staphylococcal osteomyelitis.** A central nidus is seen in each of the multiple round lytic lesions.[3]

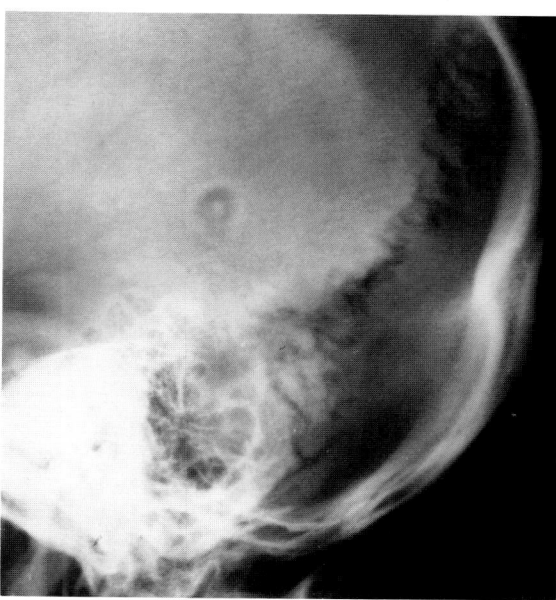

FIG SK3-4. **Doughnut lesion** containing a large density in the central area of a lucency.[4]

LOCALIZED INCREASED DENSITY OR HYPEROSTOSIS OF THE CALVARIUM

Condition	Imaging Findings	Comments
Hyperostosis frontalis interna (Fig SK4-1)	Bilateral, symmetric bony overgrowth that thickens the inner table of the frontal bone.	Almost always found in women, especially those over age 35, and generally considered to be of no clinical significance. Because the irregular thickening surrounds the venous sinuses but does not obliterate them, on frontal views the superior sagittal sinus and the veins draining into it stand out as prominent radiolucent zones surrounded by dense hyperostosis.
Meningioma (Fig SK4-2)	Localized thickening of the inner table produces an area of increased calvarial density. Dense calcification or granular psammomatous deposits may be seen in the tumor.	Benign tumor that arises from arachnoid lining cells and is attached to the dura, most commonly over the convexities of the calvarium, olfactory groove, tuberculum sellae, parasagittal region, sylvian fissure, and cerebellopontine angle. Hyperostosis is caused by an invasion of the skull vault by tumor cells that simulates osteoblastic activity. Associated radiographic findings include prominence of meningeal vascular margins and enlargement of the foramen spinosum.
Fibrous dysplasia (Fig SK4-3)	Sclerotic ground-glass appearance (more common at the base of the skull and in the facial bones than as isolated involvement of the vault).	Involvement of the facial bones causes a marked sclerosis and thickening, often with obliteration of the sinuses and orbits, that creates a leonine appearance (leontiasis ossea). May also cause multiple irregular areas of lucency with expansion of the outer table of the skull.
Metastases (Figs SK4-4 and SK4-5)	Ill-defined, often multiple areas of increased density in the calvarium.	Most originate from carcinoma of the prostate or breast carcinoma (after therapy). Tangential radiographs may show localized thickening of bone due to subperiosteal reaction. Metastases to the skull more commonly produce multiple lytic areas.
Cephalhematoma (Fig SK4-6)	Shell-like deposition of calcium beginning around the periphery of and finally bridging a well-localized soft-tissue mass under the scalp.	Result of subperiosteal hemorrhage that usually occurs over the parietal area, is limited by sutural margins, and at times is associated with a fissure fracture of the skull. Primarily found in newborns, especially those with high birth weight and following forceps delivery. The entire mass eventually may become ossified, remodeled, and assimilated into the rest of the skull, usually leaving no residual signs.
Chronic osteomyelitis	Single or multiple areas of poorly defined bone sclerosis surrounding areas of rarefaction.	Low-grade bone infections (fungus, syphilis, tuberculosis) of long duration may occasionally provoke an osteoblastic reaction in which the vault is increased by periosteal new bone. Osteomyelitis much more commonly causes lytic bone destruction. Sequestra are rare because the skull has such a rich blood supply.

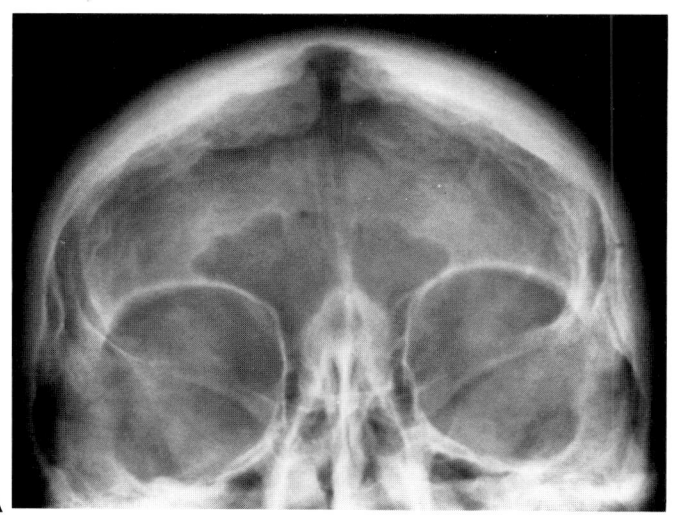 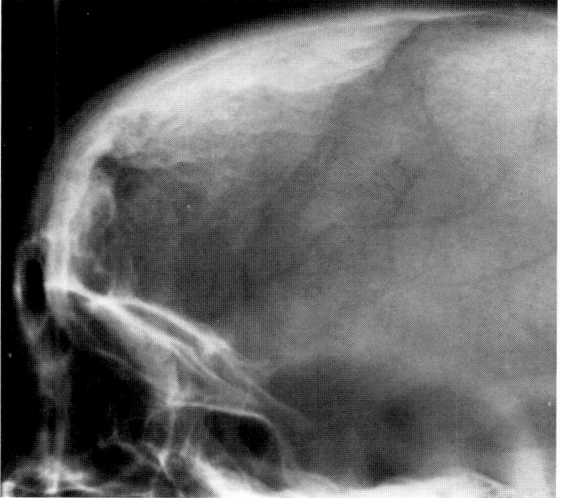

A   B

FIG SK4-1. Hyperostosis frontalis interna. (A) Frontal and (B) lateral views of the skull demonstrate bilateral symmetric osseous overgrowth that thickens the inner table of the frontal bone. Note the prominent midline lucency representing the superior sagittal sinus.

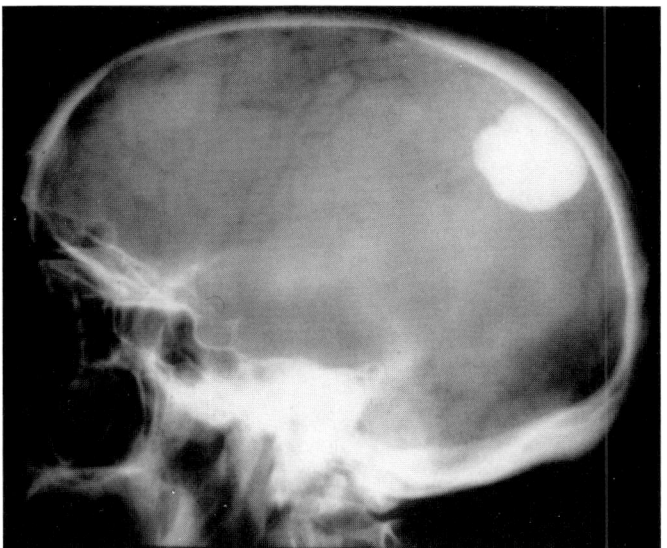

FIG SK4-2. Parietal meningioma. Dense calcification in the tumor.

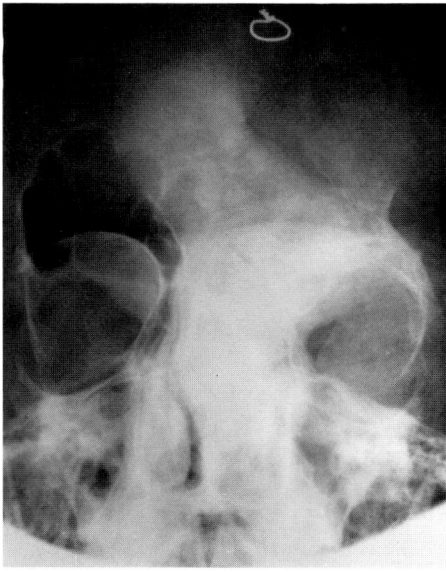

FIG SK4-3. Fibrous dysplasia. Increased density involves the left orbital region and extends to adjacent bones.[5]

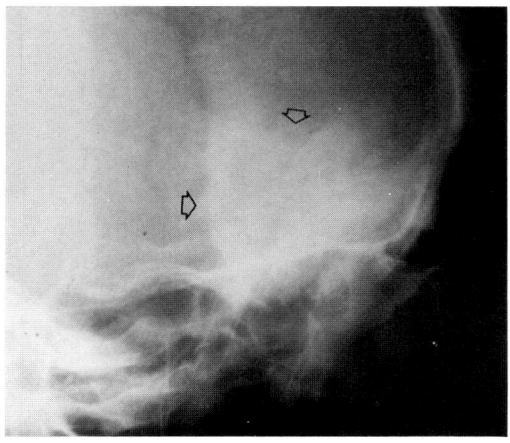

FIG SK4-4. Metastatic prostate carcinoma. Ill-defined area of increased density in the supraorbital region (arrows).

Condition	Imaging Findings	Comments
Cerebral hemiatrophy	Affected half of the skull vault is thicker and smaller than the contralateral side.	Probably due to a lack of the stimulus to bone remolding that is usually provided by the growth of the underlying cerebrum. The ipsilateral convolutional impressions of the inner table are few and shallow or are absent.
Hemangioma (Fig SK4-7)	Osseous spicules radiating from the center of a round, lucent lesion produce a typical sunburst pattern.	Pathognomonic appearance of this benign, slow-growing tumor involving the skull.
Other bone tumors (Fig SK4-8)	Various patterns of sclerosis.	Osteoma; osteochrondroma; osteosarcoma.
Radiation necrosis	Extensive area of thickened, featureless, and dense bone (often with associated lytic destruction).	Rare manifestation. Almost all the bone changes after therapeutic irradiation of an intracranial tumor are radiolucent.
Neurofibromatosis	Single or multiple areas of increased density.	Rare manifestation. Meningiomas associated with neurofibromatosis may be the cause of the hyperostosis.
Paget's disease	Localized area of dense expanded bone containing abnormally thick trabeculae.	Unusual manifestation in patients in whom the disease has remained localized but has progressed beyond the stage of lucent destruction. Most commonly a diffuse cotton-wool appearance.
Ischemic bone flap	Sclerosis may be superimposed on coalescing lytic areas at the center or margins of the flap.	May develop after surgical disruption of the blood supply to a craniotomy flap. The radiographic pattern resembles that of osteomyelitis, but the slow course and the absence of clinical signs and symptoms of infection help in making the distinction.

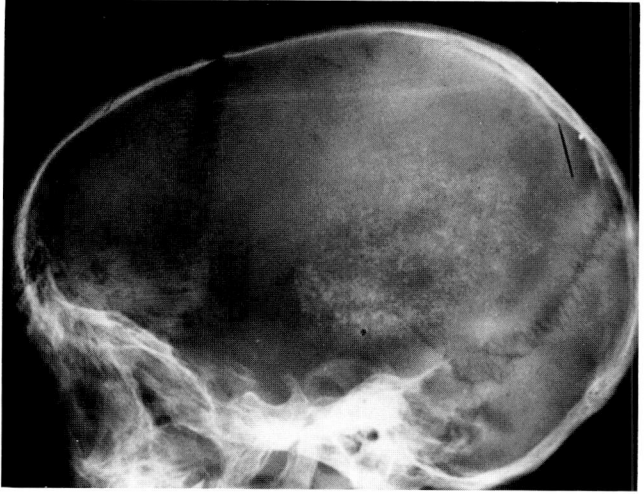

FIG SK4-5. **Metastatic neuroblastoma.** Diffuse granular calcific deposits in a metastatic lesion in the calvarium. Note the sutural widening, consistent with increased intracranial pressure.

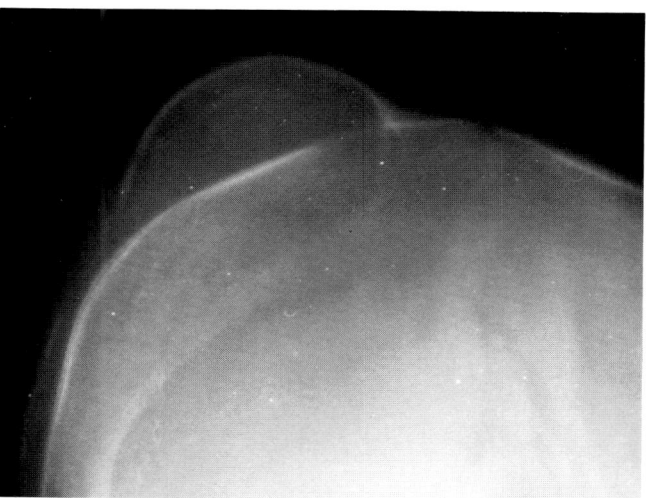

FIG SK4-6. **Calcified cephalhematoma.**

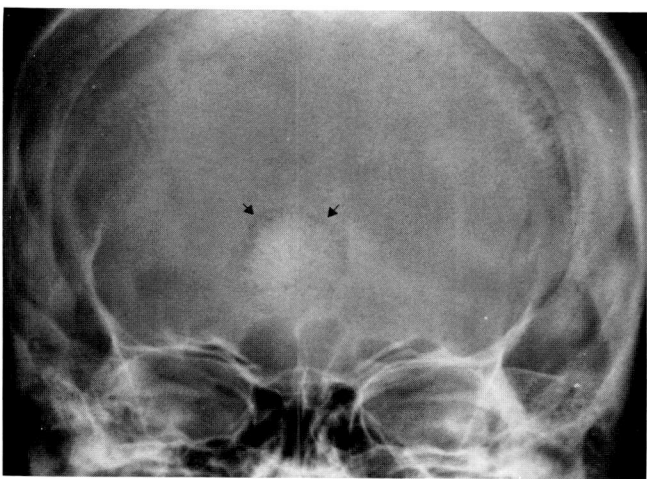

FIG SK4-7. **Hemangioma** (arrows).

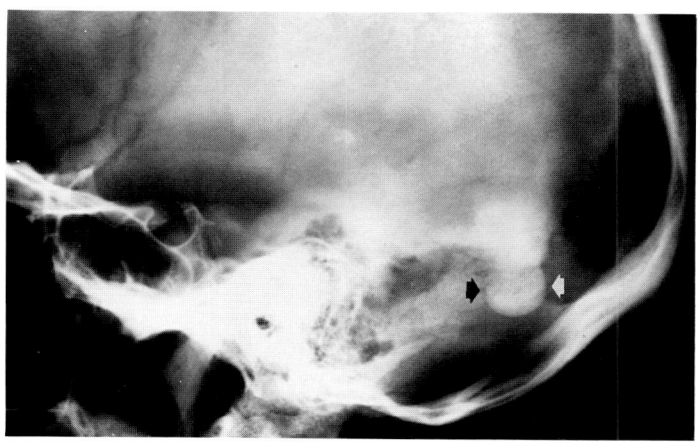

A

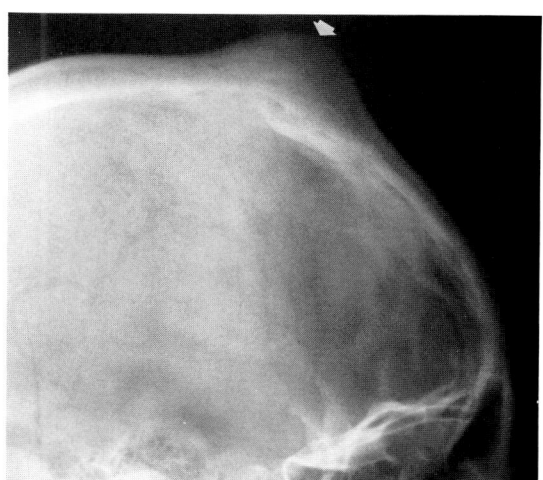

B

FIG SK4-8. **Osteoma.** (A) Lateral and (B) tangential views of the skull show sclerotic lesions (arrows) in two patients.

GENERALIZED INCREASED DENSITY OR THICKNESS OF THE CALVARIUM

Condition	Imaging Findings	Comments
Severe anemia **(Fig SK5-1)**	Hyperplastic marrow proliferating under the periosteum causes spicules of new bone to be laid down perpendicular to the inner table (characteristic hair-on-end appearance of vertical striations in a radial pattern). There is widening of the diploic space and thinning or obliteration of the outer table.	Congenital hemolytic anemias (thalassemia, sickle cell anemia, hereditary spherocytosis); less commonly, iron-deficiency anemia or long-standing cyanotic congenital heart disease. The occipital bone inferior to the internal occipital protuberance is not involved because of the lack of bone marrow in this area. In thalassemia, marrow hyperplasia in the facial bones causes lack of pneumatization of the paranasal sinuses and mastoid air cells as well as lateral displacement of the orbits and forward displacement of the upper central incisors that produce malocclusion and overbite (rodent facies).
Hyperostosis interna generalisata	Generalized calvarial thickening with irregularity of the inner table.	Condition of unknown significance that affects the entire supratentorial portion of the skull.
Paget's disease **(Fig SK5-2)**	Development of irregular islands of reparative sclerosis in the inner table followed by thickening of the diploë and later the outer table, resulting in a mottled, cotton-wool appearance.	Downward thrust of the heavy head on the softened bone of the spine may cause basilar invagination of the skull, compression of the brainstem, and numerous cranial nerve deficits.
Fibrous dysplasia **(Fig SK5-3)**	Sclerosis and thickening of the facial bones, often with obliteration of the sinuses and orbits, produce a leonine appearance (leontiasis ossea).	In the calvarium, there are usually multiple irregular areas of lucency with expansion of the outer table of the skull and only minimal involvement of the inner table.
Osteoblastic metastases **(Fig SK5-4)**	Multiple, fairly discrete, dense bony nodules of various sizes throughout the skull.	Usually secondary to carcinoma of the prostate, though almost any metastatic neoplasm may rarely produce this appearance.
Acromegaly	Generalized thickening and increased density of the bones of the skull. Most prominent in the frontal and occipital regions, leading to characteristic frontal bossing and enlargement of the occipital protuberance.	Other characteristic findings include enlargement of the sella turcica, excessive pneumatization of the paranasal sinuses (especially the frontal) and mastoids, lengthening of the mandible, and an increase in the mandibular angle (prognathous jaw).
Cerebral atrophy in childhood	Generalized calvarial thickening with few and shallow convolutional impressions in the inner table.	The greater than normal thickness is more easily recognized when it affects only half of the calvarium (cerebral hemiatrophy).
Chronic increased intracranial pressure	Generalized calvarial thickening may develop in adults.	Usually related to an intermittent congenital obstruction. Abnormal calvarial thickness may occur in children after successful relief of increased intracranial pressure (surgery for hydrocephalus).

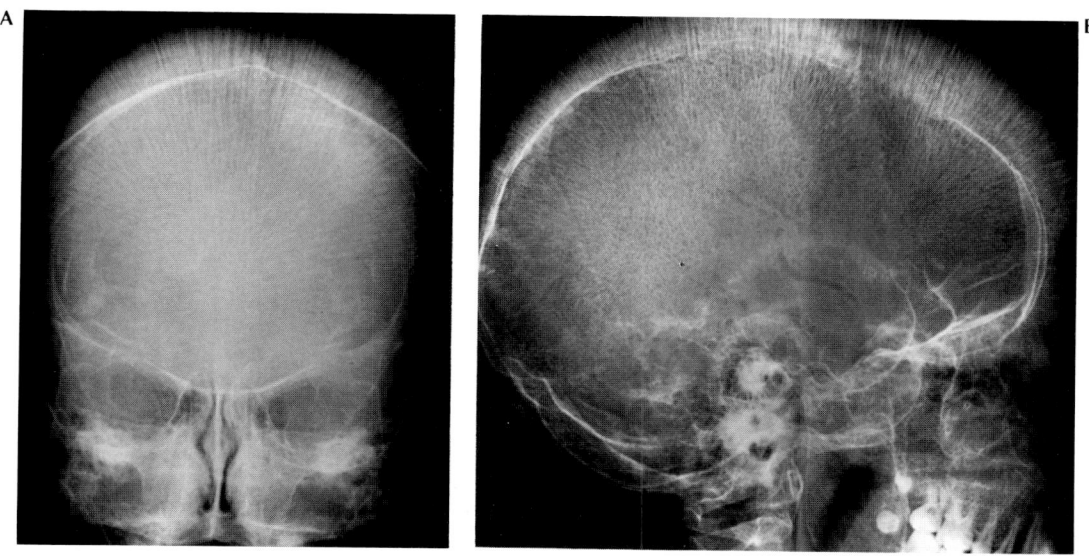

FIG SK5-1. **Thalassemia.** (A) Frontal and (B) lateral views of the skull demonstrate the hair-on-end appearance. Note the normal appearance of the calvarium inferior to the internal occipital protuberance and the poor pneumatization of the visualized paranasal sinuses.

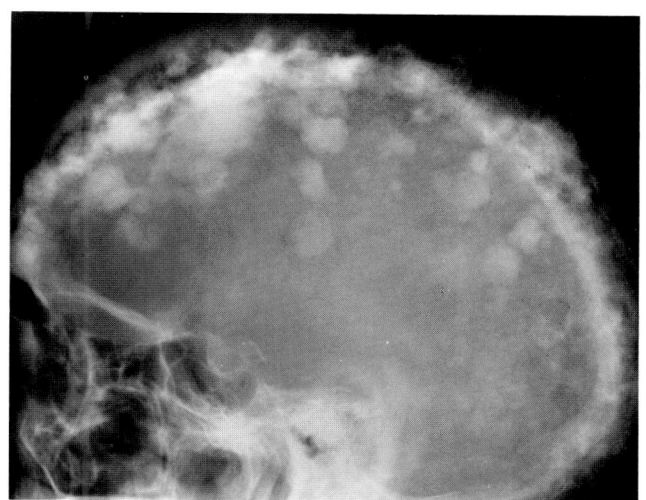

FIG SK5-2. **Paget's disease.** Typical cotton-wool appearance of the skull.

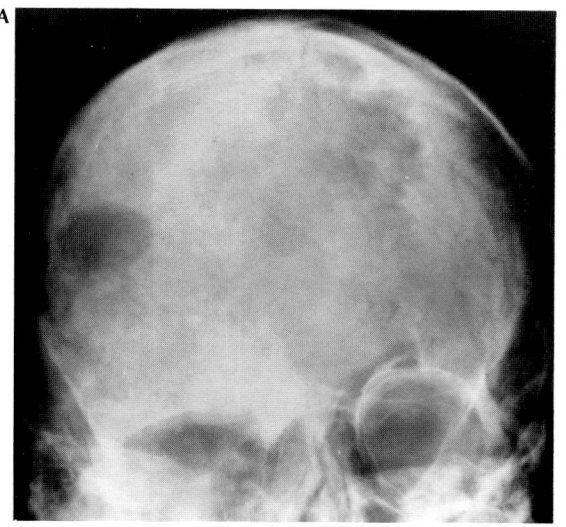
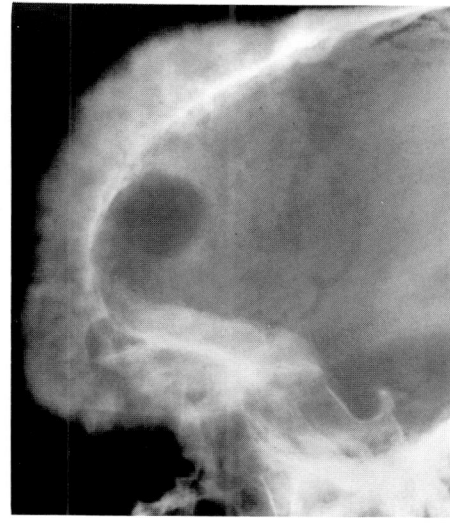

FIG SK5-3. **Fibrous dysplasia.** (A) Frontal and (B) lateral films show generalized sclerosis of the skull with a lucent area in the right frontal region. Note that the thickening primarily involves the outer table, unlike Paget's disease or osteoblastic metastases.

Condition	Imaging Findings	Comments
Dilantin therapy	Generalized calvarial thickening.	Develops after prolonged treatment with this anti-epileptic agent.
Myelosclerosis (myelofibrosis, myeloid metaplasia)	Replacement of the diploic space by dense amorphous bone.	Gradual replacement of the marrow by fibrosis produces a diffuse increase in bone density that primarily affects the spine, ribs, and pelvis.
Congenital syndromes (Fig SK5-5)	Generalized increase in calvarial density with variable amounts of bone thickening.	Osteopetrosis; pyknodysostosis; generalized cortical hyperostosis (van Buchem's disease); Engelmann-Camurati disease (progressive diaphyseal dysplasia); craniometaphyseal dysplasia; melorheostosis; dystrophia myotonica; hyperphosphatasia.
Abnormalities of calcium and phosphorus metabolism	Generalized or patchy increase in calvarial density.	Hypervitaminosis D; idiopathic hypercalcemia; hypoparathyroidism and pseudohypoparathyroidism; patients under treatment for hyperparathyroidism and rickets.
Fluorosis	Generalized increase in calvarial density.	Dense skeletal sclerosis is most prominent in the vertebrae and pelvis.
Congenital syphilis	Generalized increase in calvarial density.	Infrequent manifestation of chronic syphilitic osteitis due to congenital infection.

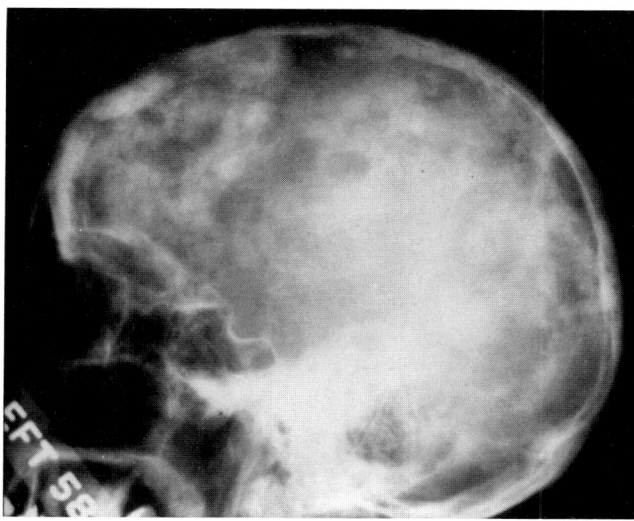

FIG SK5-4. Osteoblastic metastases. Multiple sclerotic lesions secondary to metastases from carcinoma of the breast.

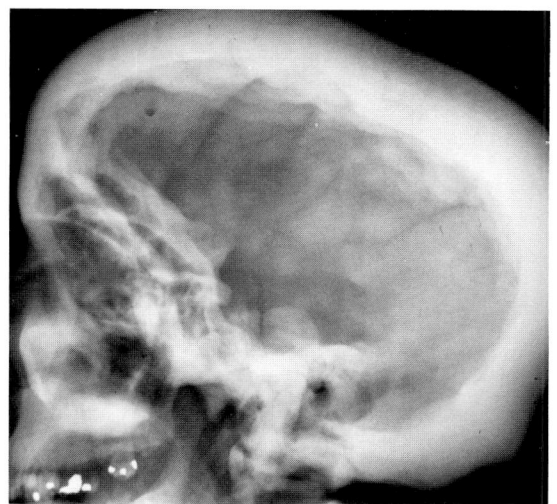

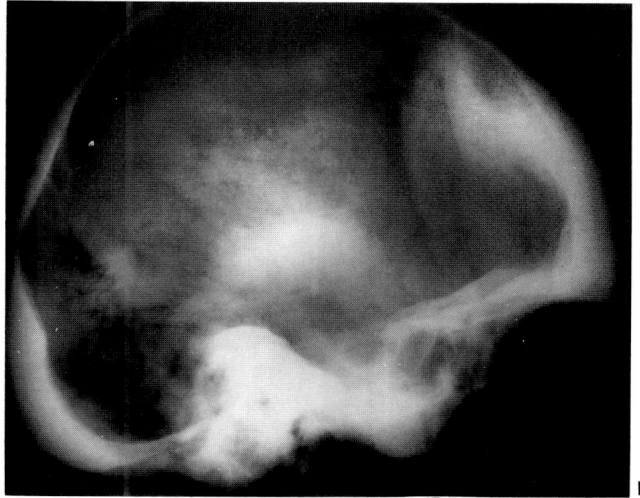

A

B

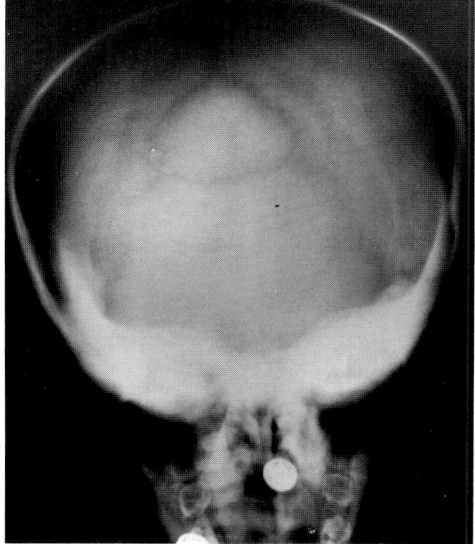

C

FIG SK5-5. Congenital syndromes. (A) Osteopetrosis. (B) Generalized cortical hyperostosis (van Buchem's disease). (C) Craniometaphyseal dysplasia. Note the unusual dense sutural bone.

NORMAL (PHYSIOLOGIC) INTRACRANIAL CALCIFICATIONS

Condition	Comments
Pineal gland **(Fig SK6-1)**	Pineal calcification is visible on lateral skull radiographs in 50% to 70% of adults (and even in 5% of children under age 10). CT scans show calcification in almost all pineal glands of adults and in a high percentage of children. The calcification is more difficult to detect on frontal views and varies from a single faint speck to a ring up to 1 cm in diameter (larger calcification in this region is probably pathologic and suggests a pinealoma or aneurysm of the vein of Galen). Pineal calcification appears about 3 cm above the highest posterior elevation of the petrous pyramids on lateral views and in the midline on frontal projections (displacement of the calcification more than 3 mm to one side of the midline suggests an intracranial mass).
Habenula **(Fig SK6-1)**	Calcification of the choroid plexus in the posterior portion of the third ventricle along the anterior surface of the habenular commissure. The typical C-shaped configuration is open posteriorly and located a few millimeters anterior and superior to the pineal gland. Although less common than pineal calcification, habenular calcification may occur in the absence of the former and provide an alternative midline indicator.
Choroid plexus **(Fig SK6-2)**	The glomus of the choroid plexus, which is located at the junction of the body of the lateral ventricle with the posterior and temporal horns, calcifies in about 20% of patients. There is a variable pattern of calcification ranging from curvilinear peripheral rings to amorphous "popcorn" nodules to a fine granularity. In lateral views the calcification is situated just posterior and superior to the pineal gland. On frontal views it is usually bilateral and reasonably symmetric, at the same level, and 2.5 to 3 cm from the midline.
Dura **(Figs SK6-3 to SK6-6)**	Dural calcification may occur along the superior sagittal sinus, falx, tentorium, petroclinoid ligaments, and interclinoid ligaments. Calcification of the falx most commonly occurs anteriorly and appears as a thin, linear opacification seen "end on" on frontal views. Calcification in the free edge of the tentorium has an inverted-V shape on frontal views, while a V-shaped appearance at the vertex reflects dural calcification around the sagittal sinus. Elderly patients often have calcification of the petroclinoid ligaments (connecting the tip of the dorsum sellae to the apex of the petrous bone) and the interclinoid ligaments (causing apparent bridging across the sella).

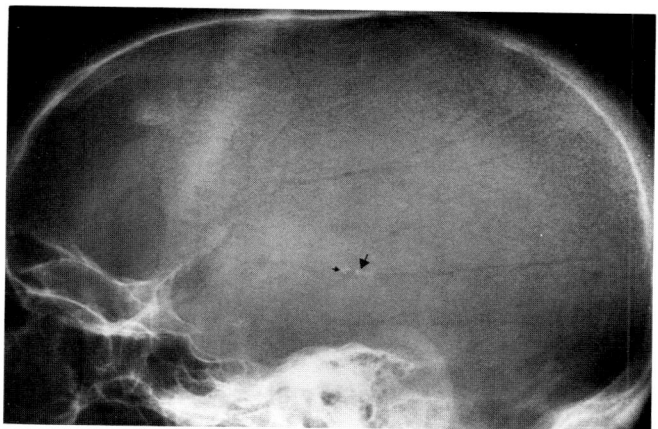

FIG SK6-1. **Pineal and habenula.** Lateral view of the skull shows calcification in the pineal gland (large arrow). Calcification in the habenular commissure (small arrow) lies a few millimeters anterior to the pineal gland and has a typical C-shaped configuration that opens posteriorly.

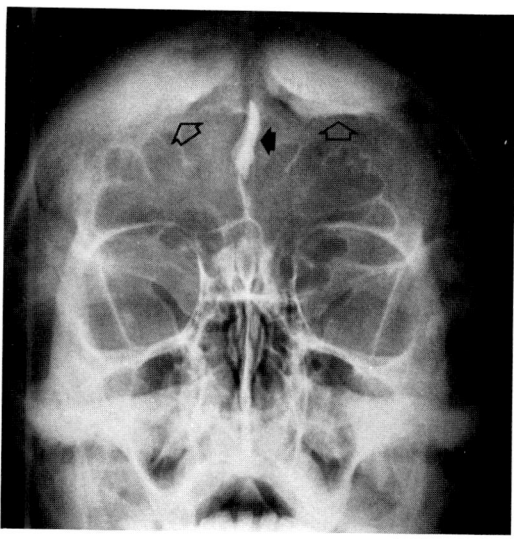

FIG SK6-3. **Falx.** Dense linear calcification in the midline (black arrow). Of incidental note is bilateral hyperostosis frontalis interna (open arrows).

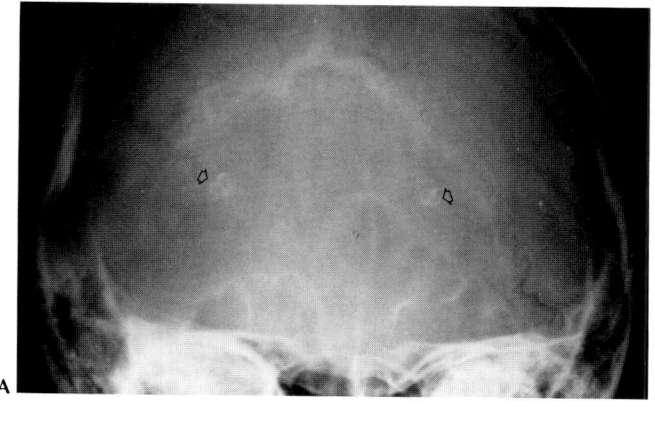

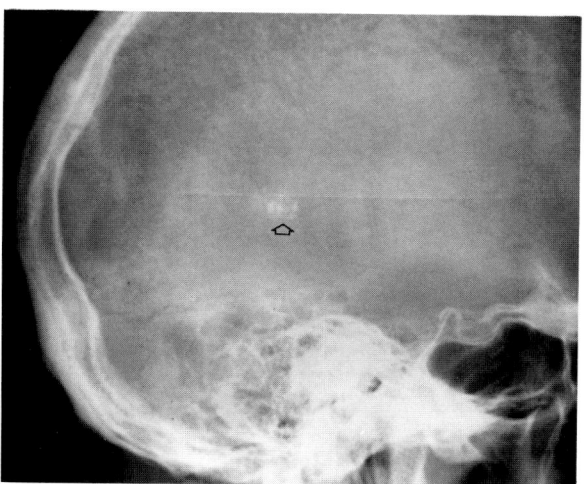

FIG SK6-2. **Choroid plexus.** (A) Frontal and (B) lateral views of the skull show the typical calcification (arrows).

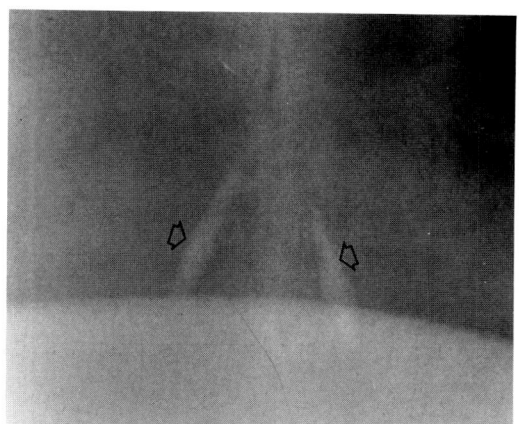

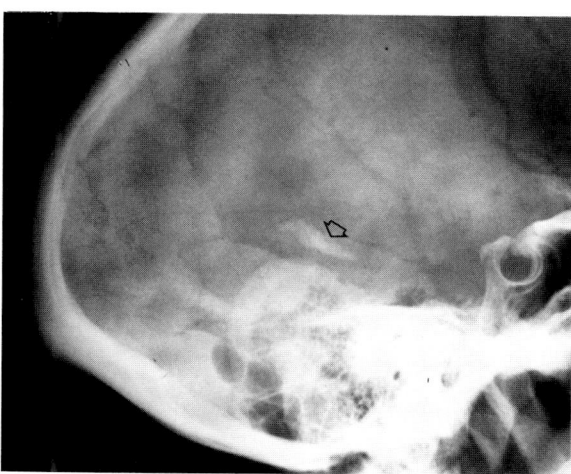

FIG SK6-4. **Tentorium.** (A) Frontal view shows the characteristic inverted-V shape of calcification (arrows) in the free edge of the tentorium. (B) Lateral view of the calcification (arrow).

Condition	Comments
"Physiologic" calcifications **Internal carotid artery** **(Fig SK6-7)**	Curvilinear streaks or dense tubular S-shaped calcification in the region of the sella turcica. Arteriosclerotic calcification is common in the internal carotid artery as it passes through the cavernous sinus. On frontal views the calcification appears as a circular ring on either side of the sella.
Basal ganglia and **dentate nucleus** **(Figs SK6-8 and** **SK6-9)**	Basal ganglia calcification appears as punctate to conglomerate densities that are symmetric and parasagittal on frontal views and may assume a gentle curve that roughly parallels the squamosal suture on lateral views. Dentate nucleus calcification is often obscured by the mastoid air cells on lateral views and is best seen on the occipital (Towne) view as symmetric crescentic densities. Calcification in the basal ganglia and, less commonly, the dentate nucleus of the cerebellum may be a normal variant or a manifestation of such conditions as hypoparathyroidism, pseudohypoparathyroidism, infections, birth anoxia, carbon monoxide poisoning, and Cockayne's syndrome (a rare form of truncal dwarfism with retinal atrophy).

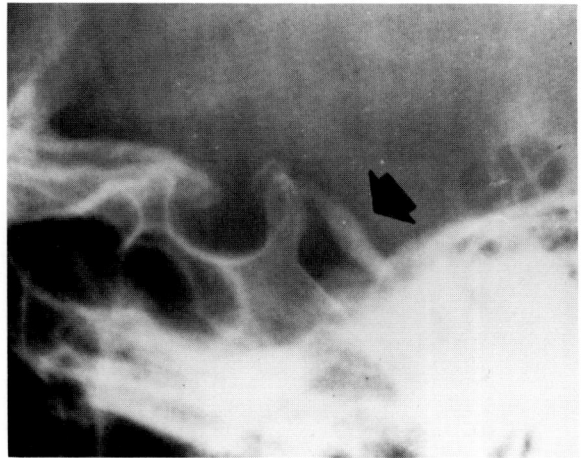

FIG SK6-5. **Petroclinoid ligament** (arrow).

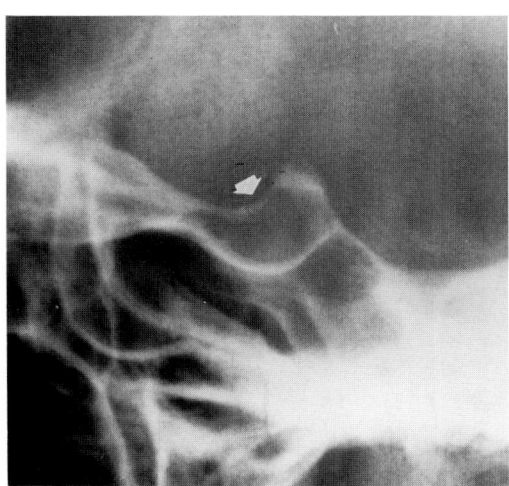

FIG SK6-6. **Interclinoid ligament** (arrow).

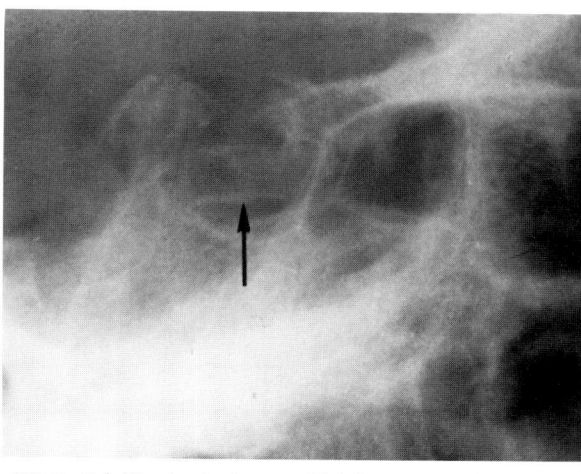
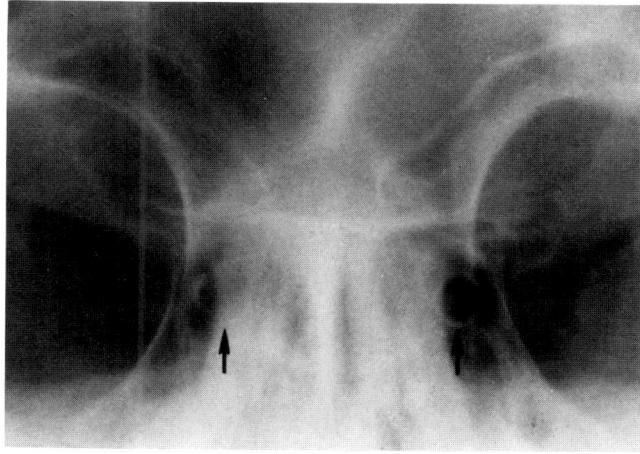

FIG SK6-7. Calcification in the carotid siphon. (A) On the lateral view the calcification appears tubular and S-shaped (arrow). (B) On an inclined posteroanterior projection, there is calcification bilaterally (arrows) that appears as circular ringlike densities lateral to and slightly above the floor of the sella.[6]

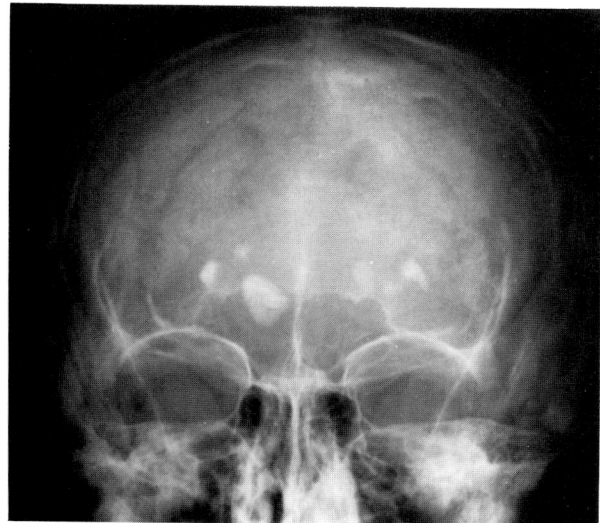
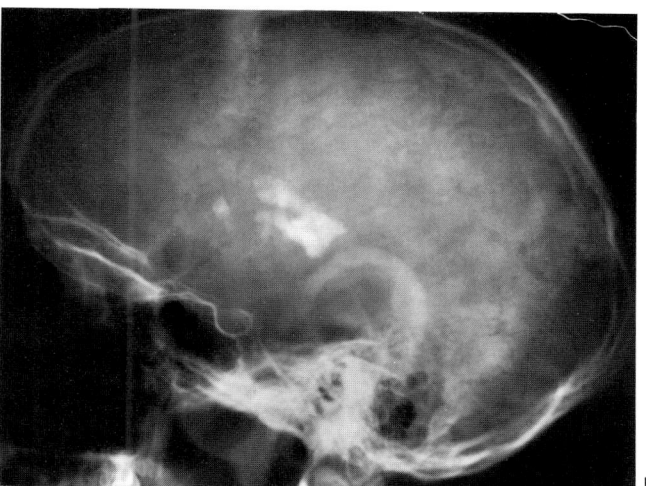

FIG SK6-8. Basal ganglia. (A) Frontal and (B) lateral views of the skull demonstrate calcification in the basal ganglia in a patient with hypoparathyroidism.

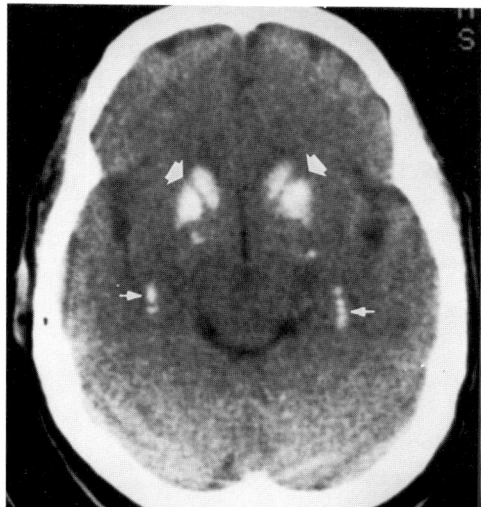

FIG SK6-9. Basal ganglia. CT scan shows characteristic bilateral calcification (broad arrows). Note also the small calcific deposits in the tail of the caudate nuclei (thin arrows).

SOLITARY INTRACRANIAL CALCIFICATIONS

Condition	Imaging Findings	Comments
Normal (physiologic) calcification (see SK6)	Various patterns and positions.	Pineal gland; habenula; choroid plexus; dura (falx, tentorium, sagittal sinus); petroclinoid and interclinoid ligaments (see page 22).
Vascular calcification		
Arteriosclerosis	Curvilinear streaks or dense tubular S-shaped calcification, primarily in the parasellar area.	Common appearance in the intracavernous portion (siphon) of the internal carotid artery. Appears as a circular ring of calcification on either side of the sella on frontal views.
Aneurysm (see Fig SK9-1)	Curvilinear ringlike calcification in the region of the circle of Willis.	Calcification is most common in atherosclerotic aneurysms of the intracavernous segment of the internal carotid artery (may be associated with erosion of the sidewall of the sella and the margins of the superior orbital fissure). There is usually partial or complete thrombosis of the aneurysm.
Vein of Galen aneurysm	Thin crescents of calcification producing a characteristic eggshell pattern.	Actually represents a variceal expansion of this vessel caused by increased blood flow from an adjacent arteriovenous malformation. The calcification is more delicate than that seen in a pineal region tumor.
Arteriovenous malformation (angioma)	Amorphous small calcific patches or flakes or a more strikingly curvilinear pattern of calcification.	About 25% of arteriovenous malformations show calcification on skull radiographs. The calcium deposits may be in the walls of component vessels (arteries and veins) or in the intervening dystrophic brain tissue.
Neoplasm		
Craniopharyngioma (Fig SK7-1)	Nodular, amorphous, or cloudlike calcification in mixed or solid lesions. Shell-like calcification along the periphery of cystic lesions. Calcification occurs in 80% to 90% of childhood tumors and 30% of tumors in adults.	Benign congenital, or rest-cell, tumor with cystic and solid components. Usually originates above the sella turcica, depressing the optic chiasm and extending up into the third ventricle. Less commonly, a craniopharyngioma lies in the sella, where it compresses the pituitary gland and may erode adjacent bony walls.
Glioma (Fig SK7-2)	Various patterns of calcification ranging from a few punctate deposits or irregular linear streaks to a densely calcified nodule.	Calcification is most commonly seen in slow-growing gliomas. Oligodendrogliomas (typically involving the frontoparietal white matter in young adults) calcify in about 50% of cases. Although low-grade astrocytomas calcify less frequently (about 20%) than oligodendrogliomas, they are much more common and therefore account for most instances of calcified gliomas.
Ependymoma	Granular or flocculent calcification, often near a ventricular surface, occurs in about 15% of cases.	Most commonly arises from the wall of the fourth ventricle in children and from a lateral ventricle in adults.

(continued page 28)

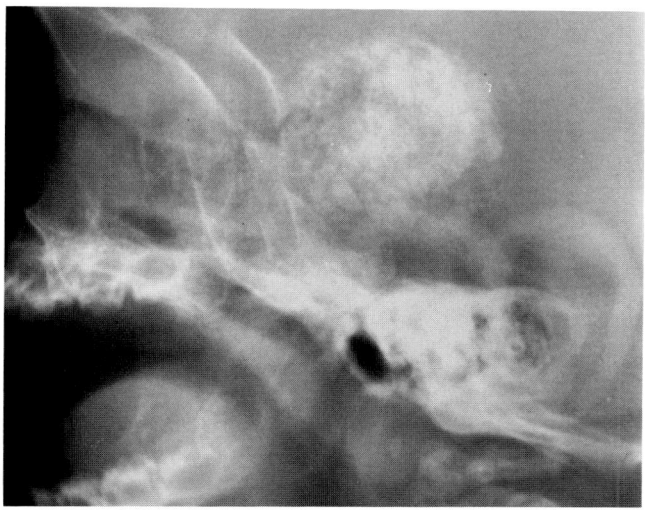

FIG SK7-1. Craniopharyngioma. Large suprasellar calcified mass in a child.

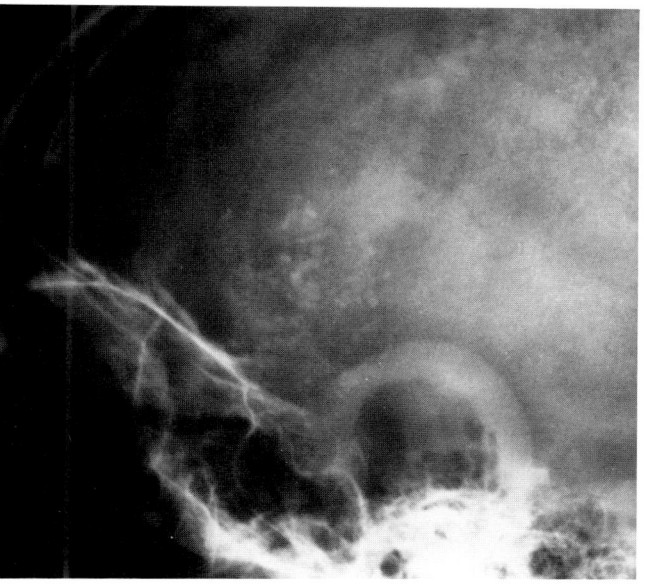

FIG SK7-2. Oligodendroglioma. Clusters of small stippled calcifications in a tumor in the inferior frontal region.[6]

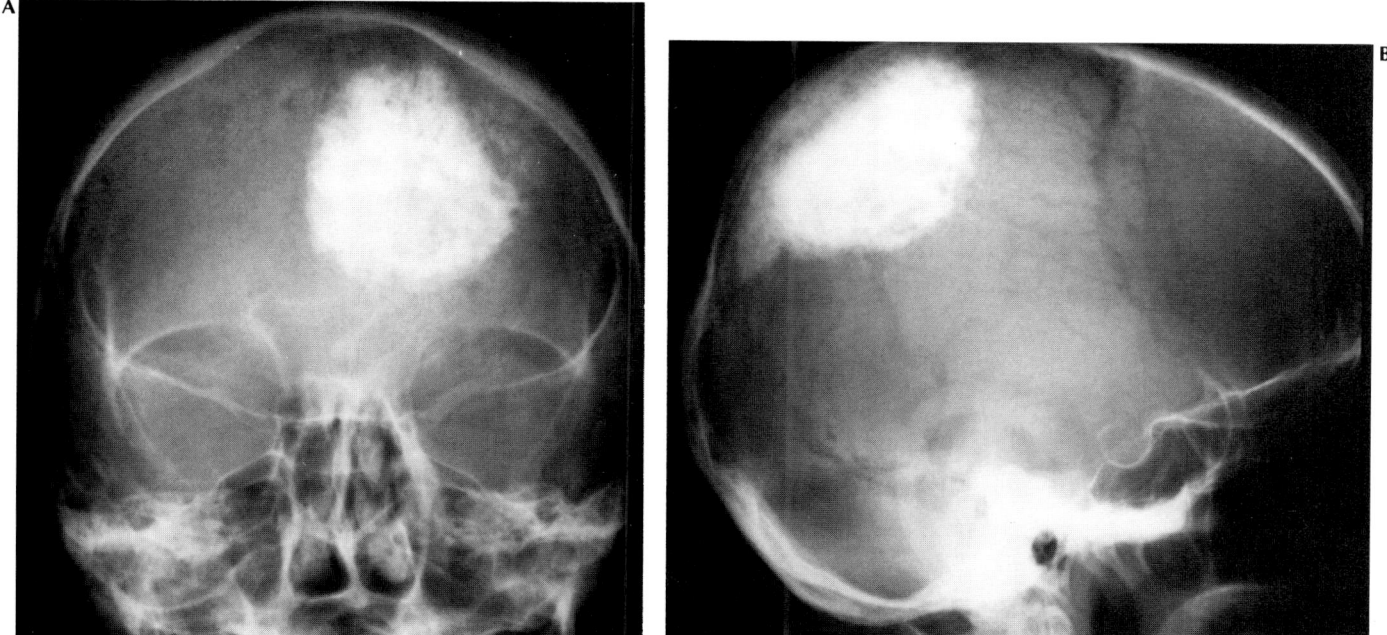

FIG SK7-3. Meningioma. (A) Frontal and (B) lateral views of the skull show dense calcification in a large left parieto-occipital tumor.

Condition	Imaging Findings	Comments
Meningioma (Fig SK7-3)	Dense calcification or granular psammomatous deposits may be visible in the tumor in about 10% of cases. Invasion of bone by tumor cells that stimulate osteoblastic activity causes hyperostosis of the calvarium.	Benign tumor that arises from arachnoid lining cells and is attached to the dura. The most common sites are the convexities of the calvarium, olfactory groove, tuberculum sellae, parasagittal region, sylvian fissure, and cerebellopontine angle. Associated radiographic findings include prominence of meningeal vascular markings and enlargement of the foramen spinosum.
Pinealoma (Fig SK7-4)	Central punctate calcification or peripheral calcific shell (> 1 cm) in about 50% of cases.	Most common tumors of the pineal region are germinomas and teratomas, both of which occur predominantly in males under 25 years of age and may be associated with precocious puberty. ''Ectopic pinealomas'' develop elsewhere in the brain, especially in the anterior aspect of the third ventricle or in the suprasellar cistern.
Pituitary adenoma	Flakes, curvilinear lines, or even complete shells of calcification develop in about 5% of cases.	Calcification occurs in large chromophobe adenomas (rarely eosinophilic adenomas) and is usually associated with ballooning or erosion of the sella. Symptoms of pituitary tumors may result from a mass effect causing compression of parasellar structures or from an alteration in pituitary trophic hormone production (increased levels with secreting adenomas; decreased levels caused by compression of the pituitary gland by a nonsecreting tumor).
Chordoma (see Fig SK9-4)	Flocculent or dense calcification in the parasellar region associated with destruction of the clivus and often extension to the sella.	Tumor arising from remnants of the notochord that most commonly involves the clivus and lower lumbosacral region. Although locally invasive, the tumors do not metastasize. Chordomas arising at the base of the skull produce the striking clinical picture of multiple cranial nerve palsies on one or both sides combined with a retropharyngeal mass and erosion of the clivus.
Lipoma of corpus callosum (Fig SK7-5)	Two symmetric curvilinear calcifications with their concavities facing the midline.	Pathognomonic appearance with the calcification actually located in adjacent cerebral tissue.
Choroid plexus papilloma (Fig SK7-6)	Intraventricular calcification in about 25% of cases.	Uncommon tumor that primarily occurs in children under 5 years of age. Unlike most tumors, choroid plexus papillomas most commonly occur in the lateral ventricles in children and in the fourth ventricle in adults. Hydrocephalus may be caused by overproduction of cerebrospinal fluid or obstruction of cerebrospinal fluid pathways.
Other brain tumors	Extremely rare calcification.	Metastases (especially osteogenic sarcoma and mucinous adenocarcinoma of the colon), angioma, neurofibroma, hamartoma.

(continued page 30)

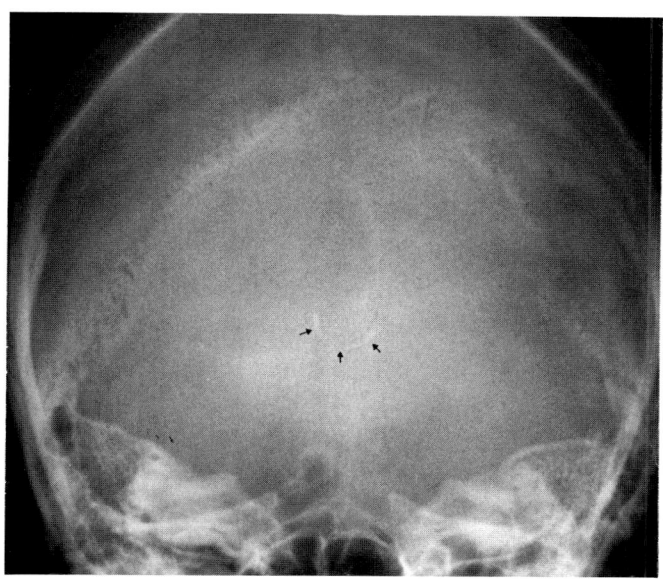

FIG SK7-4. Pinealoma. Shell of calcification (arrows) surrounding the inferior half of this 1.5-cm tumor.

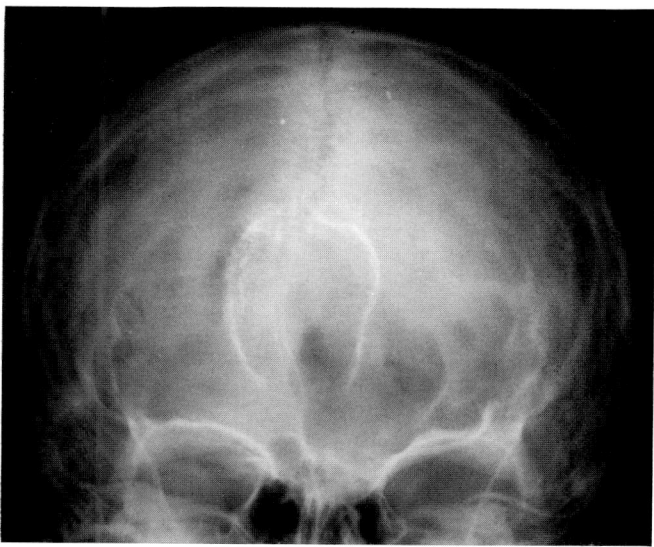

FIG SK7-5. Lipoma of the corpus callosum. Dense curvilinear calcification at the margins of a rounded midline mass anteriorly. Between the calcifications, the skull appears slightly rarefied due to the fat content of the lipoma.

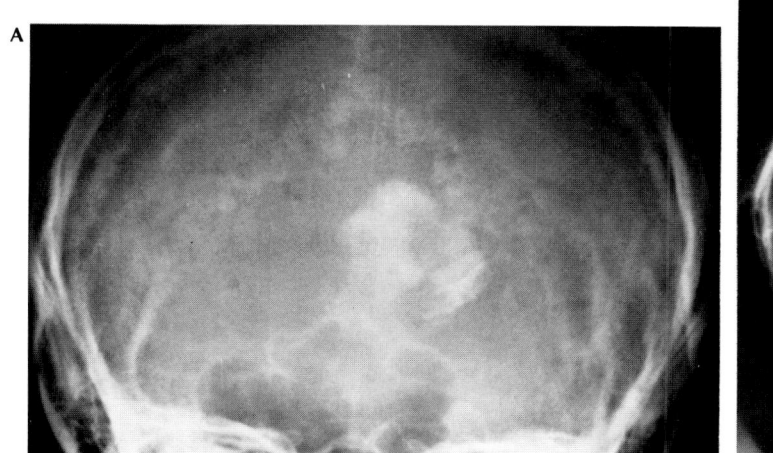

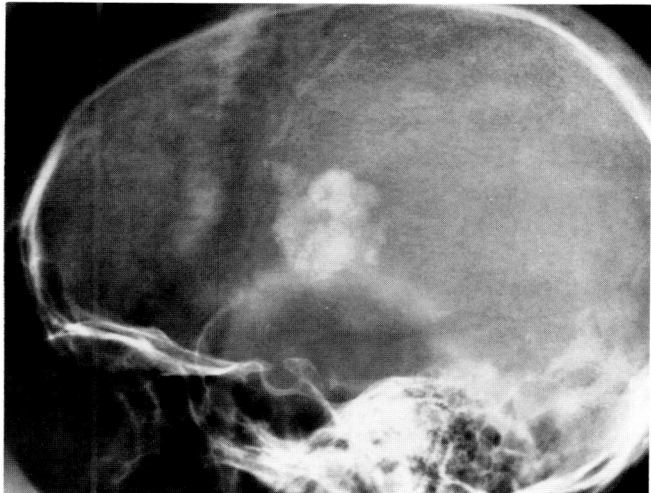

FIG SK7-6. Choroid plexus papilloma. (A) Frontal and (B) lateral views show dense calcification in the intraventricular mass.

Condition	Imaging Findings	Comments
Calvarial tumor **(see Fig SK4-7)**	Calcification may mimic meningioma or chordoma.	Enchondroma, osteochondroma, osteoma, hemangioma.
Infection		
Tuberculoma	Dense, coarsely granular calcification similar to that found in tuberculous lymph nodes. There may be multiple calcific foci.	Tuberculous infection of the brain parenchyma most commonly involves the cerebellum (especially in children) or cerebral cortex. Calcification may also develop after streptomycin treatment of tuberculous meningitis.
Healed brain abscess	Dense, irregular calcification.	Uncommon manifestation that is the end result of organization of the septic process.
Meningitis **(Fig SK7-7)**	Collections of small, not very dense, amorphous calcific nodules.	Infrequent occurrence following bacterial or tuberculous meningitis (especially after streptomycin therapy).
Hydatid (echinococcal) **cyst**	Peripheral rim or central clump of calcification.	Involvement of the brain is relatively common in endemic areas. Cerebral hydatid cysts may attain considerable size.
Torulosis	Irregular calcification in a cerebral granuloma or brain abscess.	Infection by the yeastlike fungus *Cryptococcus neoformans*, which lives in the soil, particularly that contaminated by pigeon droppings. Most frequently an opportunistic invader that infects debilitated patients or those undergoing steroid or antibiotic therapy.
Miscellaneous		
Hematoma **(Fig SK7-8)**	Large curvilinear sheets or plaques of calcification that follow the curvature of the skull.	Chronic subdural hematomas may have calcification in their membranes and margins. A nonspecific amorphous pattern of calcification rarely occurs in old intracerebral hematomas. This complication of neglected head injury is now rare because of improved diagnosis and treatment.
Radiation necrosis	Fine amorphous calcification.	Infrequent manifestation that may develop long after irradiation of the brain.
Scarring **(gliosis)**	Dense area of calcification (occasionally multiple) of variable size.	Incidental finding that may represent the end result of birth trauma or an injury later in life that has produced an intracerebral hematoma.
Cerebral infarct	Calcification that is usually in the distribution of the anterior or medial cerebral artery.	Rare manifestation that is probably related to necrosis or hemorrhage.

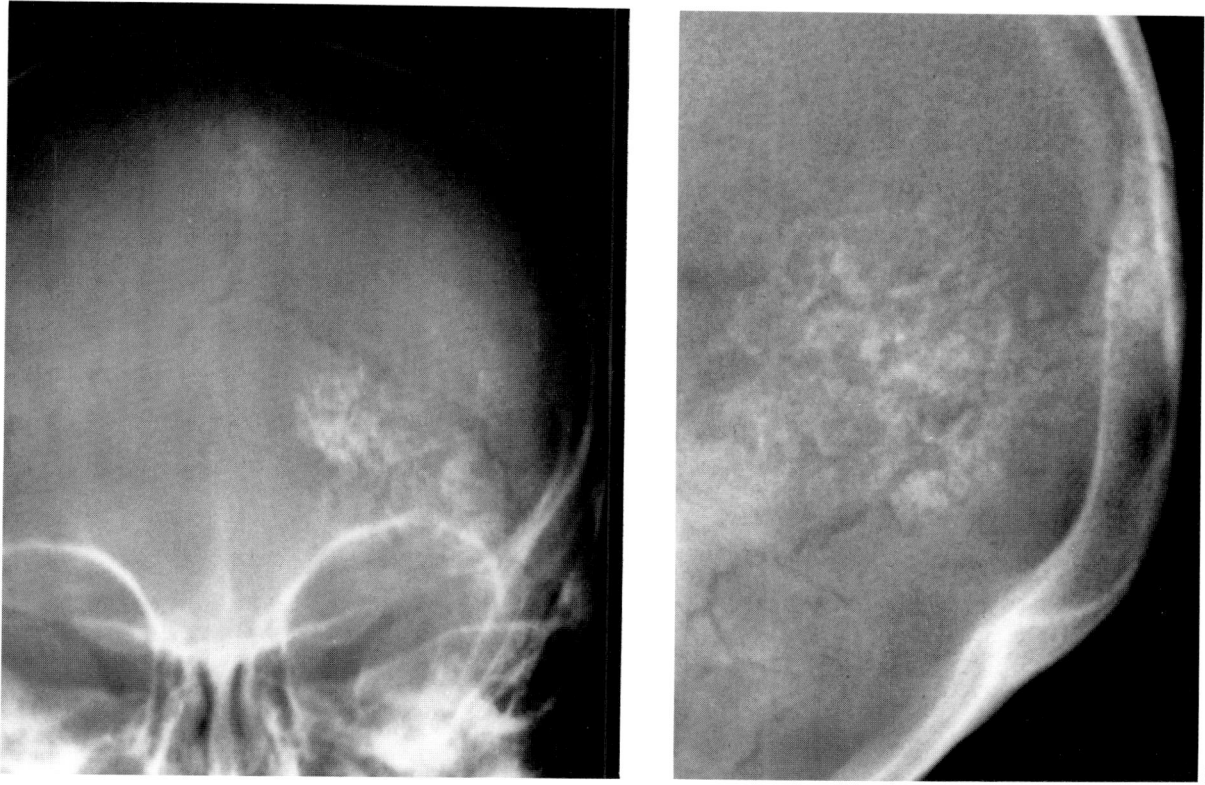

FIG SK7-7. Meningitis. (A) Frontal and (B) coned lateral views show amorphous calcification after meningococcal meningitis.

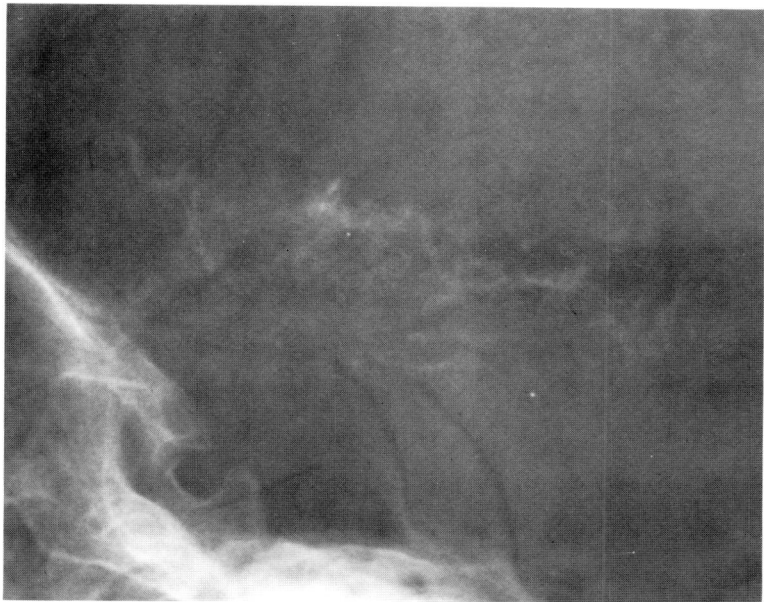

FIG SK7-8. Hematoma. Amorphous plaques of calcification after intracerebral hemorrhage.

MULTIPLE INTRACRANIAL CALCIFICATIONS

Condition	Imaging Findings	Comments
Normal (physiologic) calcification (see SK6)	Various patterns and positions.	Pineal gland; habenula; choroid plexus; dura (falx, tentorium, sagittal sinus); petroclinoid and interclinoid ligaments.
Basal ganglia calcification (Fig SK8-1)	Punctate to conglomerate densities that are symmetric and parasagittal on frontal views and may assume a gentle curve that roughly parallels the squamosal suture on lateral views.	May be a normal variant or a manifestation of such conditions as hypoparathyroidism, pseudohypoparathyroidism, infections, birth anoxia, carbon monoxide poisoning, and Cockayne's syndrome (a rare form of truncal dwarfism with retinal atrophy).
Vascular calcification	Various patterns of ringlike, curvilinear, and amorphous calcification (see page 24).	Arteriosclerosis in the intracavernous portion (siphon) of the internal carotid artery, aneurysms, and arteriovenous malformations.
Infection **Cytomegalic inclusion disease (Fig SK8-2)**	Stippled or curvilinear calcifications outlining an enlarged ventricular system.	Viral disorder that predominantly affects neonates and small infants and produces a clinical syndrome that includes jaundice, hepatosplenomegaly, purpura, and respiratory distress. In addition to the typical calcifications, there is usually marked atrophy of the brain with dilatation of the ventricular system.
Toxoplasmosis (Fig SK8-3)	Small granulomatous calcifications diffusely scattered throughout the brain parenchyma. Meningeal calcifications are plaquelike, while calcifications in the basal ganglia or thalamus tend to be striated or curvilinear.	Protozoan infection that is the most common cause of scattered intracranial calcifications in the neonate (may be indistinguishable from cytomegalic inclusion disease). In up to 80% of patients, obstruction of the aqueduct or one of the foramina by toxoplasmic granulomas causes hydrocephalus. Postinflammatory scarring with cerebral atrophy may result in microcephaly.
Viral encephalitis (Fig SK8-4)	Various patterns of calcification that may mimic toxoplasmosis or cytomegalic inclusion disease.	Rubella; neonatal herpes simplex; poliomyelitis; chickenpox; measles.
Cysticercosis (Fig SK8-5)	Multiple small oval calcifications. Dense central calcification of the larval scolex may be surrounded by an area of lucency and rimmed by calcium deposition in the overlying cyst capsule.	Infestation by the larval form of the pork tapeworm (*Taenia solium*). Central nervous system involvement commonly occurs and can produce epilepsy, mental disturbances, loss of vision, and even a fulminating disease that resembles acute encephalitis. Large cysts may mimic cerebral tumors, while cysts in the ventricles may cause hydrocephalus.
Trichinosis	Multiple small calcifications (virtually identical to cysticercosis).	Infestation by encysted larvae of *Trichinella spiralis*. Calcification in skeletal muscles is unusual in trichinosis, unlike cysticercosis, in which muscles frequently show prominent linear or oval calcifications.
Paragonimiasis (Fig SK8-6)	Intracranial calcifications appear as amorphous punctate densities, ill-defined small nodules, or aggregates of round or oval cysts that have characteristic peripheral areas of increased density ("soap bubbles"). Although individual cysts are often small, when grouped together a cluster may measure up to 10 cm in diameter.	Infestation by the liver fluke *Paragonimus westermani*, which is common in the Orient in persons who eat raw, or poorly cooked, infected crabs or crayfish. Intracranial calcifications are almost always unilateral and usually occur in the parietal and occipital lobes. Other manifestations include increased intracranial pressure, space-occupying lesions (large cysts or abscesses), subcortical atrophy, and arachnoiditis.

(continued page 34)

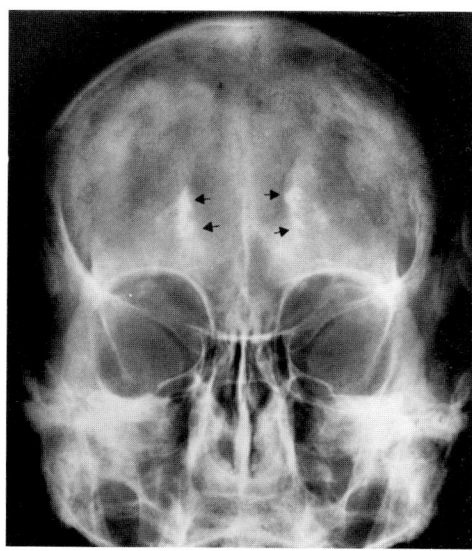

FIG **SK8-1.** **Basal ganglia calcification** (arrows) in lead poisoning.

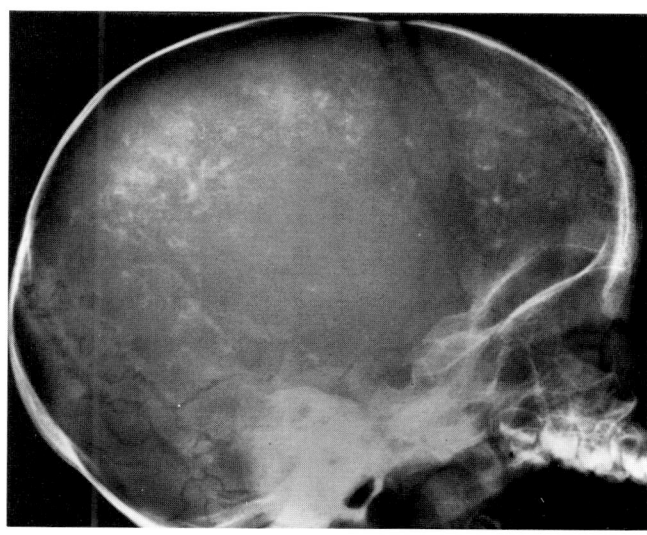

FIG **SK8-3.** **Toxoplasmosis.** Diffuse flecks, plaques, and nodules of calcification scattered throughout the brain parenchyma and meninges.

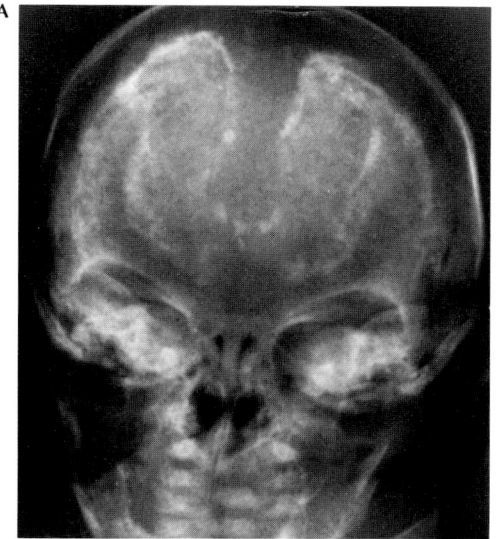

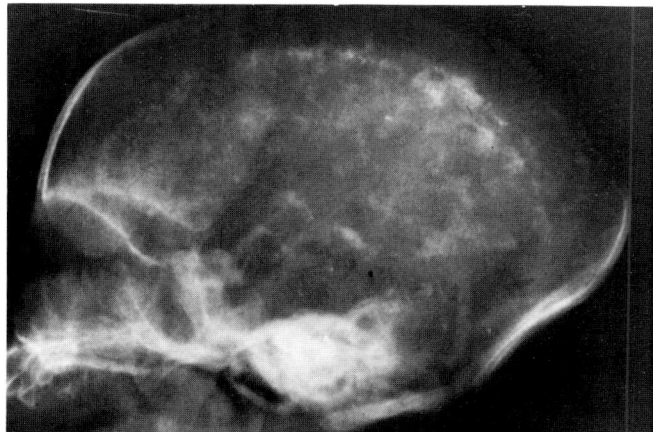

FIG **SK8-2.** **Cytomegalovirus.** (A) Frontal and (B) lateral views of the skull of a young infant demonstrate multiple intracranial calcifications with a typical periventricular distribution.

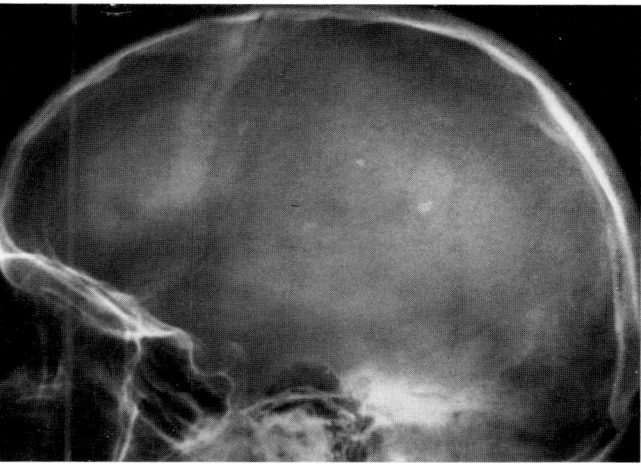

FIG **SK8-4.** **Viral encephalitis** mimicking cytomegalic inclusion disease.

FIG **SK8-5.** **Cysticercosis.** Small blebs of intracranial calcification in a young Guatemalan immigrant with headaches and seizures.

Condition	Imaging Findings	Comments
Hydatid (echinococcal) cysts	Central clumps of calcification or calcification of the peripheral rims of cysts.	Involvement of the brain is relatively common in endemic areas. Cerebral hydatid cysts may attain considerable size.
Torulosis	Irregular calcification in cerebral granulomas or brain abscesses.	Infection by the yeastlike fungus *Cryptococcus neoformans,* which lives in the soil, particularly that contaminated by pigeon droppings. Most frequently an opportunistic invader that infects debilitated patients or those undergoing steriod or antibiotic therapy.
Tuberculomas	Dense, coarsely granular calcification similar to that found in tuberculous lymph nodes.	Tuberculous infection of the brain parenchyma most commonly involves the cerebellum (especially in children) or cerebral cortex. A more plaquelike pattern of calcification may develop after streptomycin treatment of tuberculous meningitis.
Healed brain abscesses	Dense, irregular calcifications.	Uncommon manifestation that is the end result of organization of the septic process.
Tuberous sclerosis	Clusters of calcified hamartomatous nodules develop in about 75% of patients, primarily in the walls of the lateral ventricles.	Inherited disorder manifested by the clinical triad of convulsive seizures, mental deficiency, and adenoma sebaceum. The brain is typically involved with hyperplastic nodules of malformed glial-neuroglial tissue. Large lesions may obstruct the aqueduct or ventricular foramina and produce hydrocephalus. Renal angiomyolipomas occur in about half the patients.
Sturge-Weber syndrome (encephalotrigeminal angiomatosis) (Fig SK8-7)	Undulating parallel plaques of calcification in the brain cortex that appear to follow the cerebral convolutions and most often develop in the parieto-occipital area.	Congenital vascular anomaly in which a localized meningeal venous angioma occurs in conjunction with an ipsilateral facial angioma (port wine nevus). The clinical findings include mental retardation, seizure disorders, and hemiatrophy and hemiparesis. Hemiatrophy leads to elevation of the base of the skull and enlargement and increased aeration of the ipsilateral mastoid air cells.
von Hippel–Lindau disease (cerebroretinal angiomatosis)	Calcifications in retinal and, less frequently, intracranial angiomas.	Vascular malformations of the retina (usually multiple capillary angiomas) combined with one or more slow-growing hemangioblastomas of the cerebellum and spinal cord (in which calcification is rare). There may be angiomas of the liver, pancreas, and kidneys; renal tumors; and pheochromocytomas.
Multiple tumors	Various patterns of calcification (see page 26).	Meningiomas, gliomas, rare metastases.
Scarring (gliosis)	Dense calcified areas of various sizes.	Incidental finding that may represent the end result of birth trauma or injuries later in life that have produced intracerebral hematomas.
Hematoma	Large curvilinear sheets or plaques of calcification that follow the curvature of the skull.	Chronic subdural hematomas may show calcification in their membranes and margins. A nonspecific amorphous pattern of calcification rarely occurs in old intracerebral hematomas.

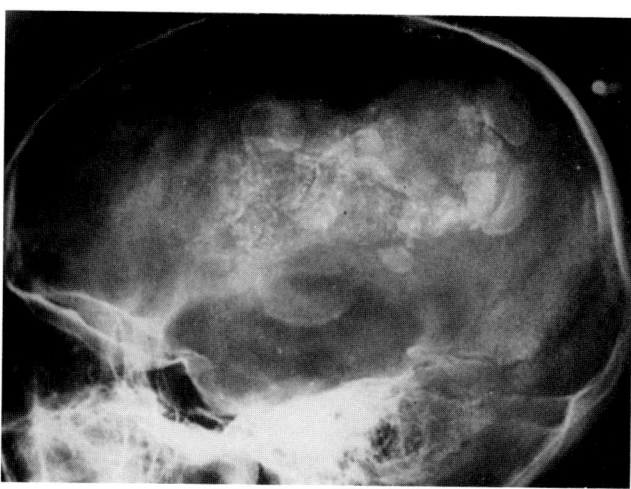

FIG SK8-6. Paragonimiasis. Characteristic soap-bubble appearance of calcification in the parietal area and posterior part of the frontal lobe. The dorsum sellae is not visible, a result of increased intracranial pressure.[7]

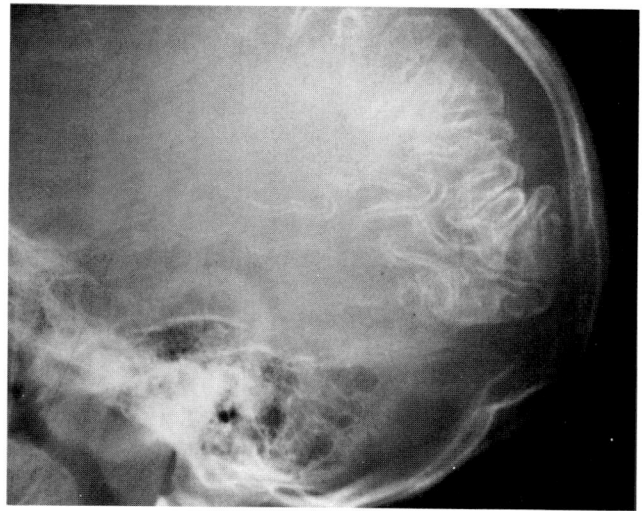

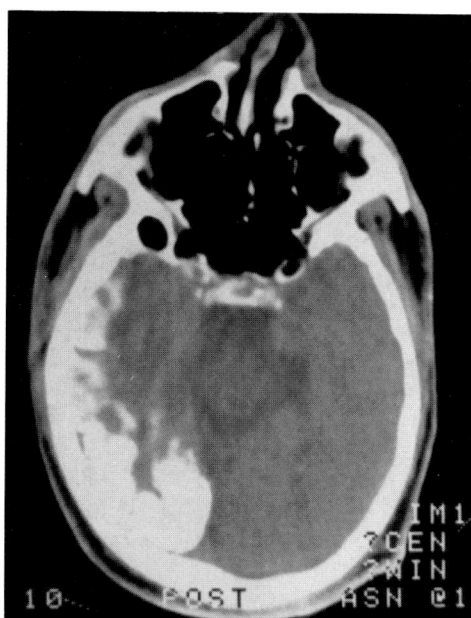

FIG SK8-7. Sturge-Weber syndrome. (A) Plain film. (B) CT scan.

SELLAR OR PARASELLAR CALCIFICATIONS

Condition	Imaging Findings	Comments
Normal structures (see Fig SK6-5)	Ligamentous calcification between the tip of the dorsum sellae and the apex of the petrous bone. Also interclinoid bridging (see Fig SK6-6).	Calcification of the petroclinoid or interclinoid ligaments commonly occurs in elderly patients.
Internal carotid artery	Calcification of the carotid siphon produces small curvilinear streaks or dense S-shaped tubular densities.	Common manifestation of arteriosclerosis involving the internal carotid artery as it passes through the cavernous sinus.
Aneurysm (Fig SK9-1)	Curvilinear or complete ring of calcification.	Most commonly in arteriosclerotic aneurysms of the cavernous portion of the internal carotid artery. May erode the sidewall of the sella and the margins of the superior orbital fissure.
Craniopharyngioma (Fig SK9-2)	Suprasellar calcification that may be nodular, amorphous, or cloudlike in mixed or solid lesions or shell-like along the periphery of cystic lesions. About 80% to 90% of childhood craniopharyngiomas show calcification (30% of adult tumors).	Benign congenital, or rest-cell, tumor with cystic and solid components. Usually originates above the sella turcica, depressing the optic chiasm and extending up into the third ventricle. Less commonly, the tumor may lie in the sella, where it compresses the pituitary gland and may erode adjacent bony walls.
Optic chiasm glioma	Speckled calcification may develop in large tumors.	Although the sella is usually normal, there may be undercutting of the anterior clinoid processes with deepening of the chiasmatic groove.
Meningioma (Fig SK9-3)	Calcification in the mass or reactive hyperostosis of adjacent bone.	Parasellar meningiomas may arise from the tuberculum sellae, diaphragma sellae, cerebellopontine angle cistern, cavernous sinus, or medial sphenoidal ridge.
Chordoma (Fig SK9-4)	Retrosellar flocculent calcification may infrequently develop in a large soft-tissue mass in association with ill-defined bone destruction or cortical expansion of the clivus.	Rare tumor, arising from remnants of the notocord, that primarily involves the clivus and lower lumbosacral region. May produce multiple cranial nerve palsies on one or both sides combined with a retropharyngeal mass and erosion of the clivus. The tumor may be locally invasive but does not metastasize.
Ectopic pinealoma	Punctate calcification in the mass.	Tumor with the histologic appearance of a pinealoma but developing elsewhere in the brain at some distance from the normal pineal gland. Generally occurs in the anterior aspect of the third ventricle or in the suprasellar cistern. The clinical triad of bitemporal hemianopsia, hypopituitarism, and diabetes insipidus may simulate a craniopharyngioma.

A

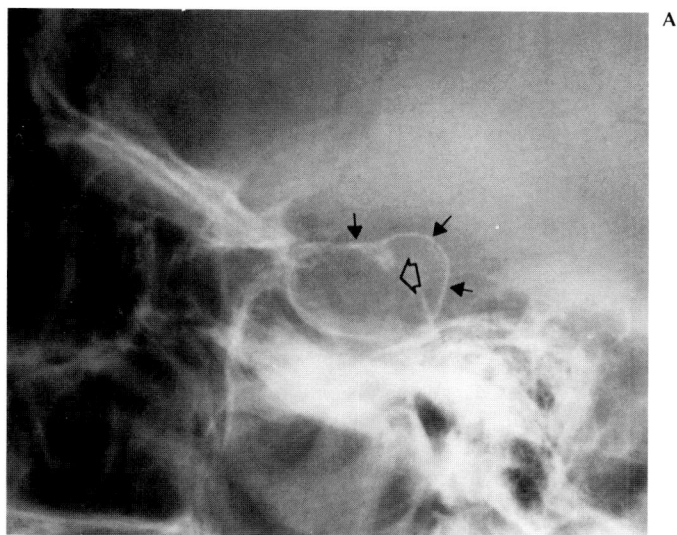

B

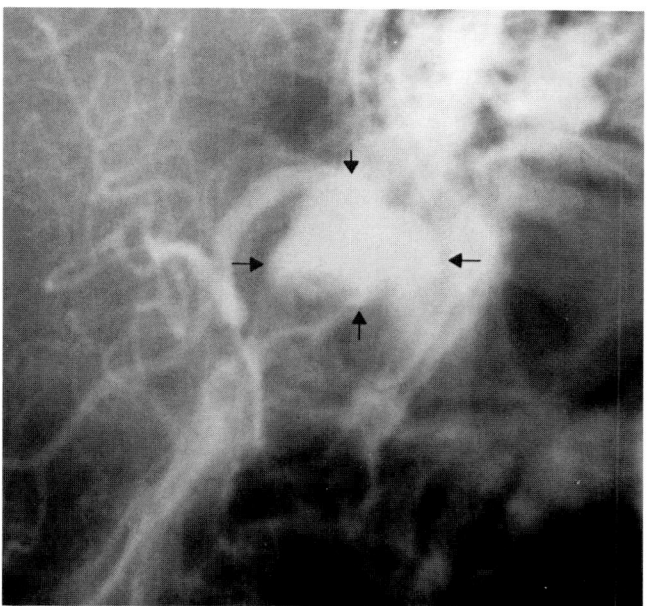

FIG SK9-1. Aneurysm simulating pituitary tumor. (A) Plain lateral view of the skull shows marked expansion of the sella turcica, with calcification (closed arrows) rimming the lesion. The open arrow points to the dorsum sellae. (B) Film from a carotid arteriogram shows the large juxtasellar aneurysm (arrows).

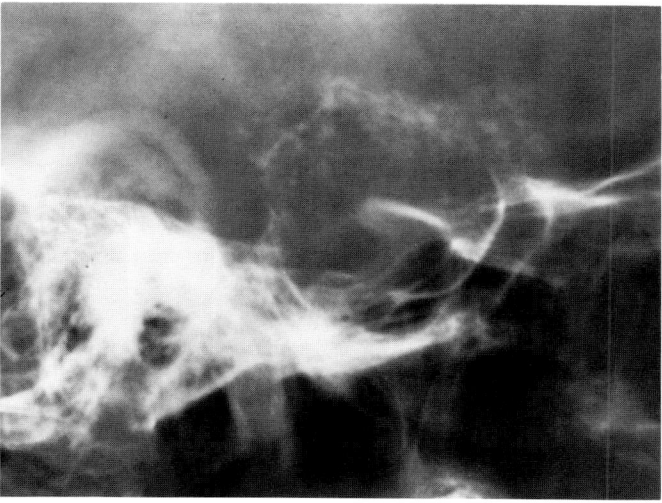

FIG SK9-2. Craniopharyngioma. Amorphous suprasellar calcification associated with enlargement and erosion of the sella turcica.

Condition	Imaging Findings	Comments
Pituitary adenoma	Calcification may develop in large chromophobe or, less frequently, eosinophilic adenomas. There is almost always associated expansion or destruction of the sella.	Pituitary adenomas, almost all of which arise in the anterior lobe, constitute more than 10% of all intracranial tumors. Symptoms may result from a mass effect causing compression of parasellar structures or from an alteration in pituitary trophic hormone production (increased levels with secreting adenomas; decreased levels caused by compression of the pituitary gland by a nonsecreting tumor).
Healed tuberculous meningitis	Collections of small, not very dense, amorphous calcific nodules.	Calcification commonly occurs in the exudate after tuberculous meningitis has been treated with streptomycin. Generally occurs in the suprasellar region, sylvian fissures, and interpeduncular cistern.
Arteriovenous malformation	Curvilinear streaks or lacelike punctate collections of calcification situated in the vessel walls.	About 25% of arteriovenous malformations exhibit calcification on skull films, though this is a rare finding in the parasellar region.
Pituitary "stones"	Small, densely calcified masses in the sella.	Calcified nodules in the sella may rarely be seen in asymptomatic persons and are thought to be the residua of small adenomas that have undergone autonecrosis.

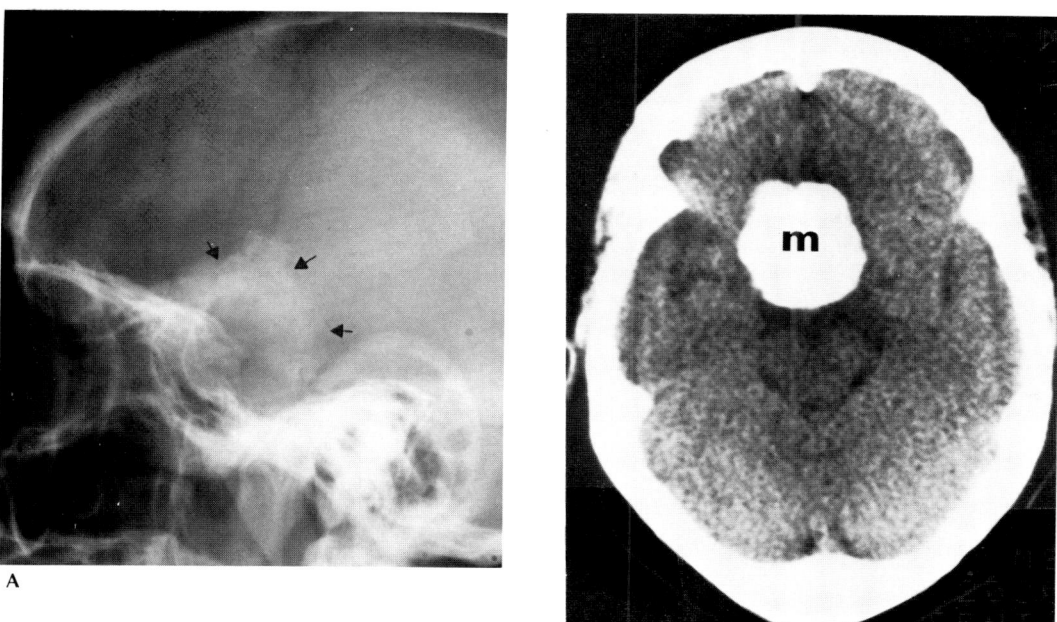

Fig SK9-3. Parasellar meningioma mimicking pituitary tumor. (A) Plain skull radiograph demonstrates a calcified mass (arrows) and destruction of the sella turcica. (B) CT scan shows the large calcified mass (m).

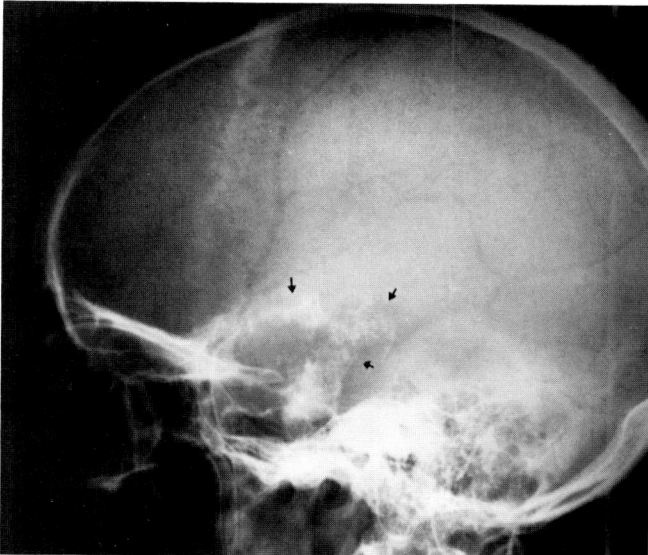

Fig SK9-4. Chordoma. Dense calcification (arrows) in a large soft-tissue mass that has eroded the dorsum sellae and the upper portion of the clivus.

ENLARGEMENT, EROSION, OR DESTRUCTION OF THE SELLA TURCICA

Condition	Imaging Findings	Comments
Chronic increased intracranial pressure	Initially, diffuse demineralization of cortical bone on the anterior aspect of the dorsum sellae and floor of the sella. Eventually, the dorsum is eroded from the top down and there may even be complete dissolution of the dorsum. The anterior and posterior clinoid processes may also be thinned or eroded.	Causes include intracranial masses, cerebral edema, hydrocephalus, and meningitis. Long-standing increased intracranial pressure (especially in children) may cause enlargement of the sella, simulating a neoplasm. If the pressure subsides to normal levels, a demineralized sella will recalcify and may appear normal on subsequent studies. Downward bulging of an expanded third ventricle acts as a pulsatile mass that causes direct sellar erosion superimposed on the bony demineralization.
Pituitary tumor (Fig SK10-1)	Ballooned sella with erosion, backward bowing, or complete destruction of the dorsum. Also unequal downward displacement of the sellar floor ("double floor") and undercutting of the anterior clinoid processes.	Pituitary adenomas primarily arise in the anterior lobe and constitute more than 10% of all intracranial tumors. Chromophobe adenomas and eosinophilic adenomas (causing acromegaly) usually produce substantial sellar enlargement, while basophilic adenomas (causing Cushing's syndrome) and prolactin-secreting microadenomas (causing amenorrhea and galactorrhea) usually do not cause any sellar abnormality. The rare carcinomas of the pituitary produce extremely rapid sellar enlargement and destruction.
Craniopharyngioma (Fig SK10-2)	Truncation or amputation of the dorsum sellae (typical of any suprasellar mass). Less commonly the tumor is intrasellar, where it compresses the pituitary gland and may erode adjacent bony walls and be indistinguishable from a pituitary tumor.	Benign congenital, or rest-cell, tumor with cystic and solid components that usually originates above the sella turcica, depressing the optic chiasm and extending up into the third ventricle. Characteristic nodular, amorphous, or cloudlike suprasellar calcification (mixed or solid lesions) or shell-like calcification along the periphery of cystic lesions is seen in 80% to 90% of childhood craniopharyngiomas (30% of adult tumors).
Other juxtasellar or suprasellar tumors	Truncation or amputation of the dorsum sellae. Occasional enlargement of the sella.	Parasellar or tuberculum sellae meningioma (calcifies in 5% to 15% of cases); optic chiasm glioma; tumor of the optic nerve sheath or hypothalamus.
Metastases	Destruction of the sella.	Rare metastases to the pituitary gland or adjacent dura and bone are usually secondary to carcinomas of the breast or lung.
Sphenoid sinus carcinoma/ mucocele (Fig SK10-3)	Soft-tissue mass in the sphenoid sinus with destruction of the sellar floor.	Rare lesions. Sphenoid sinus carcinoma develops only in elderly patients, while mucoceles may occur at any age.
Chordoma (Fig SK10-4)	Secondary invasion of the posterior aspect of the sella from a destructive lesion of the clivus.	Rare tumor arising from remnants of the notocord. There may infrequently be flocculent calcification in the retrosellar soft-tissue mass.

Condition	Imaging Findings	Comments
Aneurysm of internal carotid artery (cavernous or suprasellar segment)	Enlargement and erosion of the dorsum sellae with undercutting of the anterior clinoid processes (may mimic a pituitary tumor).	Usually asymmetric or unilateral involvement. The wall of the aneurysm frequently calcifies.
Empty sella syndrome	Slight to moderate globular enlargement of the sella without erosion, destruction, or posterior displacement of the dorsum (usually an incidental finding on plain skull radiographs).	Developmental defect in (or absence of) the diaphragma sellae that permits downward extension of the subarachnoid space into the pituitary fossa. Pulsations of cerebrospinal fluid cause remodeling and symmetric expansion of the sella that may simulate a pituitary tumor.
Generalized osteoporosis	Demineralization of the sellar floor and dorsum sellae.	Osteoporosis of aging (senile or postmenopausal osteoporosis); Cushing's disease; hyperparathyroidism.

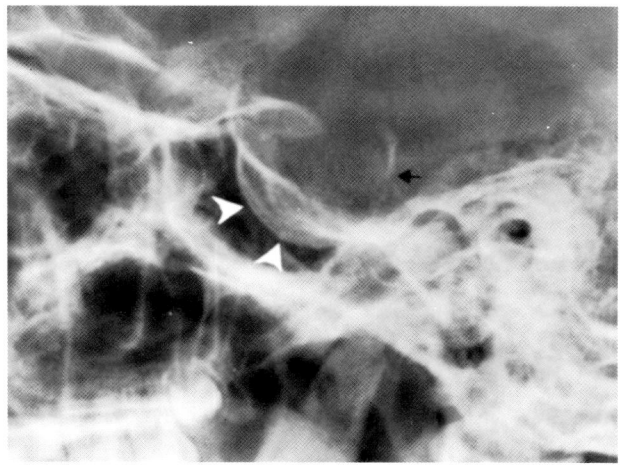

FIG SK10-1. Pituitary adenoma. Ballooning of the sella turcica with downward displacement of the floor (arrowheads) into the posterior portion of the sphenoid sinus. Note the thinning and erosion of the dorsum sellae (arrow) by the intrasellar tumor.

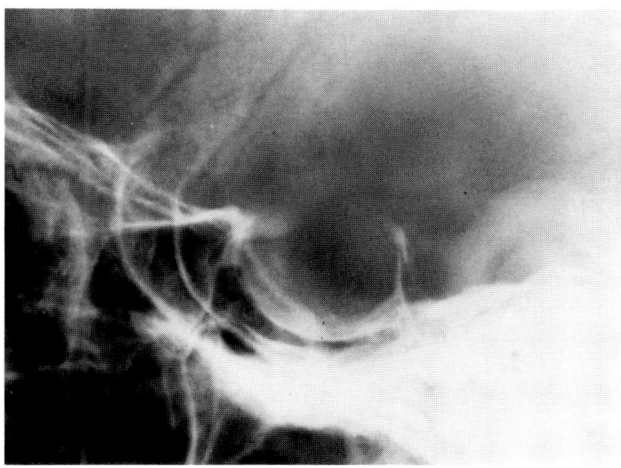

FIG SK10-2. Craniopharyngioma. Ballooning of the sella turcica with downward displacement of the floor, undermining of the anterior clinoids, and backward angulation of the dorsum.

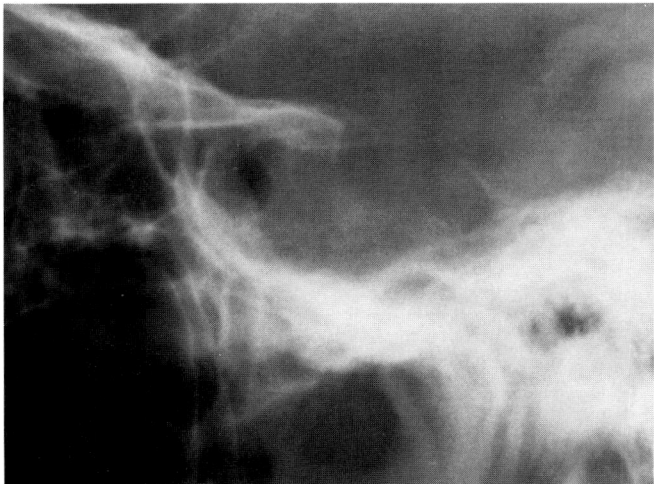

FIG SK10-3. Sphenoid sinus carcinoma. Large soft-tissue mass with complete destruction of the floor and posterior part of the sella turcica.

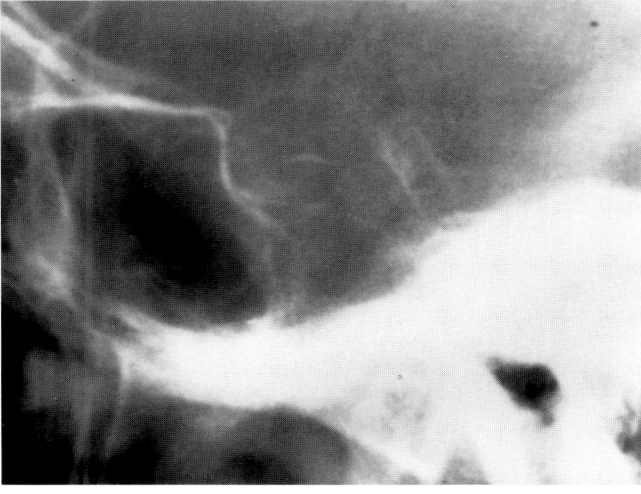

FIG SK10-4. Chordoma. Destruction of the clivus with extension into the posterior aspect of the sella.

EROSION AND WIDENING OF THE INTERNAL
AUDITORY CANAL

Condition	Comments
Normal variant (patulous canal)	Bilateral symmetry, maximum enlargement in the midportion of the canal, preservation of the porus, and a well-defined cortical margin are indicative of the true nature of the enlargement.
Acoustic neuroma (Figs SK11-1 and SK11-2)	Almost invariably the cause of pathologic widening of the internal auditory meatus and erosions near the medial aspect of the canal. Slow-growing benign tumor arising from Schwann cells in the vestibular portion of the eighth cranial nerve that represents about 85% of cerebellopontine angle tumors (usually originates in the internal auditory meatus and extends into the cerebellopontine angle cistern). CT shows a uniformly enhancing mass causing enlargement and erosion of the internal auditory canal. Small intracanalicular tumors may require CT examination after the intrathecal administration of contrast material (metrizamide or air).
Neurofibromatosis	A single enlarged auditory canal may occasionally be seen in neurofibromatosis, reflecting the widespread dural ectasia and bony malformations that can occur in this condition. More commonly, unilateral or bilateral enlargement of the internal auditory meatus in neurofibromatosis is due to an often-associated acoustic neuroma.
Other cerebellopontine angle tumors	Erosion or widening of the internal auditory canal is a rare manifestation of meningioma, epidermoid, brainstem glioma, choroid plexus papilloma, hemangioma, or other neuroma (cranial nerves V and VII).
Long-standing hydrocephalus	Rare cause of bilateral, often asymmetric, enlargement of the internal auditory canal.
Vascular	Extremely rare manifestation of an arteriovenous malformation or an aneurysm of the internal auditory canal artery.

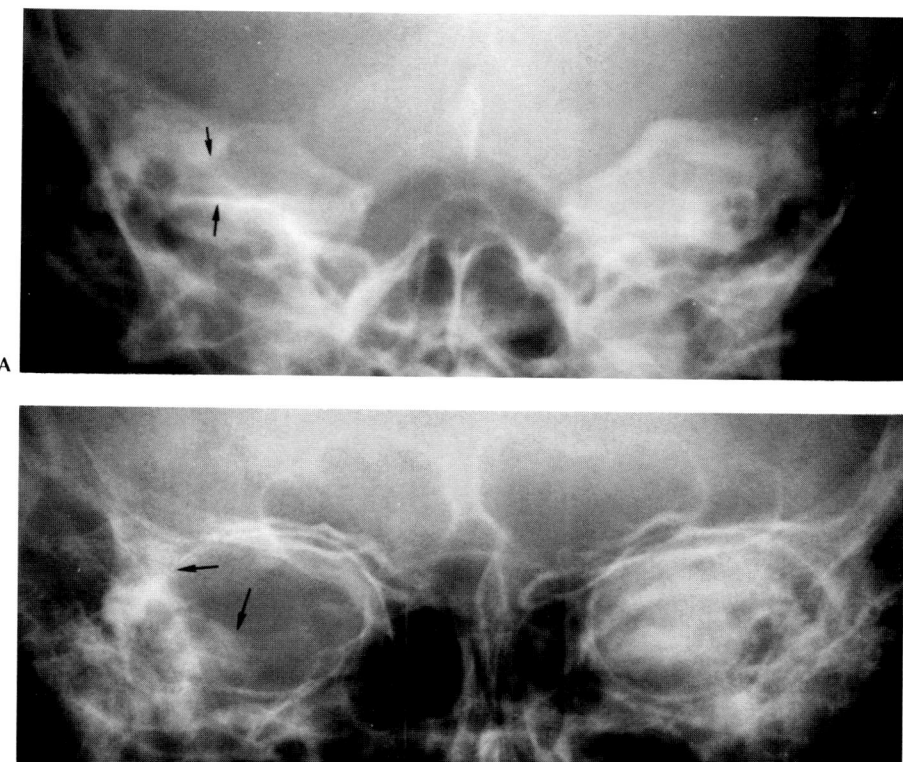

FIG SK11-1. **Acoustic neuroma.** (A) Anteroposterior (Towne) projection. There is erosion of the superior and inferior margins of the right internal auditory canal laterally (arrows). The canal, which normally has a barrel shape in this projection (note the left side), assumes the configuration of a funnel or trumpet. The angular midline density projected above the upper margin of the foramen magnum represents a calcified plaque in the falx anteriorly. (B) Posteroanterior view of an acoustic neuroma in another patient. Destruction of the medial aspect of the petrous pyramid is more advanced than in (A). The superior aspect of the medial third of the petrous pyramid has been eroded (arrows), and only the extreme lateral portion of the internal auditory canal is recognized.[6]

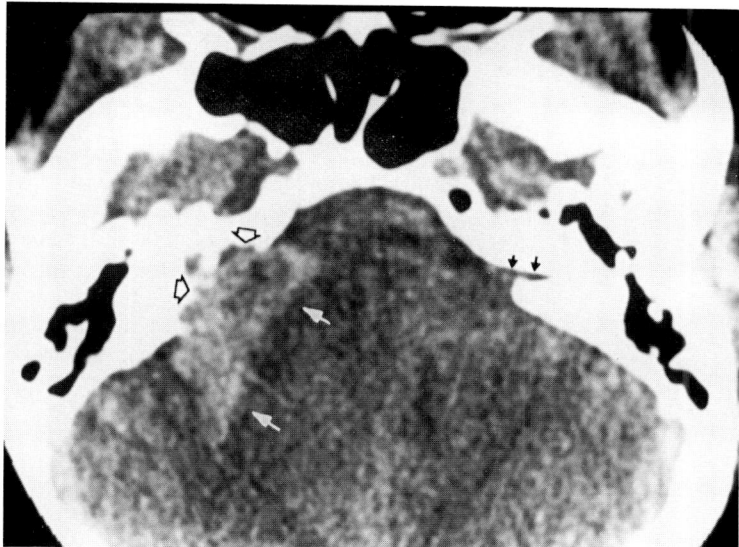

FIG SK11-2. **Acoustic neuroma.** CT scan shows widening and erosion of the right internal auditory canal (open arrows) associated with a large extra-axial mass (white arrows) in the right cerebellopontine angle. The solid black arrows point to the normal internal auditory canal on the left.

MULTIPLE WORMIAN BONES

Condition	Comments
Normal variant	A few sutural bones may be seen in normal skulls, usually in the lambdoid suture.
Cleidocranial dysostosis (Fig SK12-1)	Congenital hereditary disorder of membranous bone formation that principally involves the calvarium, clavicles, and pelvis. In the skull, there is also defective ossification of the calvarium, widening of sutures (maldevelopment of bone rather than a manifestation of increased intracranial pressure), and persistence of the metopic suture.
Osteogenesis imperfecta (Fig SK12-2)	Inherited generalized disorder of connective tissue characterized by blue sclerae, thin bones, and multiple fractures. An infant with severe disease has a paper-thin skull, and death in utero or soon after birth is usually caused by intracranial hemorrhage. If the infant survives, ossification of the skull progresses slowly, leaving wide sutures (delayed closure) with multiple wormian bones producing a mosaic appearance.
Cretinism	Hypothyroidism dating from birth that results in multiple developmental anomalies. Other skull changes are common and include increased thickness of the cranial vault, underpneumatization of the sinuses and mastoids, widened sutures with delayed closure, and a delay in the development and eruption of the teeth.
Hypophosphatasia	Inherited metabolic disorder in which a low level of alkaline phosphatase leads to defective mineralization of bone. The skull contains large unossified areas simulating severe widening of the sutures. If the infant survives and calvarial recalcification occurs, there may be premature closure of the sutures.
Pyknodysostosis	Rare hereditary dysplasia in which patients have short stature and diffusely dense, sclerotic bones. In the skull, there is failure of the cranial sutures and fontanelles to close, lack of pneumatization of the sinuses and mastoids, sclerosis and thickening of the cranial and facial bones, and characteristic mandibular hypoplasia with loss of the normal mandibular angle.

Condition	Comments
Rickets	Defective calcification of growing skeletal elements due to a deficiency of vitamin D in the diet or a lack of exposure to ultraviolet radiation. Softening of the skull bones (craniotabes) is an early finding that may be followed by frontal and parietal bossing, giving the head a boxlike appearance. The cranial sutures are widened and fontanelle closure is often delayed.
Infantile hydrocephalus	Result of ossification in the separated suture margins.

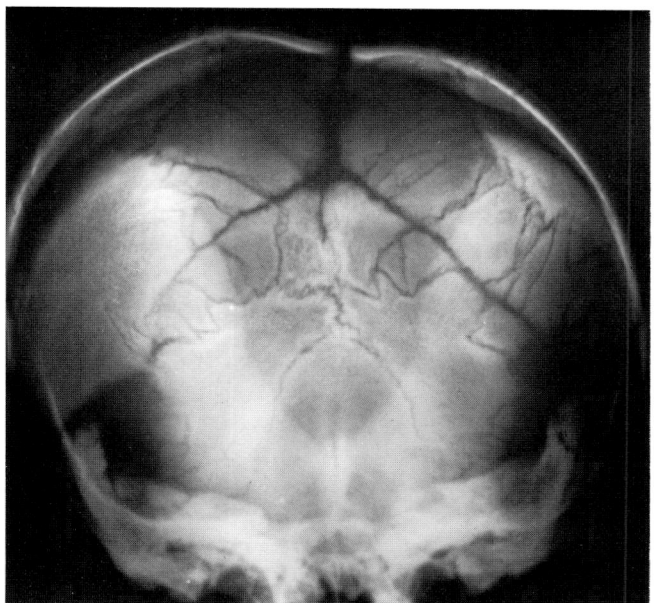

FIG SK12-1. Cleidocranial dysostosis.

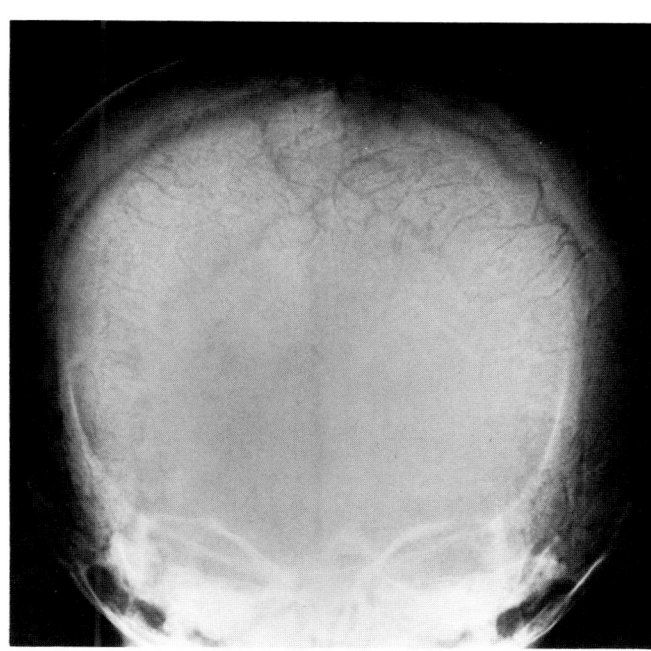

FIG SK12-2. Osteogenesis imperfecta.

BASILAR IMPRESSION

Condition	Comments
Congenital basilar impression (Fig SK13-1)	Infrequently occurs as an isolated abnormality. Usually found in association with one or more of the following defects: failure of the posterior arch of the atlas to fuse, assimilation of part or all of the atlas to the occiput, Klippel-Feil deformity, atlantoaxial dislocation, and stenosis of the foramen magnum.
Arnold-Chiari malformation	Caudal projection of the medulla and inferior-posterior portions of the cerebellar hemispheres through the foramen magnum, often to the level of the second cervical vertebra. Associated neurologic anomalies include spinal meningocele or myelomeningocele and deformities of the cervical spine and cervico-occipital junction. Occlusion of the foramina of Luschka and Magendie leads to obstructive hydrocephalus, which dominates the clinical picture in infants.
Softening of bone at the skull base (Fig SK13-2)	Paget's disease; rickets; osteomalacia; hyperparathyroidism; osteogenesis imperfecta. In these conditions the weight of the skull on the soft base permits invagination of the cervical spine.
Cleidocranial dysostosis	Congenital hereditary disorder in which faulty membranous bone formation primarily involves the calvarium, clavicles, and pelvis. Other skull anomalies include widening of the sutures, persistence of the metopic suture, and the presence of multiple accessory bones along the sutures (wormian bones).
Trauma	Trauma causing basilar impression is usually fatal.

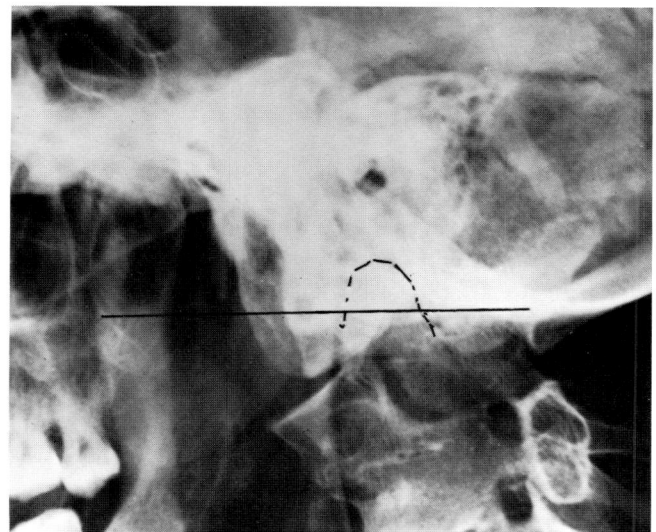

FIG SK13-1. **Congenital basilar impression** associated with assimilation of the atlas. (A) Lateral view of the skull shows fusion of C1 with the base of the occiput posteriorly and anteriorly. The odontoid process of C2 (interrupted line) projects upward into the foramen magnum and compresses its contents. Almost the entire odontoid lies above Chamberlain's line (solid horizontal line), which is drawn from the posterior margin of the hard palate to the posterior margin of the foramen magnum. (B) Frontal tomogram of the region of the craniovertebral junction shows complete fusion of the lateral mass of C1 (lower arrow) with the occipital condyle (upper arrow) bilaterally. Note the upward angulation of the petrous pyramids.[6]

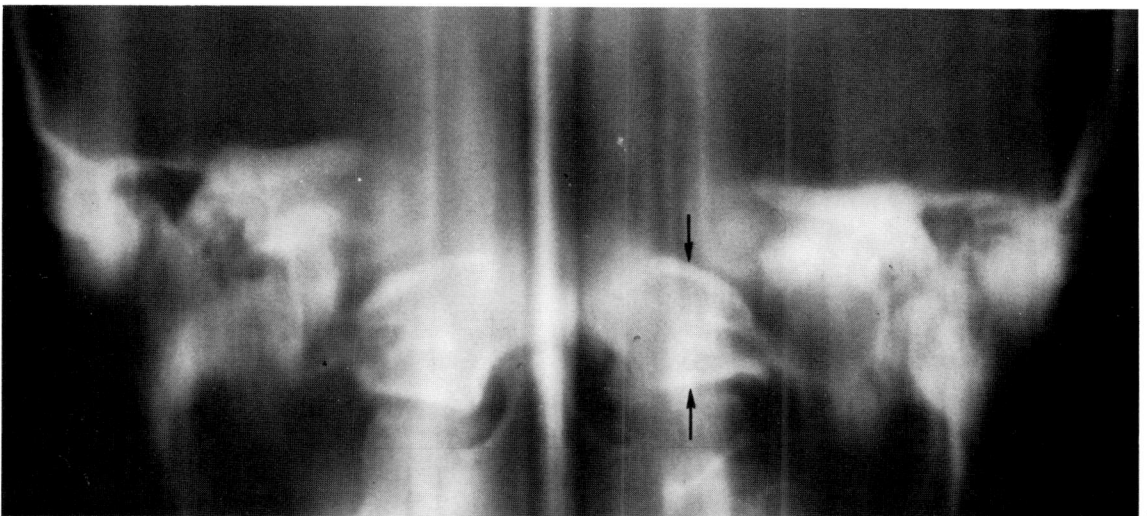

B

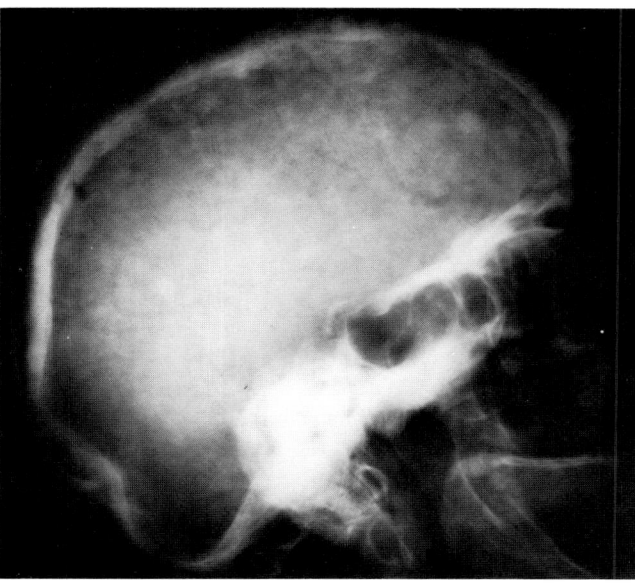

FIG SK13-2. **Basilar impression** secondary to Paget's disease. The calvarium shows a mottled thickening with nodular densities scattered throughout. Portions of the base of the skull are also sclerotic and thickened. The floor of the posterior cranial fossa is markedly depressed and slants sharply upward toward the foramen magnum. The odontoid process of C2 protrudes into the foramen magnum.[6]

CYSTLIKE LESIONS OF THE JAW

Condition	Imaging Findings	Comments
Radicular cyst (dental cyst, periodontal cyst) **(Fig SK14-1)**	Round or oval lucency with well-defined, discrete margins. Large lesions may exert uniform outward pressure on the buccal and lingual cortical plates.	Most common cyst of the mandible. Develops as a result of infection of the dental pulp and occurs at the root apex of a necrotic, nonvital tooth that has typically been gutted by caries. The radiopaque lamina dura that normally surrounds the root apex is absent. The cyst forms from epithelial remnants or cell rests in the periodontal ligament space that proliferate when stimulated by a dental inflammation.
Dentigerous cyst (follicular cyst) **(Fig SK14-2)**	Smooth, round, well-circumscribed unilocular radiolucent lesion containing the crown of an unerupted tooth. Varies in size from less than 1 cm to a huge expansile mass that fills much of the body or ramus of the mandible and expands the cortical plates.	Most commonly involves the canine and molar regions of the mandible. The cyst is derived from the dental lamina and outer enamel epithelium of developing teeth. Most are discovered in young persons during routine dental radiographic surveys or in a deliberate search for an unerupted permanent tooth.
Primordial cyst	Purely radiolucent lesion containing no tooth crown (unlike dentigerous cysts). Most commonly develops in the third molar region of the mandible and expands posteriorly into the ramus or superiorly toward the coronoid process.	Arises from special odontogenic epithelial cells that ordinarily do not participate directly in tooth development. Cysts containing keratin have a high rate of recurrence. Multiple keratin-containing primordial cysts in the mandible are a principal feature of Gorlin's syndrome (basal cell nevus syndrome).
Traumatic cyst (hemorrhagic bone cyst, solitary bone cyst) **(Fig SK14-3)**	Unilocular lucent cavity with no internal trabeculation that is fairly well defined at its periphery but is usually without a complete cortical border. A characteristic feature is its tendency to extend upward between the teeth toward the alveolar crest without causing splaying, movement, or erosion of the teeth (the scalloped superior border seems to undulate around the roots and up into the intradental bone).	Fluid-containing structure without an epithelial lining. Generally found in older children and adolescents (rare over age 35). Usually asymptomatic and an incidental radiographic finding.
Periapical rarefying osteitis (periapical granuloma, periapical abscess) **(Fig SK14-4)**	Localized round lucency at the apex of a nonvital tooth with associated discontinuity of the opaque lamina dura. Usually fairly well circumscribed, though it may be ill defined in an acute infection.	General term that includes periapical abscess and periapical granuloma, both of which may produce the same radiographic appearance and are treated identically (root canal filling or tooth extraction).
Ameloblastoma (adamantinoma) **(Fig SK14-5)**	Initially, a round unilocular cavity in the interdental or periapical bone. With increasing size, a characteristic multiloculated mass containing multiple round cystic cavities with curved septa. Large lesions cause irregular and undulating expansion of the adjacent cortex. Resorption of tooth roots is common.	Most common benign tumor of the mandible. Usually develops in the body of the mandible at its junction with the ramus. Lesions larger than 5 cm often contain one or two larger central cavities surrounded by numerous small daughter cysts. Adenoameloblastoma and ameloblastic fibroma are rare tumors occurring in the first two decades of life that are clinically less aggressive than ameloblastomas and may contain clusters of calcification and retained teeth.

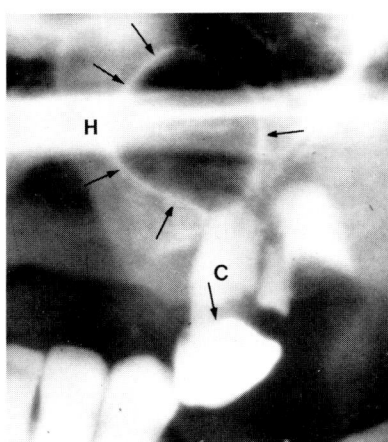

FIG SK14-1. Radicular cyst. Regular, well-circumscribed lucent lesion (arrows). The involved tooth has gross caries (C). The shadow of the hard palate (H) is superimposed across the cyst.[8]

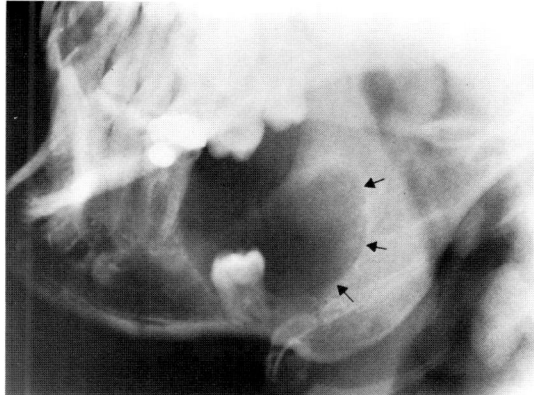

FIG SK14-2. Dentigerous cyst. Smooth, well-circumscribed lucent cavity (arrows) containing the crown of an unerupted tooth.

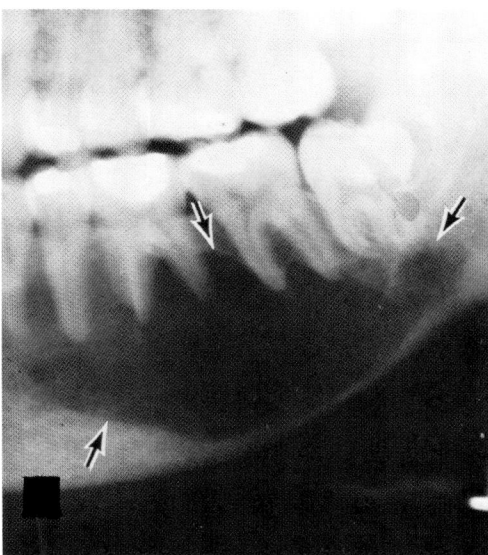

FIG SK14-3. Traumatic cyst. Note the thinning of the inferior border of the mandible and the characteristic scalloping of the superior border of the lesion around the roots of the teeth (arrows).[8]

FIG SK14-4. Periapical rarefying osteitis. The lamina dura can be seen around the canine root apex but not around the apex of the lateral incisor (arrows). Radiographically, it is impossible to distinguish among granuloma, cyst, or abscess in this lesion.[8]

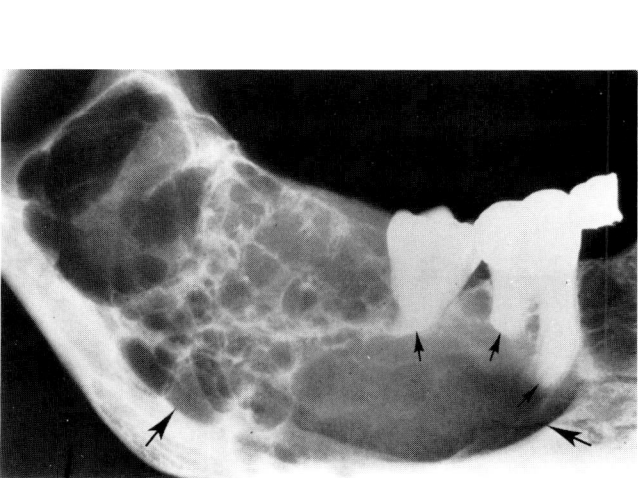

FIG SK14-5. Ameloblastoma. Plain radiograph of an excised specimen shows a lesion extending from the molar region to the superior portion of the ramus (upper left). Note particularly the multilocularity of the lesion, the heterogeneity in the size of various loculations, the well-defined margins (large arrows), and the resorption of tooth roots (small arrows).[8]

Condition	Imaging Findings	Comments
Fibrous dysplasia **(Figs SK14-6 and SK14-7)**	Expansile, lytic to sclerotic, fairly well-circumscribed lesion. Usually unilateral and most commonly involves the posterior portion of the maxilla.	Jaw involvement occurs in about 10% of cases (more common in the polyostotic form). In children, bilateral lesions (frequently with a familial pattern) can produce a multiloculated and bubbly cystic expansion of the mandible, termed *cherubism*.
Fissural developmental cyst	Lucent lesion that most commonly arises in the midline of the mandible or maxilla (incisive canal or nasopalatine cyst). Infrequently located laterally (globulomaxillary cyst) between the lateral incisor and canine tooth.	Arises from epithelial remnants at lines of embryonic fusion of the frontonasal process and the two maxillary processes.
Cementoma (cementifying fibroma) **(see Fig SK15-3)**	Initially, a radiolucent periapical lesion resembling a radicular cyst (though the involved tooth is usually healthy). Primarily involves the mandible and is often multiple.	Mesodermal tumor that arises from proliferation of connective tissue of the periodontal membrane and may reflect a localized form of fibrous dysplasia. In the late stage of development, complete calcification of the lesion results in an ovoid or round radiopaque mass surrounded by a lucent space that separates it from surrounding normal bone.
Giant cell (reparative) granuloma **(Fig SK14-8)**	Unilocular or multilocular expansile lesion that occurs twice as frequently in the mandible as the maxilla and usually arises anterior to the first molars.	Nonneoplastic reactive type of bone disease that is initiated by some unknown stimulus and is virtually identical histopathologically to giant cell tumor of the skeleton. Primarily affects adolescents and young adults.
Paget's disease	Diffuse lytic, mixed, or sclerotic process with gross enlargement of the entire mandible (unlike fibrous dysplasia, which is almost always unilateral).	Jaw involvement (most commonly in the maxilla) occurs in about 15% of patients. There is almost always concomitant involvement of the skull.
Histiocytosis X	Osteolytic area in or near the alveolar process. Characteristic "floating teeth" appearance.	Eosinophilic granuloma (often multiple) destroys the bony support of one or more teeth (especially in the posterior alveolar ridge) while leaving the tooth structures intact.
Hyperparathyroidism **(Fig SK14-9)**	Generalized loss of the lamina dura without widening of the periodontal membrane. Brown tumors (often multiple) appear as well-defined, round cystic lucencies that may expand the affected bone.	Resorption of the lamina dura is a much less sensitive radiographic indicator of hyperparathyroidism than the basically analogous subperiosteal cortical resorption of the phalanges. This appearance is also nonspecific, since it can occur in Paget's disease, fibrous dysplasia, and osteomalacia.
Metastases and nonodontogenic benign and primary malignant tumors	Variable appearance similar to the counterparts of these processes occurring elsewhere.	Metastases may be hematogenous or may spread directly from tumors of the oral or nasal cavity, salivary glands, or skin. Rare instances of aneurysmal bone cyst, hemangioma, neurofibroma, fibrosarcoma, osteosarcoma (see Fig SK15-6), chondrosarcoma, and multiple myeloma.

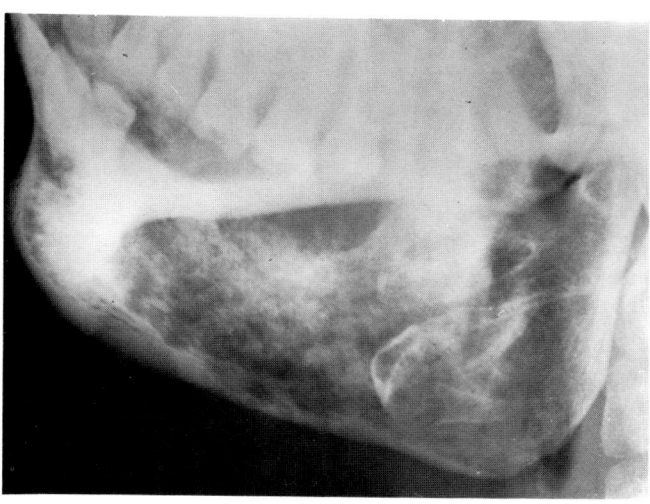

FIG SK14-6. **Fibrous dysplasia.** Large mixed lytic and sclerotic lesion involving most of one mandibular ramus.

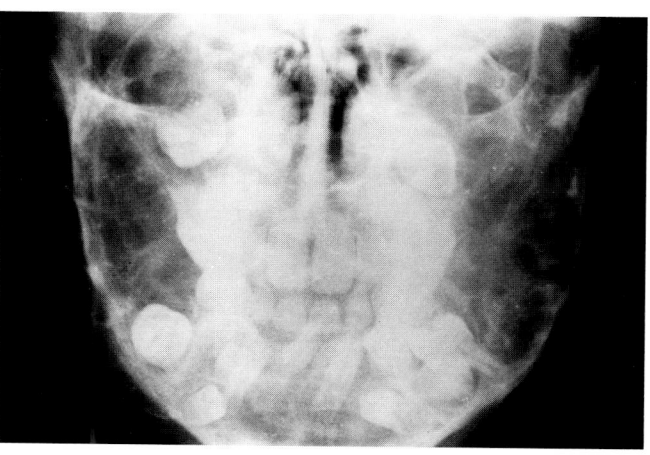

FIG SK14-7. **Cherubism.** Typical multiloculated appearance and associated malpositioning of teeth in a patient with bilateral fibrous dysplasia.[8]

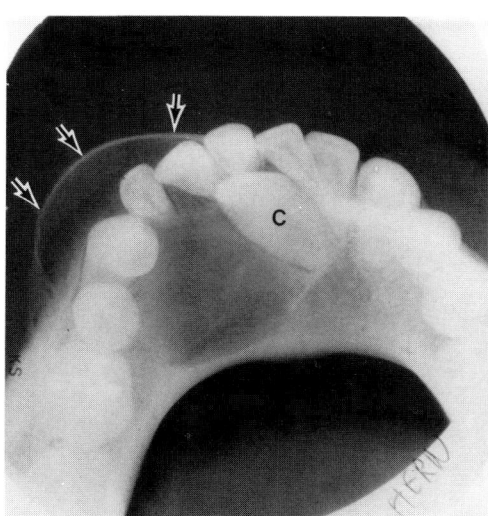

FIG SK14-8. **Giant cell granuloma.** Occlusal view demonstrates an expansile radiolucency in the anterior portion of the mandible producing even, regular swelling of the buccal cortical plate (arrows) and intrusion of a canine tooth (C).[8]

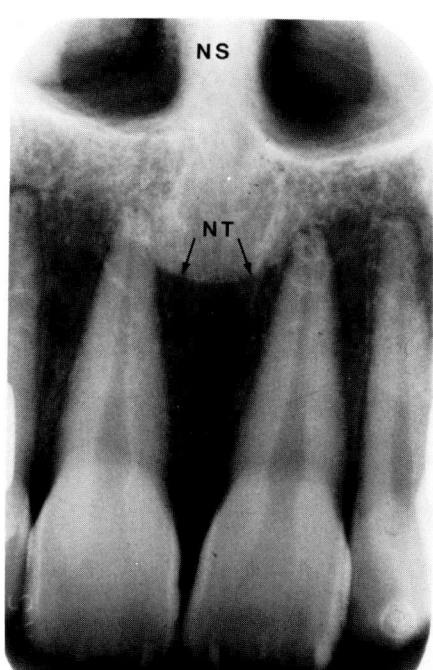

FIG SK14-9. **Primary hyperparathyroidism.** The overall bone density between the teeth is overly radiolucent, indicating severe demineralization. There was loss of lamina dura from around the roots, which causes the roots to have the appearance of accentuated tapering. (NT, tip of nose and NS, nasal septum).[8]

RADIOPAQUE LESIONS OF THE JAW

Condition	Imaging Findings	Comments
Odontoma **(Fig SK15-1)**	*Compound* odontoma appears as a small bundle of numerous dwarfed, misshapened rudimentary teeth surrounded by a thin radiolucent line representing the fibrous capsule. *Complex* odontoma appears as a uniformly opaque, irregular mass surrounded by a thin but intact radiolucent line.	More common *compound* type originates from proliferation of fetal dental lamina and usually contains 3 to 36 (up to 2,000) tiny teeth. *Complex* odontoma is generally a single tumor mass composed of two or more hard dental tissues (enamel, dentin, or cementum) in various proportions. The jumbled mass does not even remotely resemble normal teeth.
Torus mandibularis and palatinus **(Fig SK15-2)**	Opaque exostosis or bony protuberance that occurs along the midline of the palate or along the lingual surface of the mandible. Almost always bilateral and usually symmetric.	Benign, static growths that do not become malignant and have no clinical significance (unless denture construction is contemplated). *Torus mandibularis* occurs on the lingual surface of both sides of the mandible above the myelohyoid ridge, primarily in the canine-premolar region. *Torus palatinus* occurs on both midline margins of the hard palate of the maxilla.
Paget's disease	Various patterns of sclerosis in the later stages.	Round, radiopaque foci of abnormal bone may produce a ''cotton wool'' appearance. As the fluffy, opacified areas enlarge and become more numerous, they tend to coalesce.
Fibrous dysplasia **(see Fig SK14-6)**	May produce a unilateral, primarily sclerotic, fairly well-circumscribed lesion.	Jaw involvement occurs in about 10% of cases and may produce an expansile, lytic appearance.
Cementoma **(cementifying fibroma)** **(Fig SK15-3)**	In the late stage of development, there is almost complete opacification of the previously lucent lesion. This results in an ovoid or round dense mass surrounded by a lucent space separating it from normal bone.	Mesodermal tumor that is initially completely lucent and may reflect a localized form of fibrous dysplasia. Often multiple and most frequently involves the mandible.
Ossifying fibroma **(Fig SK15-4)**	Various amounts of calcified material in a unilocular, well-marginated mass.	Probably arises from primitive mesenchymal tissue surrounding the tooth. The dense material formed by the tumor may be typical bone or resemble cementum.
Osteoma **(Fig SK15-5)**	Island of dense bone that grows very slowly. Primarily involves the mandible below the lower molars and protrudes inferiorly.	Generally does not produce symptoms or signs until its size causes notable deformity. May be multiple in the skull, face, or jaw and associated with multiple colonic polyps in Gardner's syndrome.
Osteosarcoma **(Fig SK15-6)**	Central, ill-defined area of bone destruction with variable amounts of opacification that may resemble a mass of cotton wool.	Represents about 7% of all osteosarcomas. The most common symptoms are bone swelling and bleeding around the necks of the teeth. A bizarre pattern of periosteal response occasionally occurs.

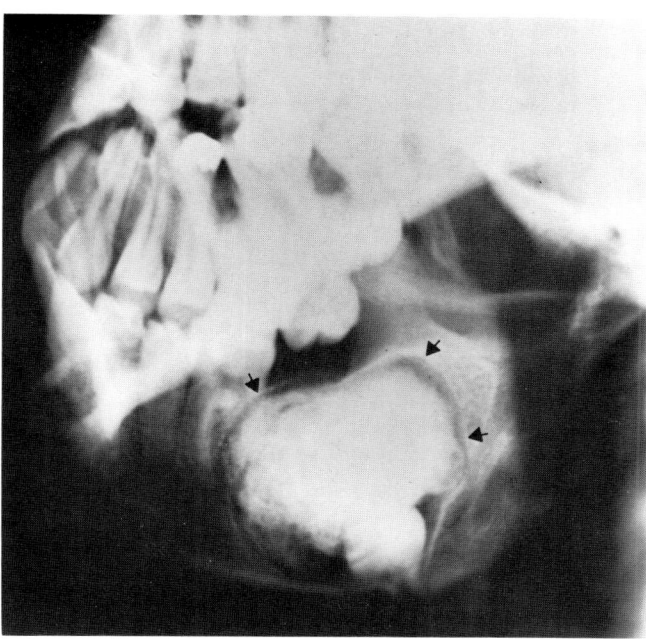

FIG SK15-1. Odontoma. Densely calcified mandibular mass surrounded by a thin radiolucent line (arrows) representing the fibrous capsule.

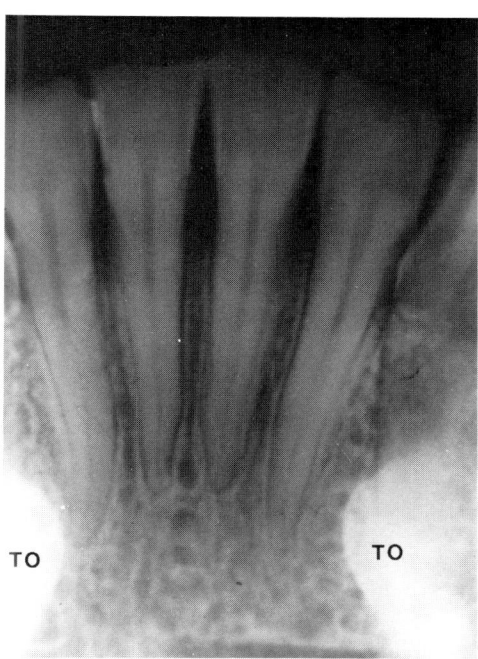

FIG SK15-2. Torus mandibularis. On this periapical view of the anterior teeth, tori (TO) appear bilaterally as convex radiopaque protuberances pointing medially from the sides of the film. These bony exostoses could be easily seen and palpated intraorally.[8]

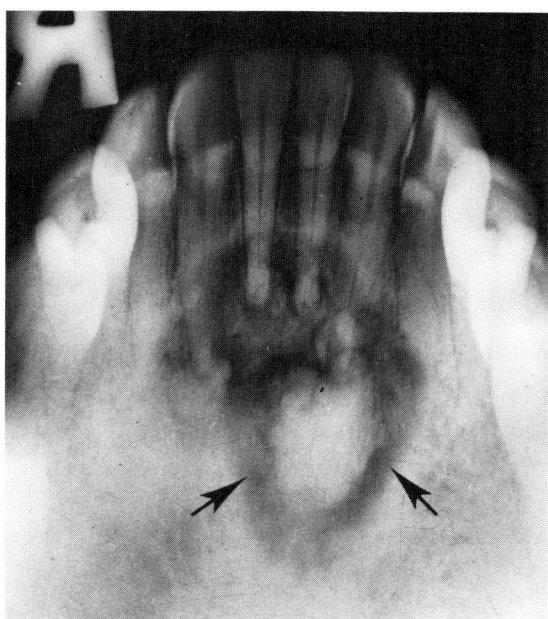

FIG SK15-3. Cementoma. Occlusal view reveals a calcified mass with a lucent zone separating it from the surrounding palate (arrows). Note the small radiopaque densities surrounding tooth roots.[8]

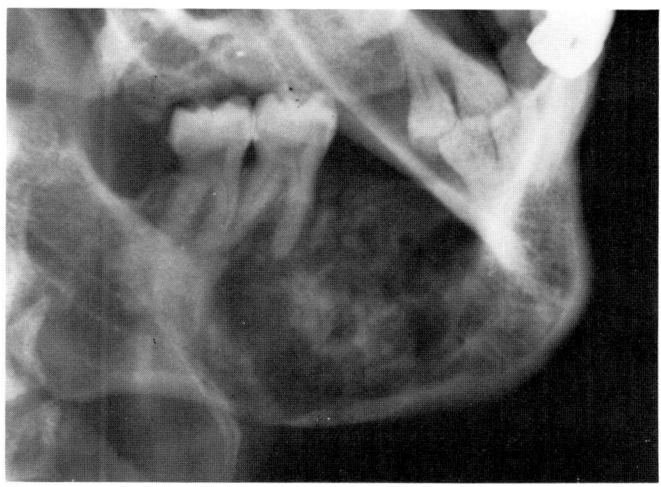

FIG SK15-4. Ossifying fibroma. Amorphous calcification with a large, well-marginated lucent mass.

Condition	Imaging Findings	Comments
Osteopetrosis	Mandible may be involved in the generalized bony sclerosis.	Rare hereditary bone dysplasia in which failure of the resorptive mechanism of calcified cartilage interferes with its normal replacement by mature bone.
Garré's sclerosing osteomyelitis	Exuberant sclerotic periosteal reaction and cortical thickening that usually involves the lower border of the mandible.	Response to a mandibular infection that is secondary to necrotic teeth in children and adolescents. There may be surprisingly little intraosseous bone destruction.
Infantile cortical hyperostosis (Caffey's disease) (Fig SK15-7)	Bilateral thickening of the inferior mandibular cortex. The deposition of layers of new bone may sometimes produce a laminated appearance.	Mandible is the most common bone involved in this condition, which occurs within the first 5 months of life.

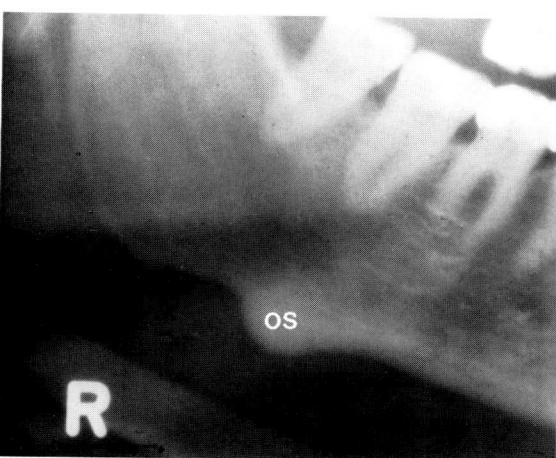

FIG SK15-5. Osteoma. The lesion (OS) is at its usual location at the inferior mandibular border just anterior to the angle. This sessile type of osteoma is seen as bulging of the cortex inferiorly.[8]

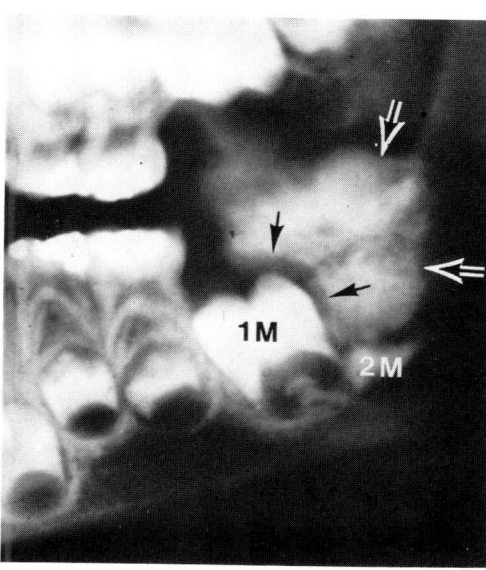

FIG SK15-6. Osteosarcoma of the mandible. The outlined arrows indicate the superior and posterior limits of the tumor, which has a fluffy radiopaque character. Superiorly, the lesion had extended past the occlusal surface of the teeth and had perforated the oral mucosa. Note that the lesion has not yet eroded through the radiolucent follicle (black arrows) of the unerupted first molar tooth (1M). (2M, second molar).[8]

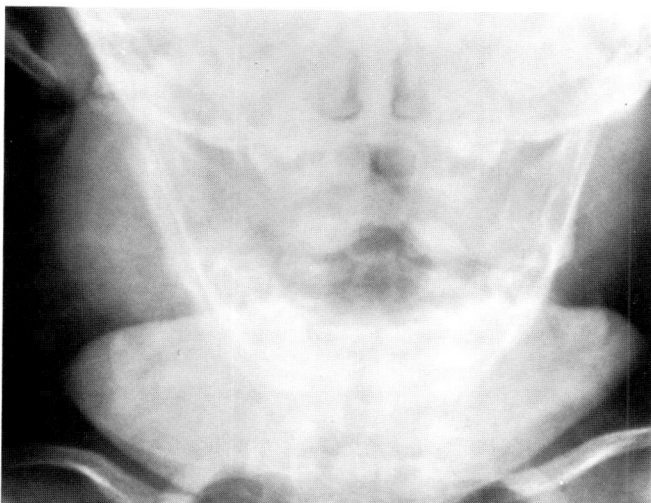

FIG SK15-7. Infantile cortical hyperostosis (Caffey's disease). Bilateral thickening of the mandibular cortex, more prominent on the right.

MASS IN A PARANASAL SINUS

Condition	Imaging Findings	Comments
Mucous or serous retention cyst	Homogeneous soft-tissue mass that usually involves the floor or lateral wall of the maxillary sinus. A dome-shaped or spherical configuration is usually diagnostic, though some cysts are broad-based and can simulate an air-fluid level.	Most common sinus complication of inflammatory sinusitis. A mucous retention cyst results from obstruction of a seromucinous gland with resulting cystic expansion (its wall is lined by epithelium of the specific gland involved). A serous cyst results from fluid accumulation and loculation in the submucosal layers of the mucoperiosteum and thus does not have an epithelial lining (the two conditions are radiographically indistinguishable).
Mucocele (Fig SK16-1)	Initially, clouding of the involved sinus with effacement of the normal mucoperiosteal line and reactive bone sclerosis. The net effect of bone destruction (with resulting decreased density) and the increased soft-tissue density of the mucocele itself makes most frontal sinus mucoceles appear radiolucent when compared to the adjacent frontal bone.	Complication of inflammatory disease that probably reflects obstruction of the ostium of the sinus and the accumulation of mucous secretions. The most clinically important cystic complication of inflammatory disease because it can expand and destroy adjacent structures. Primarily involves the frontal sinuses (65%). About 25% affect the ethmoid sinuses and 10% the maxillary sinuses. Infection of the lesion is termed a pyocele.
Sinusitis (Figs SK16-2 and SK16-3)	Soft-tissue density (mucosal thickening) lining the walls of the involved sinuses. An air-fluid level in the sinus indicates acute inflammatory disease. Most commonly affects the maxillary sinuses.	Viral infection or allergic reaction involving the upper respiratory tract may lead to the obstruction of drainage from one or more of the paranasal sinuses and the development of localized pain, tenderness, and fever. Destruction of the bony sinus wall is an ominous sign indicating secondary osteomyelitis.
Granulomatous disease (Fig SK16-4)	Various patterns of soft-tissue swelling, polypoid lesions, bone destruction, and sclerosis involving the sinuses.	Infectious causes include tuberculosis, syphilis, leprosy, glanders (*Pseudomonas mallei*), yaws, and fungal disorders (mucormycosis, actinomycosis). Granulomatous involvement of the sinuses also occurs in sarcoidosis and erythema nodosum.
Wegener's granulomatosis (Fig SK16-5)	Thickening of the mucous membranes of the paranasal sinuses that may progress to destruction of the nasal bones, orbits, mastoids, and base of the skull.	Necrotizing vasculitis and granulomatous inflammation that primarily affects the upper and lower respiratory tracts and the kidneys. The paranasal sinuses are involved in more than 90% of patients.
Midline granuloma (Fig SK16-6)	Granulomatous masses in the nose and sinuses cause clouding or complete obliteration of the air space. May progress to extensive destruction of the nasal bone and the medial walls of the maxillary antra.	Uncommon disease characterized by local inflammation, destruction, and often mutilation of the tissues of the upper respiratory tract and face. The sinus involvement is similar to Wegener's granulomatosis (but there are no pulmonary or renal lesions).
Fracture with hemorrhage	Localized submucosal hematoma may simulate a polyp (eg, blowout fracture of the orbit producing a polypoid mass on the roof of the maxillary sinus).	Partial or complete sinus opacification may be a manifestation of an acute fracture or the sequela of an old fracture.

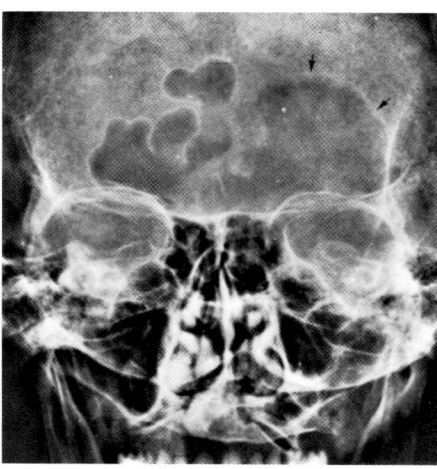

FIG SK16-1. **Mucocele** of left frontal sinus. The right frontal sinus has a normal scalloped margin with a sharp mucoperiosteal line. On the left, the frontal sinus is slightly clouded when compared to the normal right side; however, the overall appearance on the left is that of a "lucent" defect. The contour is smooth and the mucoperiosteal line is hazy or absent (arrows).[8]

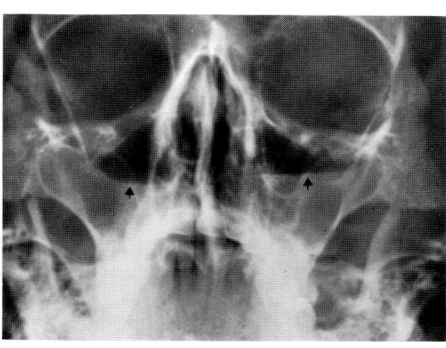

FIG SK16-2. **Acute sinusitis.** There is mucosal thickening involving most of the paranasal sinuses, and air-fluid levels (arrows) appear in both maxillary antra.

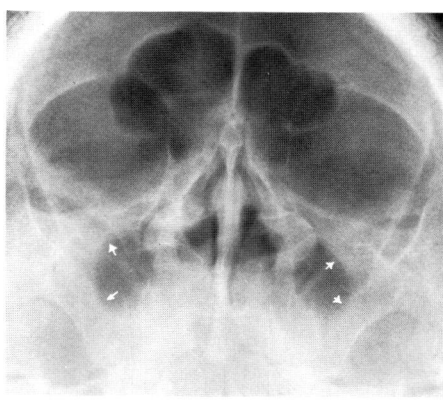

FIG SK16-3. **Chronic sinusitis.** Mucosal thickening appears as a soft-tissue density (arrows) lining the walls of the maxillary antra.

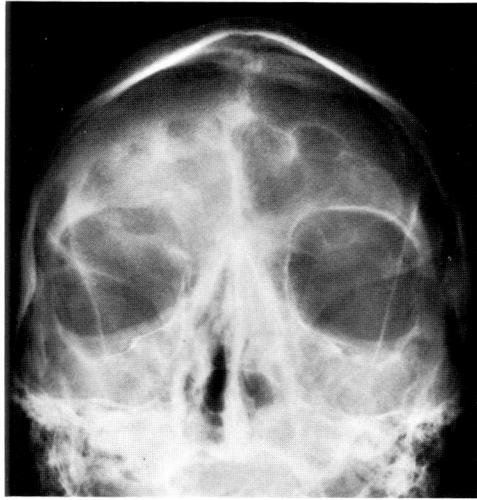

FIG SK16-4. **Mucormycosis** causing pansinusitis with osteomyelitis. There is destruction of the roof of the right orbit with a loss of the mucoperiosteal line of the right frontal sinus.

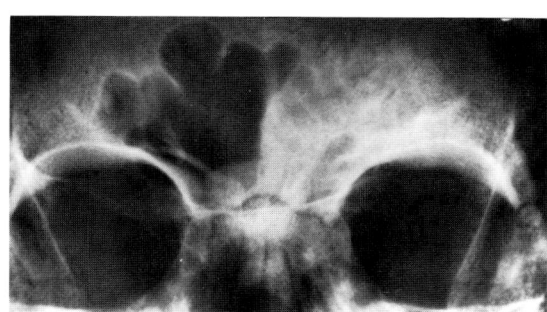

FIG SK16-5. **Wegener's granulomatosis.** Obliteration of the left frontal sinus, which has become densely opaque.[9]

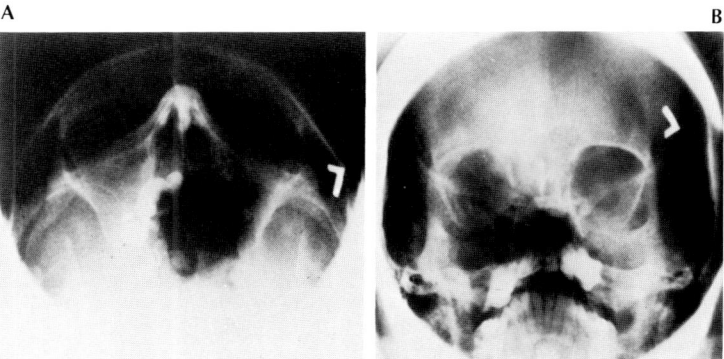

FIG SK16-6. **Midline granuloma.** (A) Extensive destruction of the palate and the left maxillary sinus with involvement of the floor of the left orbit. (B) In another patient, there is destruction of the nasal septum and the right maxillary sinus.[10]

Condition	Imaging Findings	Comments
Barotrauma	Mucosal thickening (often nodular) that may progress to complete opacification of the involved sinus.	Complication of sudden markedly negative intrasinus pressure (in airplane pilots and deep-sea divers) that causes rupture of mucosal vessels and results in subepithelial hematomas as well as free intrasinus bleeding. The radiographic changes primarily involve the maxillary sinuses (though the frontal sinuses are clinically affected more often) and may take 3 to 10 weeks to completely return to normal.
Encapsulated fluid/polyp	Localized soft-tissue mass along the wall of a sinus.	Encapsulated exudate, pus, or blood or localized inflammatory hypertrophic swelling of the mucosa.
Carcinoma (Fig SK16-7)	Soft-tissue mass with diffuse bone destruction but no sclerotic reaction.	Some 90% are squamous cell carcinomas, which are usually found in patients over age 40. About 80% arise in the maxillary sinuses.
Other malignant neoplasms (Fig SK16-8)	Appearance identical to that of carcinoma (there may be new bone formation in osteosarcoma).	Rare manifestation of sarcoma, lymphoma, extramedullary plasmacytoma, mixed salivary tumor, or melanoma.
Benign neoplasm (Figs SK16-9 and SK16-10)	Various patterns ranging from a soft-tissue mass to a dense bony lesion.	Chondroma; hemangioma; dermoid; lipoma; osteoma. Juvenile nasopharyngeal angiofibroma produces characteristic anterior bowing of the posterior wall of a maxillary sinus.
Odontogenic lesion	Mass at the base of a maxillary sinus.	Various types of cysts and tumors (see pages 48 and 52).
Extrinsic neoplasm invading sinus	Soft-tissue mass with destruction of sinus walls.	Pituitary, orbital, oral, or nasopharyngeal tumor; chordoma; Burkitt's lymphoma.
Fibrous dysplasia	Expansion and nonhomogeneous opacification of the involved sinuses with marked sclerosis and thickening of the facial bones.	Similar appearance may occur in ossifying fibroma (considered a localized form of fibrous dysplasia in the facial bones).
Surgical ciliated cyst	Various patterns (fibrosis simulating mucosal disease, a soft-tissue mass, or complete opacification of the sinus).	Follows the Caldwell-Luc procedure, in which an anterior opening is made into the maxillary sinuses between the roots of the upper canine and first molar teeth.

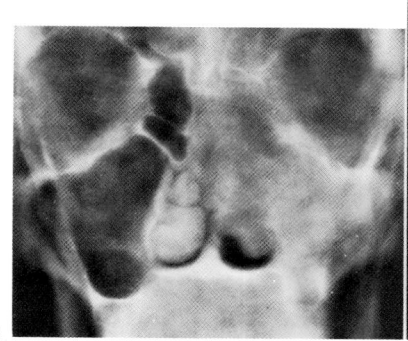
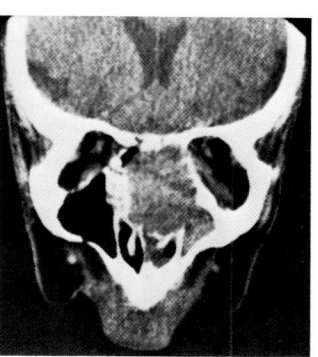

A   B

FIG SK16-7. **Malignant tumors of the paranasal sinuses.** (A) Coronal tomogram reveals a tumor mass in the left nasal cavity and ethmoid and maxillary sinuses. The lamina papyracea, orbital floor, and most of the remaining antral margins are intact (mixed tumor of minor salivary gland origin). (B) Coronal CT scan shows an expansile nonenhanced tumor of the left nasal cavity and ethmoid and maxillary sinuses (cylindroma).[8]

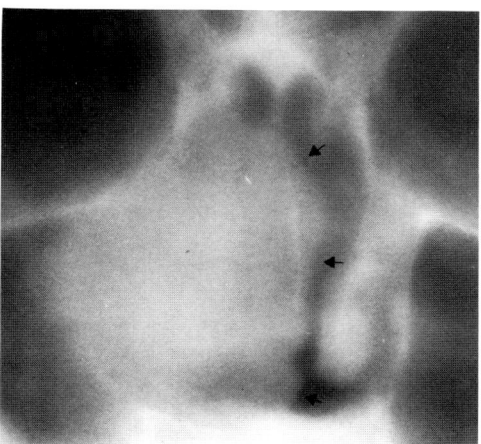

FIG SK16-8. **Extramedullary plasmacytoma.** A large lesion of the right nasal cavity (arrows) causes destruction of the medial wall of the right maxillary antrum.[11]

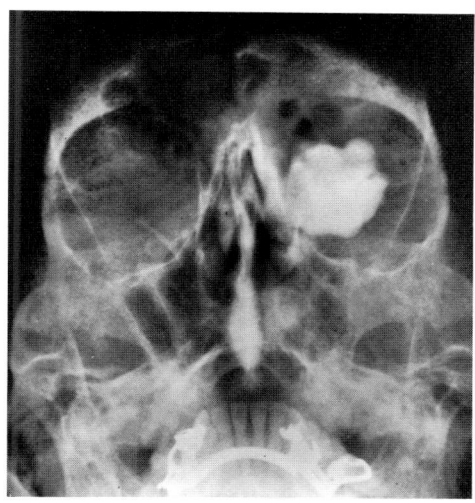

A

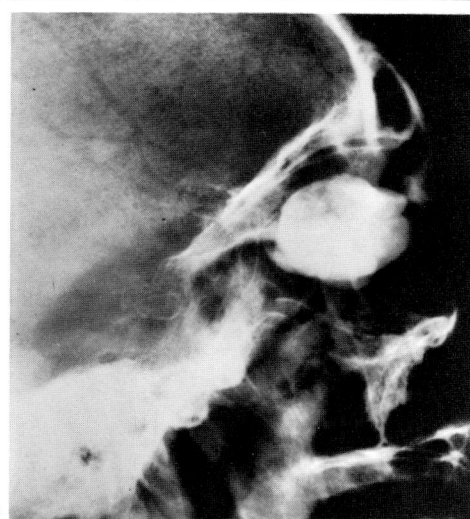

B

FIG SK16-9. **Osteoma** of the ethmoid sinus. (A) Frontal and (B) lateral views of the skull demonstrate a large, extremely dense osteoma filling and expanding the left ethmoid sinus.

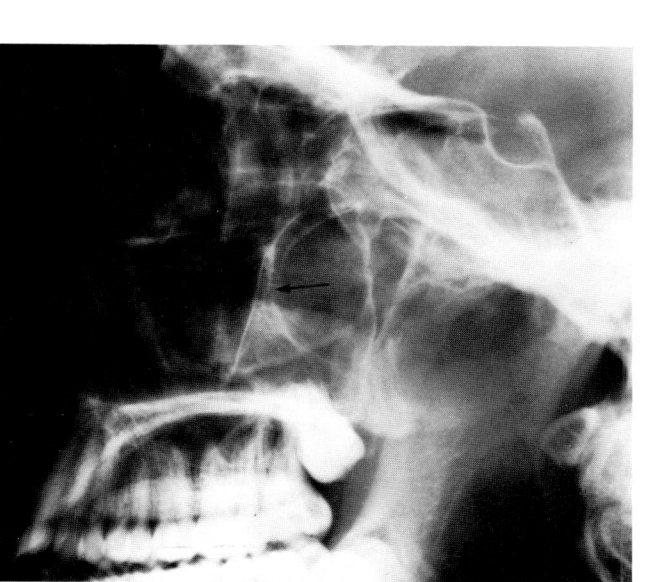

FIG SK16-10. **Juvenile nasopharyngeal angiofibroma.** Pronounced anterior bowing (arrow) of the posterior wall of the maxillary sinus.[12]

DILATED CEREBRAL VENTRICLES

Condition	Imaging Findings	Comments
Noncommunicating (obstructive) hydrocephalus	Symmetric distention of the ventricular system proximal to the obstruction and a ventricular system of normal or less than normal size distal to the obstruction.	Possible site of obstruction should be examined in detail with thin CT slices and, if necessary, overlapping cuts to establish the pathogenesis of the obstruction.
Level of foramen of Monro (Fig SK17-1)	Enlargement of the lateral ventricles with normal-sized third and fourth ventricles.	Colloid cyst; suprasellar tumors (especially craniopharyngioma); intraventricular tumors; arachnoid cysts of the suprasellar cistern; intraventricular hemorrhage (trauma, arteriovenous malformation, hemophilia). Unilateral tumors, such as those arising in the hypothalamus, basal ganglia, or cerebral parenchyma, may obstruct only one side and cause dilatation of the opposite ventricle and mass compression of the ipsilateral ventricle.
Level of aqueduct (Fig SK17-2)	Enlargement of the lateral and third ventricles with a normal-sized fourth ventricle.	Most common causes are congenital aqueduct stenosis or occlusion (most commonly associated with the Arnold-Chiari malformation) and neoplasm (pinealoma, teratoma). Other underlying conditions include cyst of the quadrigeminal cistern, brainstem edema, aneurysmal dilatation of the vein of Galen, hemorrhage, and acute infection.
Level of outlet of fourth ventricle (Fig SK17-3)	Enlargement of the entire ventricular system (with the fourth ventricle often dilated out of proportion).	Atresia of fourth ventricle foramina (Dandy-Walker cyst); Arnold-Chiari malformation; basilar arachnoiditis (eg, tuberculous meningitis); tonsilar herniation; neoplasm (medulloblastoma, ependymoma); basilar impression (eg, Paget's disease); arachnoid cyst.
Communicating hydrocephalus (Fig SK17-4)	Generalized ventricular enlargement with normal or absent sulci.	Obstruction of the normal cerebrospinal fluid pathway distal to the fourth ventricle (usually involves the subarachnoid space at the basal cisterns, cerebral convexity, or foramen magnum). Causes include infection (meningitis, empyema), subarachnoid or subdural hemorrhage, congenital anomalies, neoplasm, and dural venous thrombosis. A similar pattern is seen in "normal-pressure" hydrocephalus, a syndrome of gait ataxia, urinary incontinence, and dementia associated with ventricular dilatation and relatively normal cerebrospinal fluid pressure.

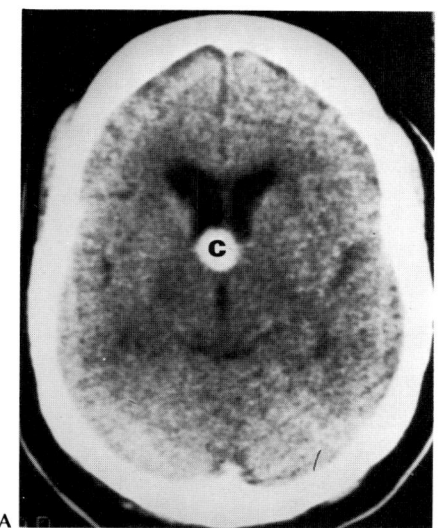

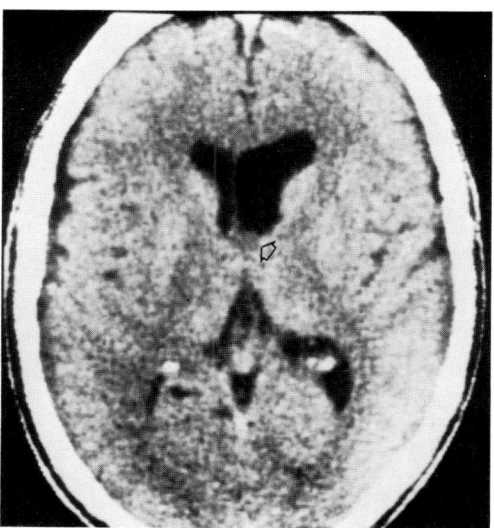

FIG SK17-1. Level of the foramen of Monro. (A) Bilateral enlargement of the frontal horns with a normal-sized third ventricle in a patient with a hyperdense colloid cyst (c). (B) Unilateral enlargement of the left frontal horn caused by a tiny hypodense unilateral tumor (arrow).

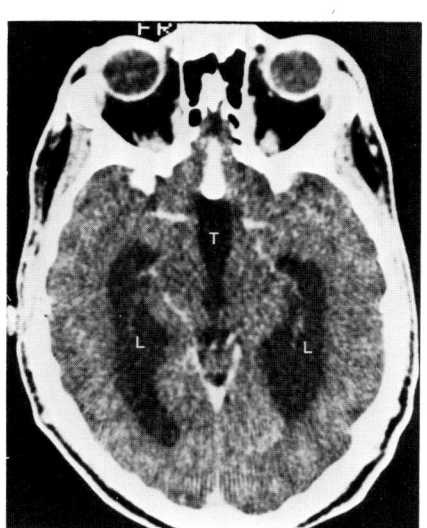

FIG SK17-2. Level of the aqueduct. Dilatation of the lateral (L) and third (T) ventricles in a patient with congenital hydrocephalus. The symptoms of headache and papilledema resolved after ventricular shunting.

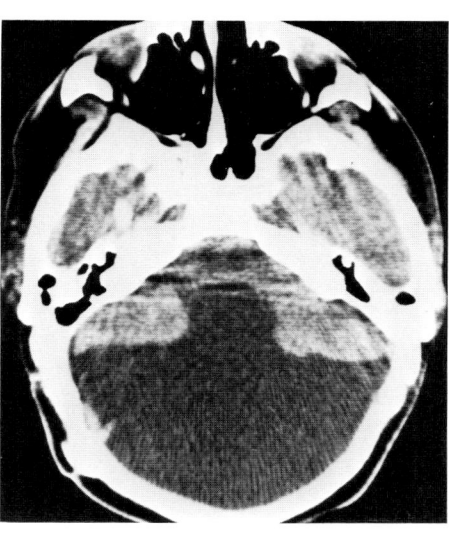

FIG SK17-3. Dandy-Walker cyst. Huge low-density cyst that occupies most of the enlarged posterior fossa and represents an extension of the dilated fourth ventricle.

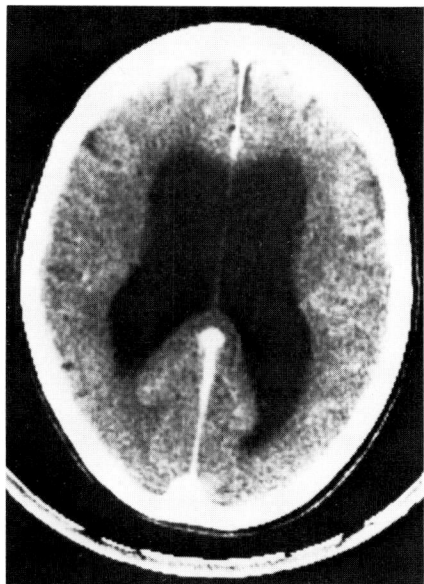

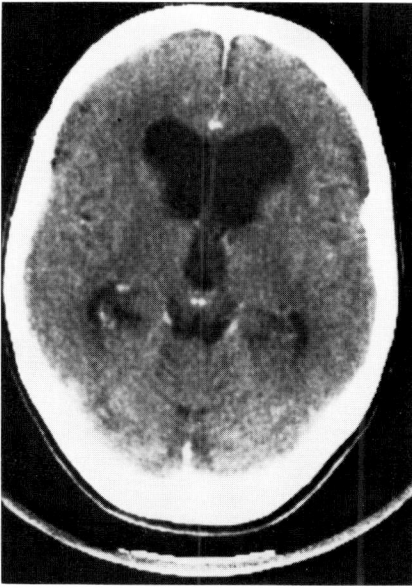

FIG SK17-4. Communicating hydrocephalus. Generalized ventricular enlargement in a 69-year-old patient with ataxia, dementia, and incontinence. Note the absence of the dilated sulci seen in obstructive hydrocephalus.[13]

Condition	Imaging Findings	Comments
Overproduction of cerebrospinal fluid (Fig SK17-5)	Generalized enlargement of the ventricular system.	Choroid plexus papilloma or carcinoma that causes overproduction of cerebrospinal fluid. This rare tumor usually occurs in the fourth ventricle in adults and the lateral ventricle in children. Differentiation from other intraventricular masses is made by the CT demonstration of its choroid location and the typical choroidal pattern of contrast enhancement.
Atrophy (atrophic hydrocephalus) (Figs SK17-6 to SK17-8)	Diffuse dilatation of the lateral and third ventricles as well as the cisterns. The sulci over the surfaces of the cerebral hemispheres are prominent and appear as wide linear lucent stripes.	Multiple causes including normal aging, degenerative diseases (Alzheimer's, Pick's, Jakob-Creutzfeldt, Binswanger's), Huntington's disease, congenital inflammatory disease (eg, toxoplasmosis, torulosis, cytomegalic inclusion disease), vascular disease (multifocal infarct, arteriovenous malformation).
Atrophy of one cerebral hemisphere (Fig SK17-9)	Enlargement of the ipsilateral lateral ventricle and sulci and a shift of midline structures to the affected side.	Usually the result of complete occlusion of the ipsilateral middle cerebral artery. If the occlusion occurs in early childhood, the affected half of the skull is underdeveloped.
Localized atrophy (Fig SK17-10)	Focal enlargement of a part of one ventricle or a group of sulci.	Usually a late residual of previous insult to the brain (eg, infarct, hematoma, severe contusion, abscess).

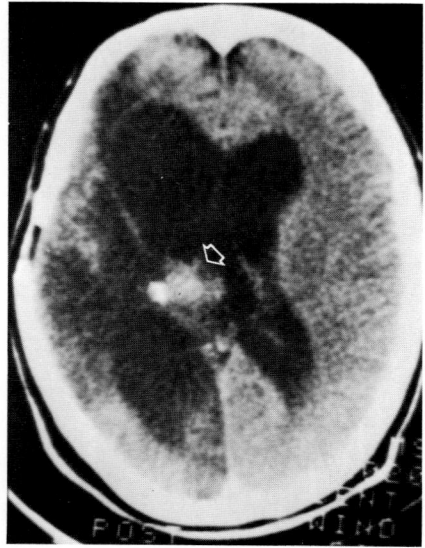

FIG SK17-5. Choroid plexus papilloma. Enhancing ventricular mass (arrow) causing pronounced generalized enlargement of the ventricular system.

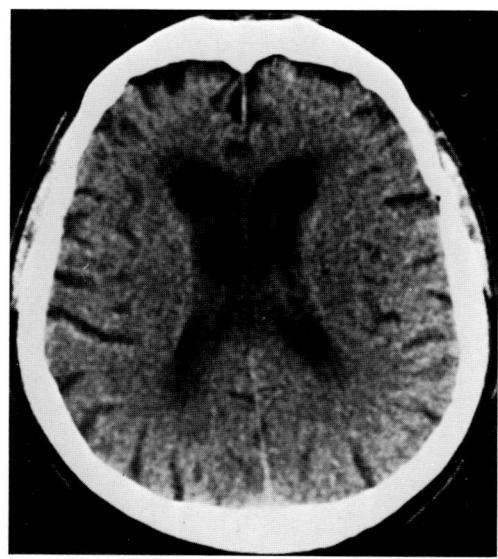

FIG SK17-6. Normal aging. CT scan of a 70-year-old man shows generalized ventricular dilatation with prominence of the sulci over the surfaces of the cerebral hemispheres.

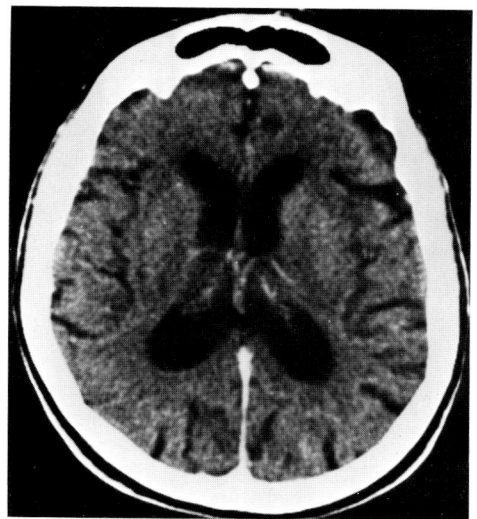

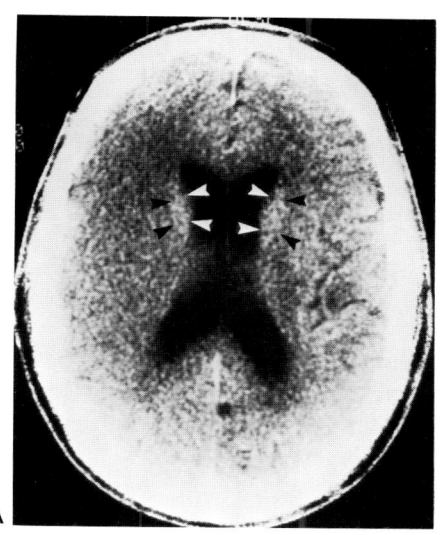

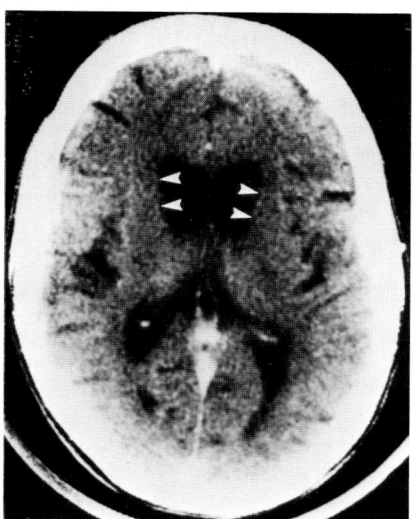

FIG SK17-7. Alzheimer's disease. Noncontrast scan of a 56-year-old woman with progressive dementia shows generalized enlargement of the ventricular system and sulci.

FIG SK17-8. Huntington's disease. (A) CT scan in a normal patient shows the heads of the caudate nucleus (black arrows) producing a normal concavity of the frontal horns (white arrows). (B) In a patient with Huntington's disease, atrophy of the caudate nucleus causes a characteristic loss of the normal concavity (white arrowheads) of the frontal horns.

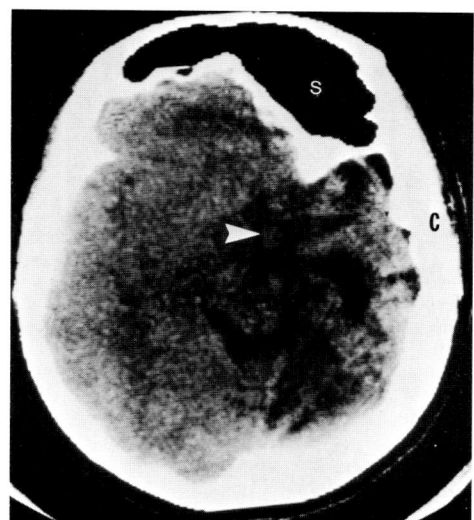

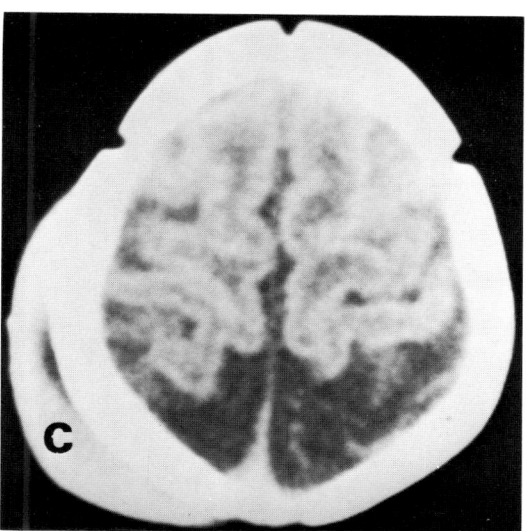

FIG SK17-9. Cerebral hemiatrophy (Davidoff-Dyke syndrome). CT scan of a 5-year-old boy who had intrauterine difficulties demonstrates extensive loss of brain volume in the left hemisphere. There is also enlargement of the left hemicalvarium (C), enlargement of the left frontal sinus (S), and a shift of midline structures such as the third ventricle (arrowhead) from right to left. The low density in the remainder of the hemisphere represents encephalomalacia.

FIG SK17-10. Localized atrophy. Contrast-enhanced scan of an infant with intrauterine infection shows bilateral occipital atrophy. Note the cephalhematoma (C) on the right.

RING-ENHANCING LESION

Condition	Comments
Glioblastoma multiforme (Figs SK18-1 and SK18-2; see Figs SK20-2 and SK22-2)	Thick, irregular ring enhancement in a solitary lesion that tends to be situated in a deep hemispheric location and associated with surrounding low-attenuation edema and glial cell infiltration. May occasionally have a relatively uniform rim of enhancement that mimics the capsule of an abscess.
Metastases (Fig SK18-3)	Irregular rim enhancement with a relatively lucent center due to tumor necrosis. Typically located at the gray matter–white matter junction and usually associated with surrounding low-density edema that tends to be relatively concentric and uniform in the adjacent white matter (unlike glial cell infiltration with glioblastoma multiforme, which is usually eccentric and irregular in both gray and white matter).
Lymphoma (Fig SK18-4)	Single or multiple ring-enhancing lesions that primarily affect transplant recipients (high incidence of central nervous system lymphoma in these patients).
Abscess (Figs SK18-5 to SK18-8)	Usually a relatively thin, uniform ring of enhancement associated with considerable reactive edema and a strongly suggestive clinical picture of fever, leukocytosis, obtundation, extracranial infection, or a previous operation. Some pyogenic or fungal abscesses may develop a relatively thick capsule, which resembles the periphery of a high-grade glioma or metastasis. The relatively poor inflammatory response of deep hemispheric white matter may cause the capsule of an abscess to be less developed along the medial wall than along the lateral margin, a feature that may aid in distinguishing an abscess from a neoplasm.
Resolving intracerebral hematoma (3 to 6 weeks old) (Fig SK18-9)	Thin, uniform ring of contrast enhancement that initially represents perivascular inflammation and defects in the tight capillary junctions and eventually reflects the collagenous capsule. Causes of intracerebral hematoma include trauma, surgery, hypertensive vascular disease, vascular malformation, mycotic aneurysm, and berry aneurysm.
Nonacute subdural hematoma	Occasionally produces a pattern of thick rim enhancement with loculation, reflecting its richly vascular surrounding membrane.

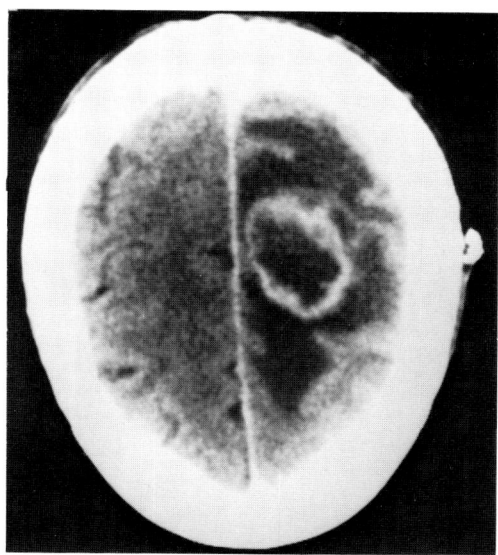

FIG SK18-1. Glioblastoma multiforme. Thick irregular ring-enhancing lesion associated with a large amount of surrounding low-attenuation edema.

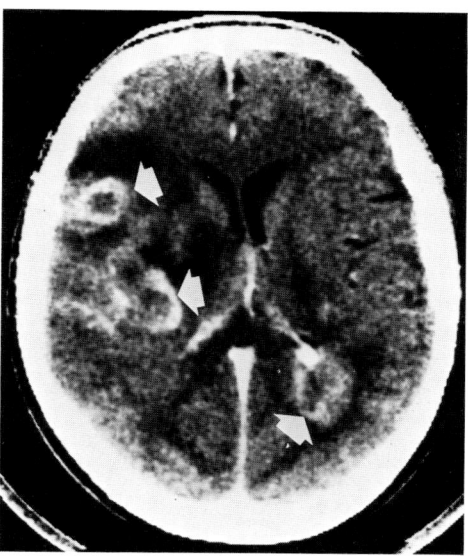

FIG SK18-2. Multicentric glioblastoma multiforme. Bilateral irregular enhancing masses (arrows) with surrounding low-density edema.

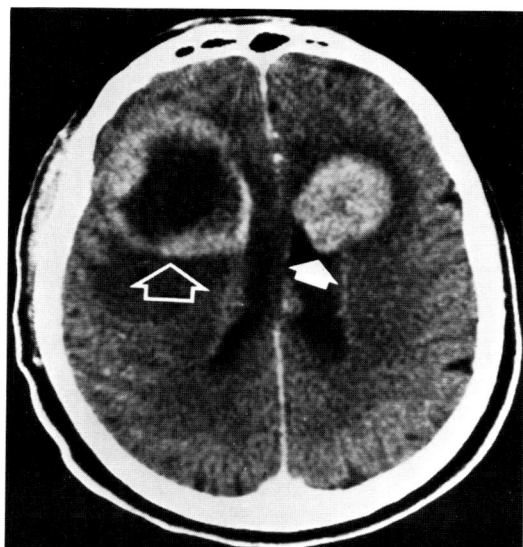

FIG SK18-3. Metastases. Enhancing metastases from squamous cell carcinoma of the lung that are both ring-enhancing (open arrow) and solid (solid arrow).

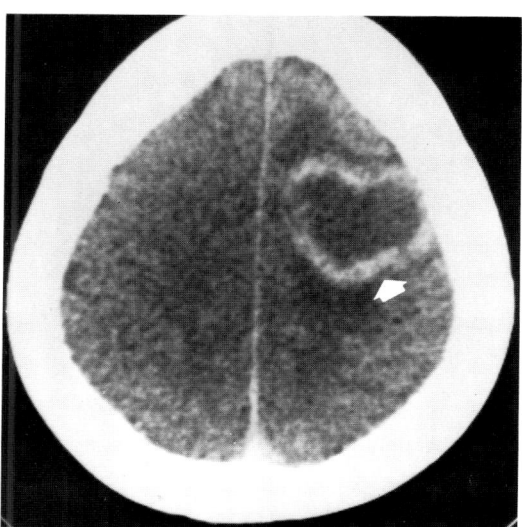

FIG SK18-4. Lymphoma developing after renal transplantation. Heart-shaped, peripherally enhancing, central lucent lesion (arrow) situated in the frontoparietal region. There is moderate surrounding edema.[14]

Condition	Comments
Atypical meningioma **(Fig SK18-10)**	A few meningiomas contain low-attenuation, non-enhancing areas (necrosis, old hemorrhage, cyst formation, or fat in the meningioma tissue) that produce a thick, often irregular, rim. This pattern, especially if associated with prominent edema, may mimic a malignant glioma or metastasis. Coronal scans demonstrating that the mass arises from a dural base suggest the diagnosis of meningioma, though superficial gliomas may invade the dura and dural-based metastases may occur.
Radiation necrosis **(Fig SK18-11)**	Occasional manifestation. Develops in the tumor bed 9 to 24 months after radiation therapy and may be impossible to differentiate from recurrent or residual tumor.

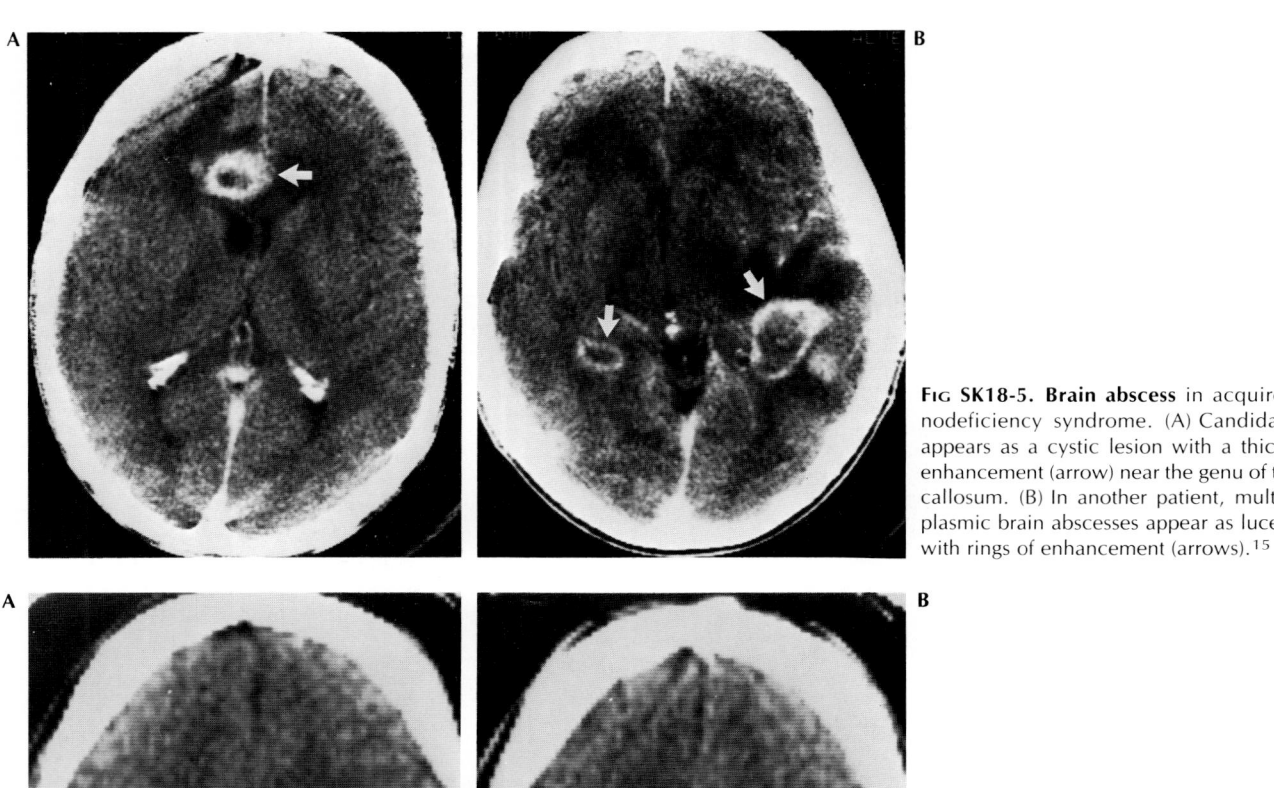

FIG **SK18-5. Brain abscess** in acquired immunodeficiency syndrome. (A) Candidal abscess appears as a cystic lesion with a thick zone of enhancement (arrow) near the genu of the corpus callosum. (B) In another patient, multiple toxoplasmic brain abscesses appear as lucent lesions with rings of enhancement (arrows).[15]

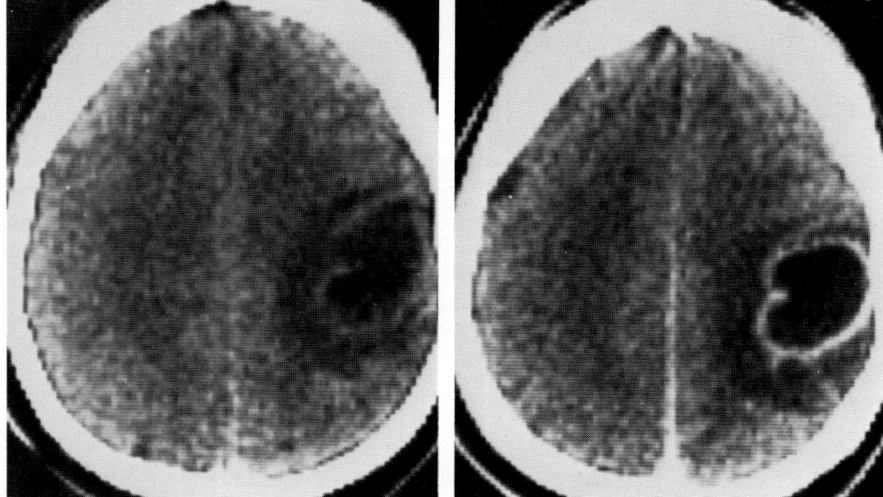

FIG **SK18-6. Cysticercosis.** (A) Precontrast CT scan shows a primarily low-density area in the right frontoparietal region. The ring of increased density around the lesion is vaguely evident initially, but becomes readily apparent after contrast enhancement (B).[16]

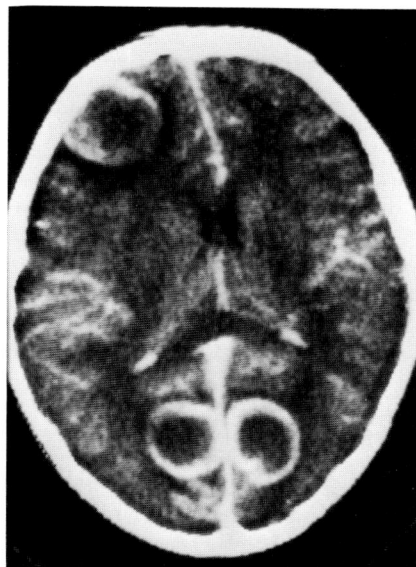

FIG SK18-7. Pyogenic brain abscesses. One frontal and two occipital lesions with relatively thin, uniform rings of enhancement.

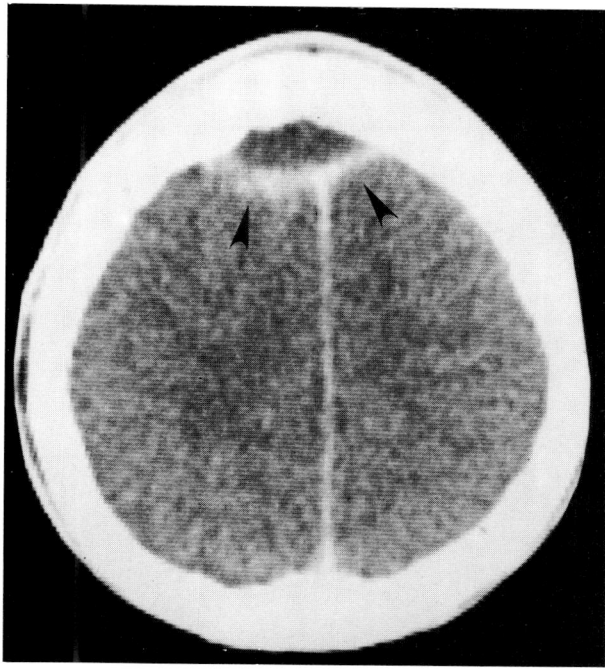

FIG SK18-8. Epidural abscess. Biconvex hypodense lesion with contrast-enhanced dural margin (arrowheads) that crosses the falx and displaces the falx away from the inner table of the skull.[17]

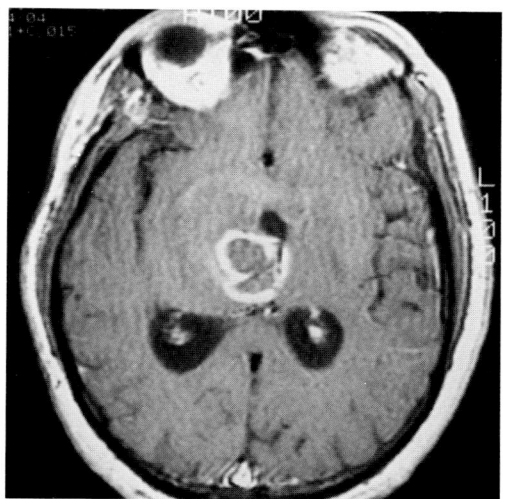

FIG SK18-9. Resolving intracerebral hematoma. Five weeks after the initial episode of bleeding, there is peripheral contrast enhancement of the thalamic lesion.

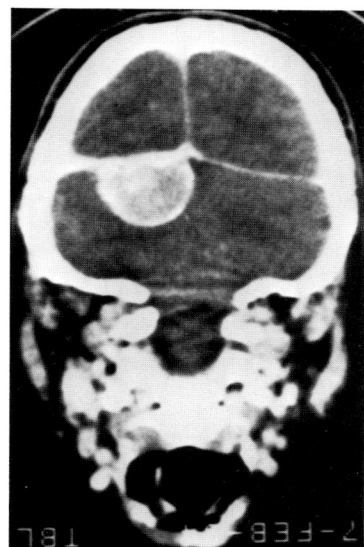

FIG SK18-10. Atypical meningioma. The contrast enhancement is predominantly peripheral, with the area of central necrosis remaining relatively nonenhanced. The correct diagnosis is indicated by the origin of the tumor from the thickened tentorium.

FIG SK18-11. Radiation necrosis. Lesion with ring enhancement and surrounding edema that could represent a primary or metastatic tumor. At autopsy the mass was found to represent postradiation necrosis with sarcomatous changes in a patient who had undergone surgery for a solitary metastasis.[17]

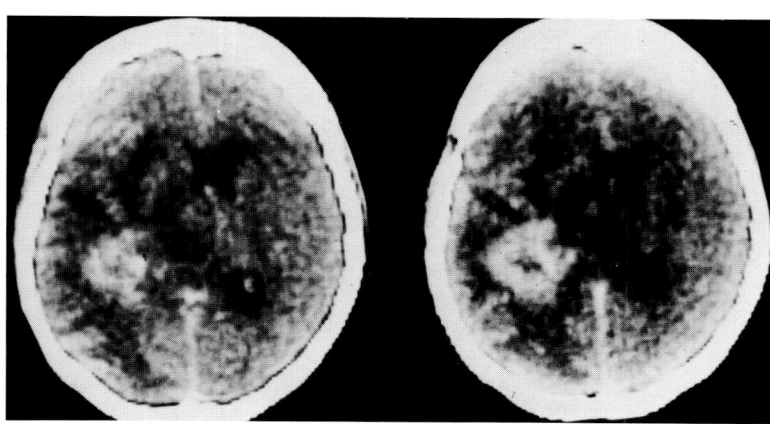

MULTIPLE ENHANCING CEREBRAL AND CEREBELLAR NODULES

Condition	Comments
Metastases **(Figs SK19-1 and SK19-2)**	Round, well-marginated, homogeneously enhancing nodules that are typically located at the gray matter–white matter junction and are often associated with some peritumoral edema. The major malignant tumors causing intracranial metastases are, in decreasing order of frequency, lung, breast, skin (melanoma), colon, rectum, and kidney.
Primary lymphoma **(Fig SK19-3)**	Homogeneously and often intensely enhancing masses that most commonly occur in the basal ganglia, corpus callosum, or periventricular region. Peritumoral edema is usually slight. Primary lymphoma of the brain is rare in otherwise healthy individuals and is much more common in patients who are immunosuppressed (especially organ transplant recipients).
Multiple sclerosis **(Figs SK19-4 and SK19-5)**	Contrast enhancement in plaques of demyelination is unusual except in rapidly evolving ones with surrounding inflammatory changes. The plaques in multiple sclerosis usually have a more central or periventricular location, unlike the more peripheral position of metastases near the gray matter–white matter junction.

Disseminated infection
  Cysticercosis
  (Figs SK19-6 and
  SK19-7)
	Multiple small, homogeneously enhancing nodules may develop after infection by the larvae of the pork tapeworm (*Taenia solium*). Usually associated with much more extensive edema than are metastases. May demonstrate multiple enhancing rings, some of which contain focal calcification representing the scolices of degenerated larvae.

Tuberculosis	Homogeneously enhancing nodules or small rings with central punctate lucencies representing foci of cavitation surrounded by a rim of inflammatory cells.
Histoplasmosis	Pattern identical to that of multiple tuberculous abscesses.
Toxoplasmosis	Multiple densely enhancing nodules (or ring-enhancing lesions) that occur at both the gray matter–white matter junction and in a periventricular location.

Subacute, multifocal infarction
  Arterial
  (Fig SK19-8)
	Small focal enhancing lesions distributed along vascular watersheds. Underlying causes include hypoperfusion, multiple emboli, cerebral vasculitis (eg, systemic lupus erythematosus), and meningitis.

(continued page 70)

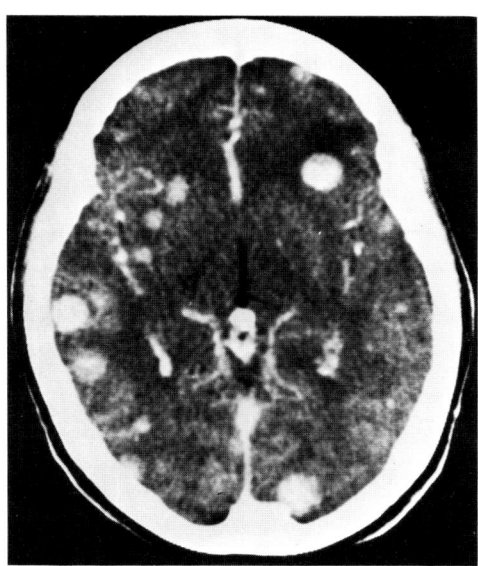

FIG SK19-1. Metastatic carcinoma. Multiple enhancing masses of various shapes and sizes representing hematogenous metastases from carcinoma of the breast.

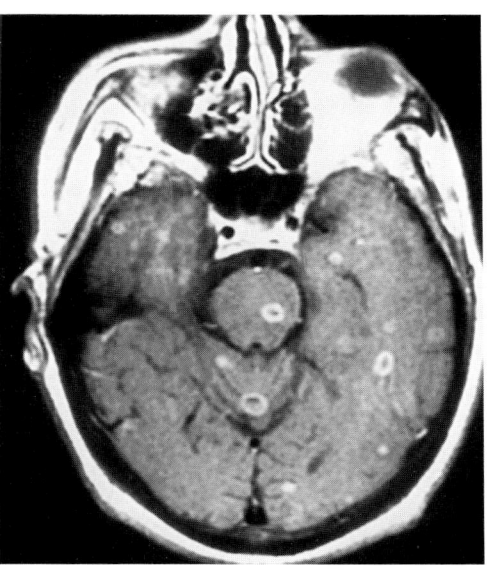

FIG SK19-2. Metastatic carcinoma. Multiple enhancing masses representing hematogenous metastases from carcinoma of the lung.

FIG SK19-3. Primary lymphoma. (A) Homogeneous enhancement of multiple periventricular nodules (arrows). (B) Another section shows additional enhancing lymphomatous nodules in the basal ganglia (large arrows) and posterior fossa (small arrows). Note the cystic cavum septum pellucidi (open arrow).[13]

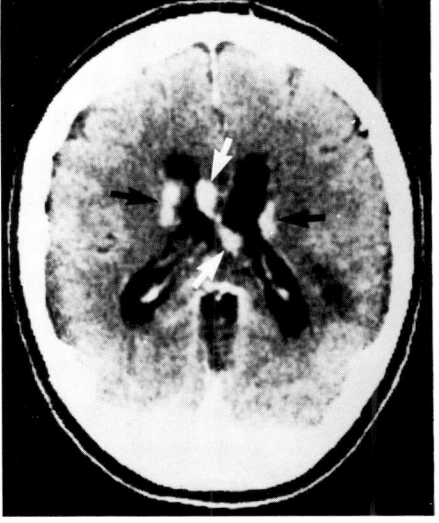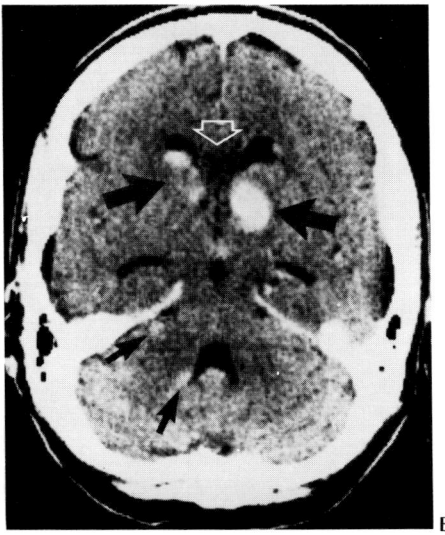

A B

FIG SK19-4. Multiple sclerosis simulating metastases. Nodular enhancement in periventricular and subcortical white matter resulting from demyelination.[13]

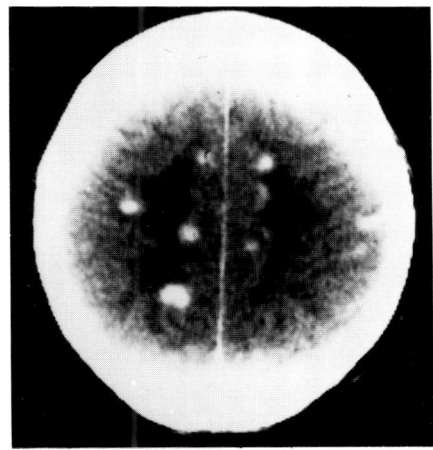

Condition	Comments
Venous	Parasagittal hemorrhages due to cortical venous infarction are a highly specific secondary finding in superior sagittal sinus thrombosis.
Sarcoidosis (Fig SK19-9)	Homogeneous enhancement of the noncaseating granulomas (more often affects the meninges than the brain).

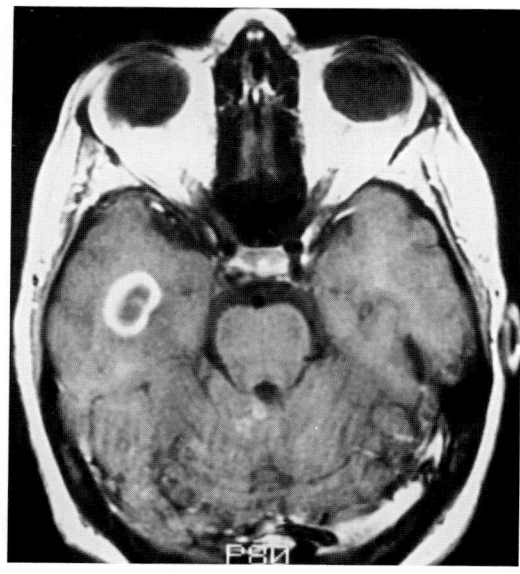

FIG SK19-5. **Multiple sclerosis.** Single large ring-enhancing lesion.

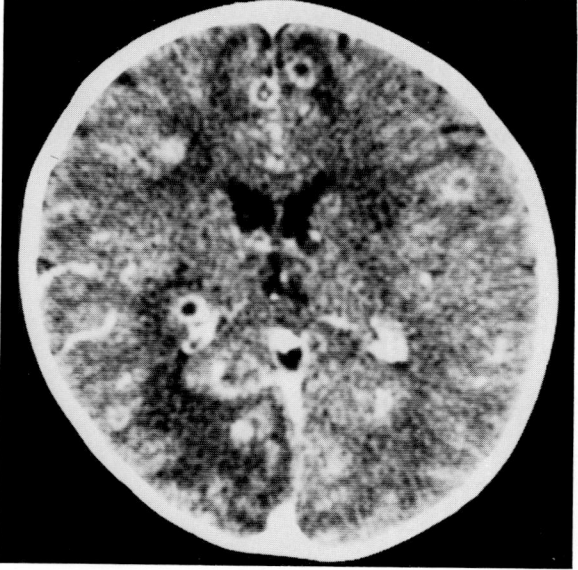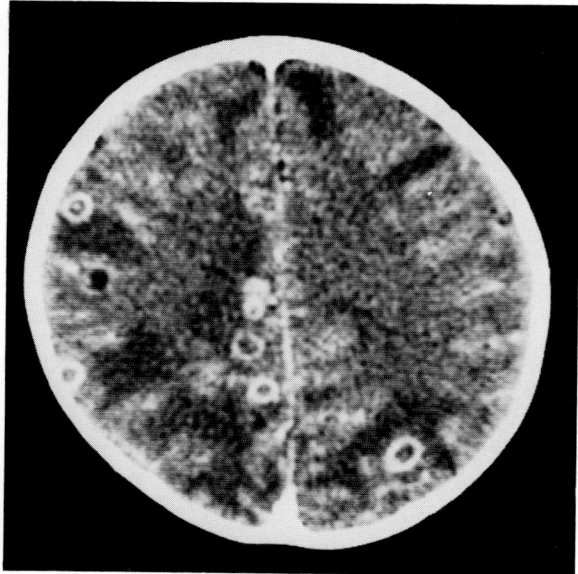

FIG SK19-6. **Cysticercosis.** Multiple enhancing nodules or rings, some of which contain focal calcification representing the scolices of erupted larvae. Note the zones of surrounding edema.[13]

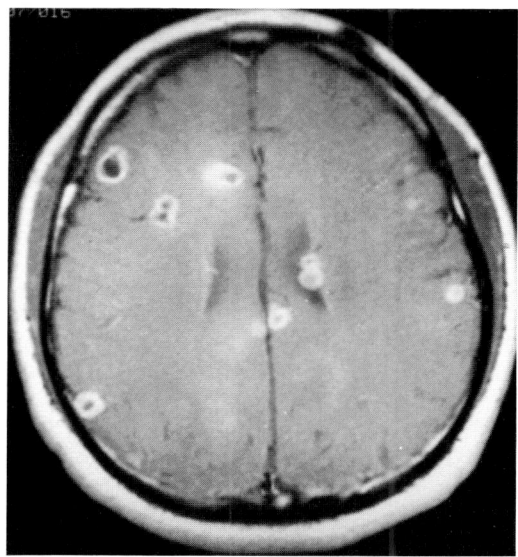

FIG SK19-7. **Cysticercosis.** Multiple enhancing nodules.

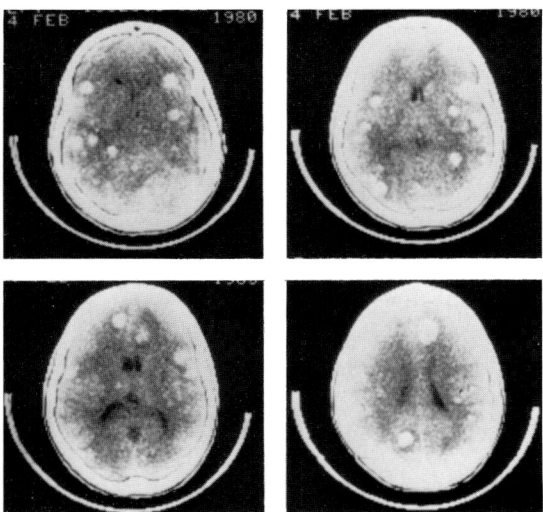

FIG SK19-8. **Subacute, multifocal infarction.** Multiple enhancing nodules producing a pattern mimicking metastases.

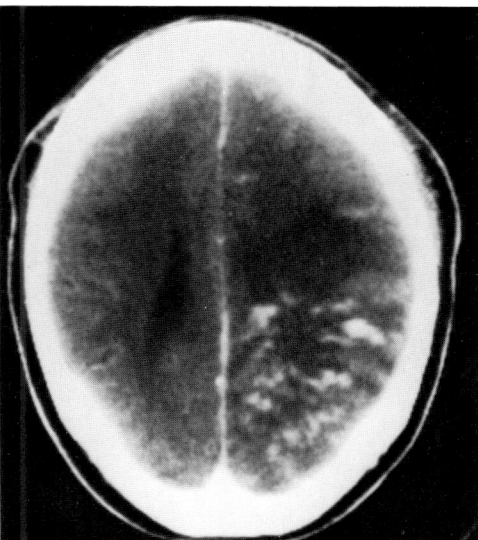

FIG SK19-9. **Sarcoidosis.** Multiple linear and nodular areas of increased density in the posterior half of the left cerebrum extending from the meninges to the deep white matter. This appearance represents infiltration of the Virchow-Robin space by granulomatous disease, in this case sarcoidosis. Note the associated encephalomalacia.[18]

HYPODENSE SUPRATENTORIAL MASS ON COMPUTED TOMOGRAPHY

Condition	Imaging Findings	Comments
Astrocytoma (Fig SK20-1)	Hypodense lesion with little contrast enhancement or peritumoral edema. Calcification frequently occurs.	Slowly growing tumor that has an infiltrative character and can form large cavities or pseudocysts.
Glioblastoma multiforme (Fig SK20-2)	Large inhomogeneous mass with irregular, poorly defined margins and central hypodense zones. Contrast enhancement is usually intense and inhomogeneous, and a ring with thickened irregular walls or nodules of enhancement is common.	Highly malignant lesion that is predominantly cerebral in location. Typically has low-attenuation tissue consisting of edema and malignant glial cells surrounding the enhancing portion of the tumor.
Oligodendroglioma (Fig SK20-3)	Large, irregular, inhomogeneous mass containing calcification and hypodense zones. Variable peritumoral edema and contrast enhancement.	Slow-growing tumor that originates from oligodendrocytes in the central white matter (especially the anterior half of the cerebrum). Calcification (peripheral or central, nodular or shell-like) occurs in about 90% of tumors.
Metastasis (Fig SK20-4)	Hypodense mass surrounded by edema (which usually exceeds tumor volume). Variable contrast enhancement depending on the size and type of tumor.	The density of a metastasis depends on its cellularity and neovascularity and the presence of central necrosis or hemorrhage. Epithelial tumors are typically hypodense; melanoma, choriocarcinoma, and osteosarcoma are usually hyperdense.
Ganglioglioma/ ganglioneuroma	Small, well-defined hypodense or ill-defined isodense mass. Calcified and cystic areas are frequent and most tumors show homogeneous contrast enhancement.	Rare, relatively benign, slow-growing tumors containing mature ganglion cells and stromal elements derived from glial tissue. Typically occur in adolescents and young adults in the temporal and frontal lobes, basal ganglia, and anterior third ventricle.
Epidermoid (primary cholesteatoma) (Fig SK20-5)	Round, sharply marginated, nearly homogeneous hypodense mass. May have extremely low attenuation due to a high fat content. No contrast enhancement.	The result of inclusion of ectodermal germ layer elements in the neural tube during its closure between the third and fifth weeks of gestation. Ectodermal inclusion early in this period produces a midline tumor, while later inclusion produces an eccentrically located lesion. More common in the cerebellopontine angle and suprasellar region.
Dermoid	Inhomogeneous midline mass that often contains focal areas of fat, mural or central calcification, or bone. No contrast enhancement.	Congenital inclusion of both ectodermal and mesodermal germ layer elements at the time of neural tube closure. Contains hair follicles and sebaceous and apocrine glands (derived from mesoderm) that produce a thick, buttery mixture of sweat and sebum.

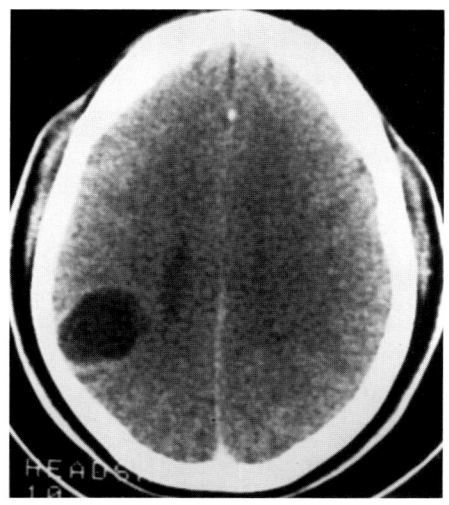

FIG SK20-1. Cystic astrocytoma. Hypodense mass with a thin rim of contrast enhancement. ◄

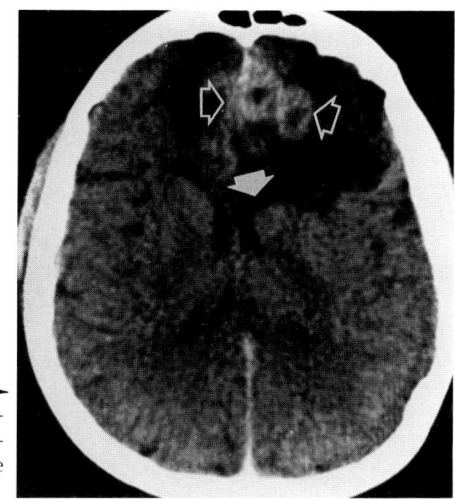

FIG SK20-2. Glioblastoma multiforme. Irregular enhancing lesion (open arrows). The substantial mass effect of the tumor distorts the frontal horns (closed arrow). ►

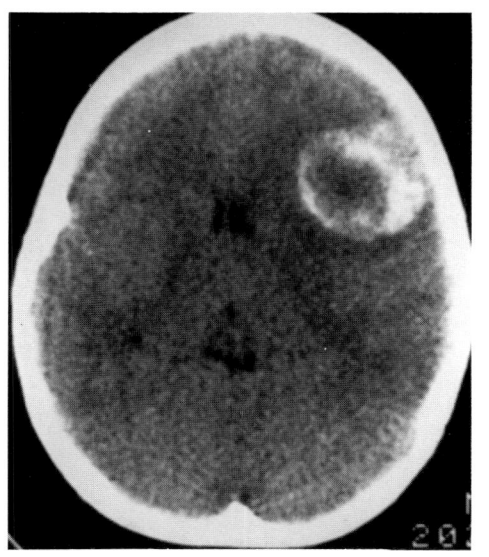

A

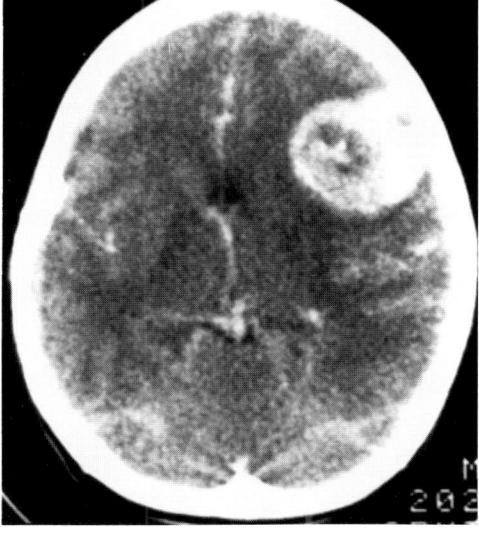

B

FIG SK20-3. Oligodendroglioma. (A) Nonenhanced scan showing a hypodense mass containing amorphous areas of calcification. (B) After the intravenous injection of contrast material, there is marked contrast enhancement.

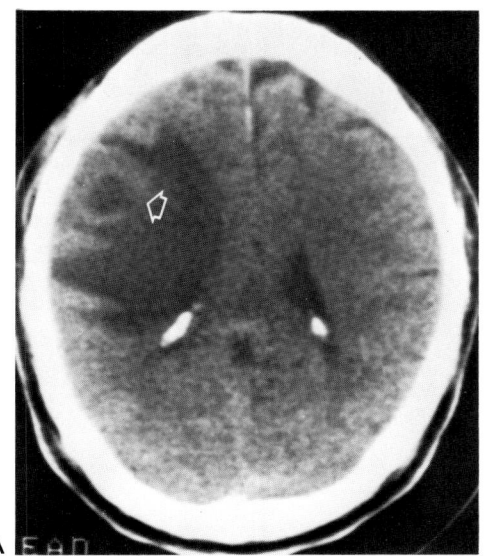

A

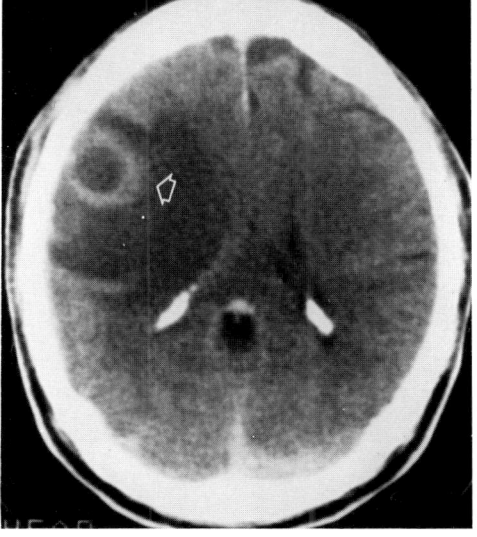

B

FIG SK20-4. Metastasis. (A) Nonenhanced scan shows a small hypodense mass with an isodense rim (arrow) surrounded by extensive edema. (B) After the intravenous injection of contrast material, there is prominent ring enhancement (arrow) about the metastasis.

Condition	Imaging Findings	Comments
Lipoma **(Fig SK20-6)**	Well-defined, homogeneously hypodense fatty mass that occurs in the midline. No contrast enhancement.	Uncommon congenital tumor resulting from inclusion of mesodermal adipose tissue at the time of neural tube closure. Most commonly involves the corpus callosum (often with dense, curvilinear mural calcification).
Radiation necrosis **(see Fig SK22-11)**	Deep, focal, hypodense mass that is usually in or near the irradiated tumor bed. May show an irregular ring of contrast enhancement.	Develops 9 to 24 months after radiation therapy and may be impossible to differentiate from recurrent or residual tumor.
Cerebral infarction **(Figs SK20-7 to SK20-10)**	Triangular or wedge-shaped area of hypodensity involving the cortex and the underlying white matter down to the ventricular surface.	Unlike a hypodense glioma, an infarct has a distinctive shape that corresponds to the distribution of a specific vessel or vessels and has a characteristic pattern of peripheral, rarely central, enhancement. The clinical diagnosis is usually obvious because of the abrupt onset of symptoms.
Pyogenic abscess **(Fig Sk20-11)**	Central hypodense zone (pus, necrotic tissue) surrounded by a thin, isodense ring (fibrous capsule) and peripheral low-density tissue (reactive edema).	Unlike intermediate-grade and highly aggressive gliomas, where enhancement is often ringlike but irregular in thickness, a cerebral abscess is characterized by a thin uniform ring of enhancement. There also is usually a strongly suggestive clinical picture of fever, leukocytosis, obtundation, extracranial infection, or a previous operation.
Hytadid (echinococcal) cyst **(Fig SK20-12)**	Round, sharply marginated, smooth-walled hypodense mass.	Rare manifestation of this parasitic infection. The parenchymal cysts tend to be large and multiple, with no reactive edema or contrast enhancement.
Herpes simplex encephalitis **(Fig SK20-13)**	Poorly defined, frequently bilateral areas of decreased attenuation, especially involving the temporal and parietal lobes.	Most common cause of nonepidemic fatal encephalitis in the United States. The putamen, which is spared by this infection, often forms the sharply defined, slightly concave or straight medial border of the low-density zone. Various patterns of contrast enhancement develop in about half the patients.
Cerebritis	Irregular, poorly marginated hypodense area (representing edema) in the white matter or basal ganglia that may behave as a mass and result in effacement of the adjacent sulci or ventricle. Unlike most cerebral abscesses, there is no discrete ringlike capsule on unenhanced scans in patients with cerebritis.	Focal inflammatory process in the brain, usually resulting from bacteria or fungi, which may progress to abscess formation (requires about 10 to 14 days). After administration of contrast material, may show a well-defined ring that tends to increase in thickness on serial scans.
Resolving intracerebral hematoma **(3 to 6 weeks old)** **(see Fig SK22-9)**	Hypodense region with a thin uniform ring of enhancement that mimics a neoplasm.	Usually a history of previous intracerebral hematoma.

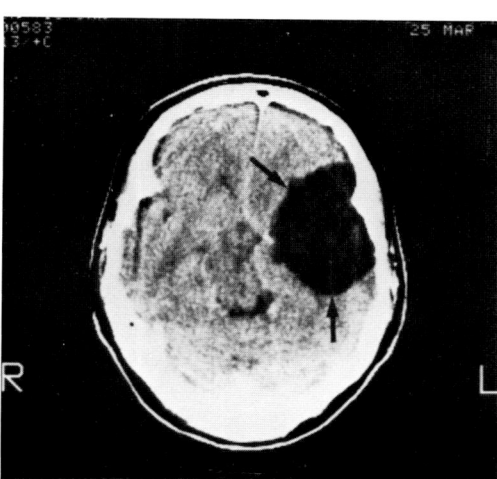

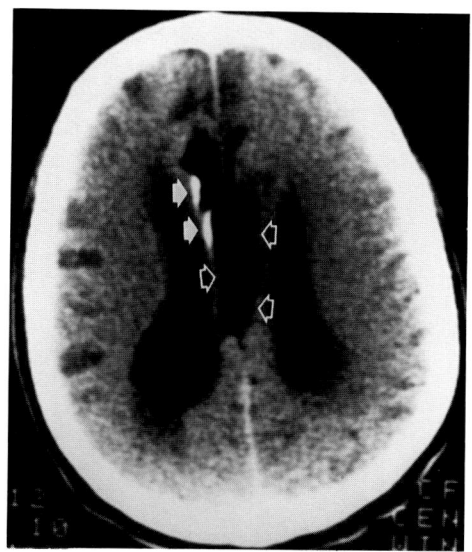

FIG SK20-5. Epidermoid. Enhanced scan shows a large, sharply marginated, low-attenuation, extra-axial sylvian mass (arrows).[13]

FIG SK20-6. Lipoma of the corpus callosum. Extremely low-density mass (open arrows) involving much of the corpus callosum. Note the peripheral calcifications (closed arrows).

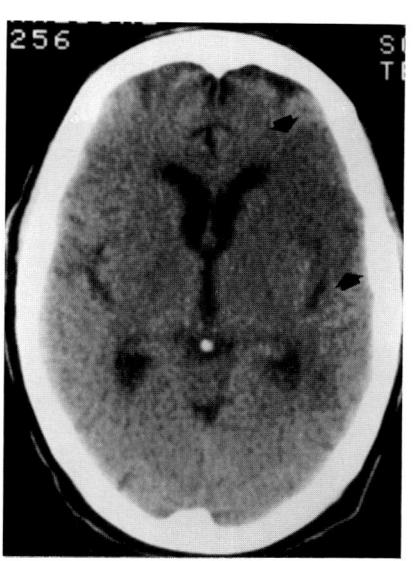

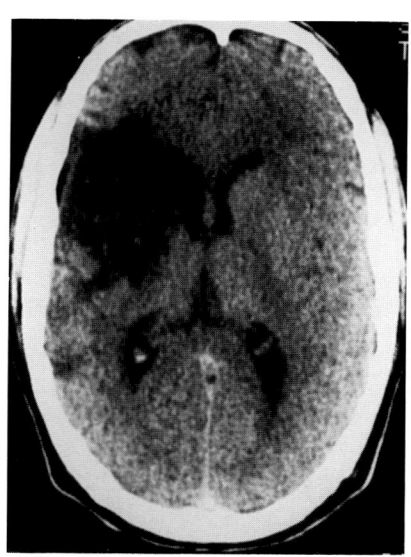

FIG SK20-7. Acute left middle cerebral artery infarct. Scan obtained 20 hours after the onset of acute hemiparesis and aphasia shows obliteration of the normal sulci (arrows) in the involved hemisphere. There is low density of the gray and white matter in the distribution of the left middle cerebral artery.

FIG SK20-8. Chronic right middle cerebral artery infarct. Low-attenuation region with sharply defined borders and some dilation of the adjacent ventricle.

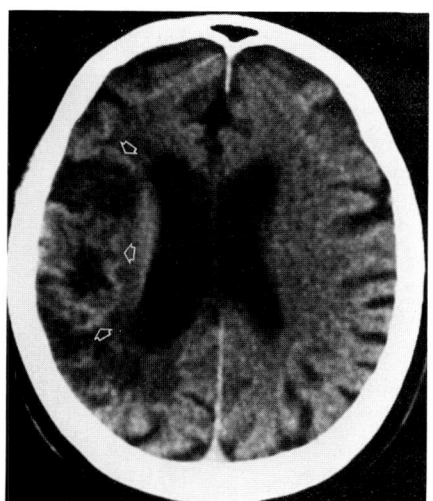

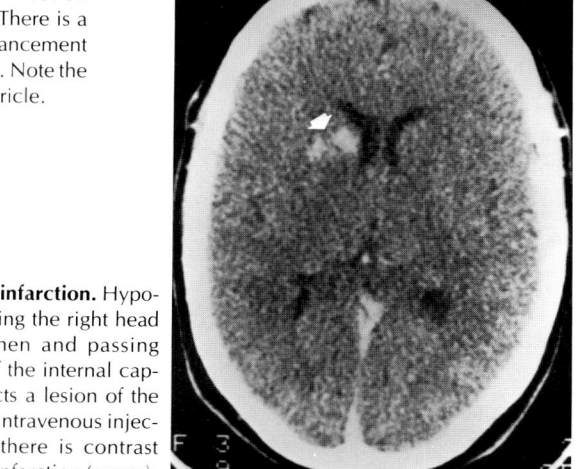

FIG SK20-9. Old infarct in the distribution of the right middle cerebral artery. There is a thin peripheral rim of contrast enhancement (arrows) about the hypodense region. Note the enlargement of the right lateral ventricle.

FIG SK20-10. Basal ganglia infarction. Hypodense region (arrow) involving the right head of the caudate and putamen and passing through the anterior limb of the internal capsule. This distribution reflects a lesion of the artery of Heubner. After the intravenous injection of contrast material, there is contrast enhancement of the area of infarction (arrow).

Condition	Imaging Findings	Comments
Resolving subdural hematoma (Figs SK20-14 and SK20-15)	Well-defined, hypodense, crescentic mass adjacent to the inner table of the skull.	After the injection of contrast material there is characteristic enhancement of the richly vascular membrane that forms around a subdural hematoma 1 to 4 weeks after injury. Occasionally, contrast material seeps into the hematoma and produces a fluid-fluid level.
Subdural empyema (Fig SK20-16)	Crescentic or lentiform, extra-axial hypodense collection (representing pus) adjacent to the inner border of the skull. After administration of contrast material, a narrow zone of enhancement of relatively uniform thickness separates the hypodense extracerebral collection from the brain surface.	Suppurative process in the cranial subdural space that is most commonly the result of the spread of infection from the frontal or ethmoid sinuses. Less frequent causes include mastoiditis, middle ear infection, purulent meningitis, penetrating wounds to the skull, craniectomy, or osteomyelitis of the skull. Often bilateral and associated with a high mortality rate, even if properly treated.
Epidural abscess (see Fig SK22-8)	Poorly defined area of low density adjacent to the inner table of the skull. There may be an adjacent area of bone destruction or evidence of paranasal sinus or mastoid infection. After the intravenous injection of contrast material, the inflamed dural membrane appears as a thickened zone of enhancement on the convex inner side of the lesion.	Almost invariably associated with cranial bone osteomyelitis originating from an infection in the ear or paranasal sinuses. The infectious process is localized outside the dural membrane and beneath the inner table of the skull. The frontal region is most frequently affected because of its close relation to the frontal sinuses and the ease with which the dura can be stripped from the bone.
Multiple sclerosis (Fig SK20-17)	Multifocal, nonconfluent, low-attenuation regions with distinct margins near the atria of the lateral ventricles.	Contrast enhancement in the plaques is unusual except in rapidly evolving ones with surrounding inflammatory changes.
Necrosis of the globus pallidus	Bilaterally symmetric areas of low attenuation in the basal ganglia.	Causes include carbon monoxide poisoning, barbiturate intoxication, cyanide or hydrogen sulfide poisoning, hypoglycemia, hypoxia, hypotension, and Wilson's disease.

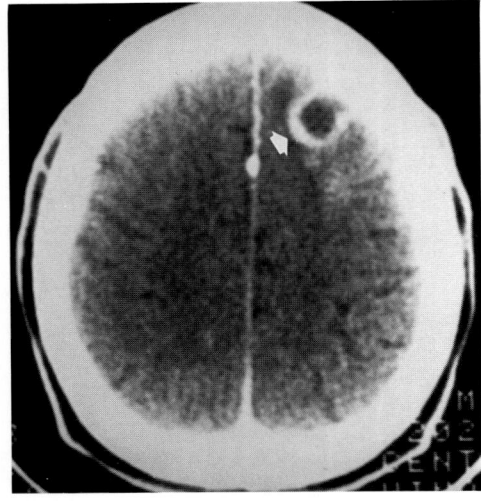

FIG SK20-11. **Pyogenic abscess.** Hypodense lesion surrounded by a uniform ring of contrast enhancement (arrow).

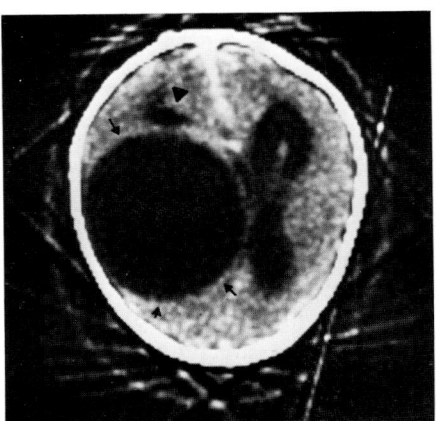

FIG SK20-12. **Echinococcal cyst.** Huge right supratentorial hypodense mass (arrows). The right ventricle is partially visible posterior and medial to the cyst (arrowhead), and the left ventricle is enlarged.[19]

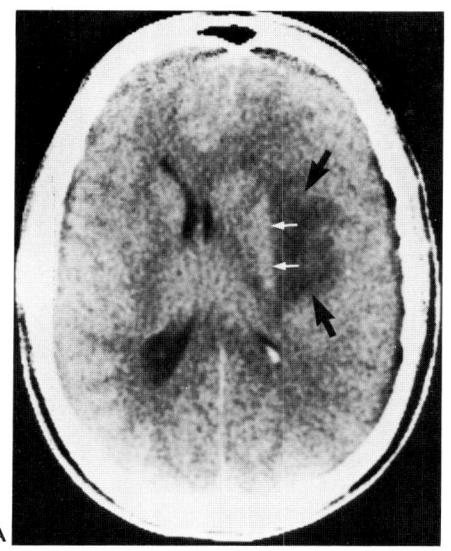

A

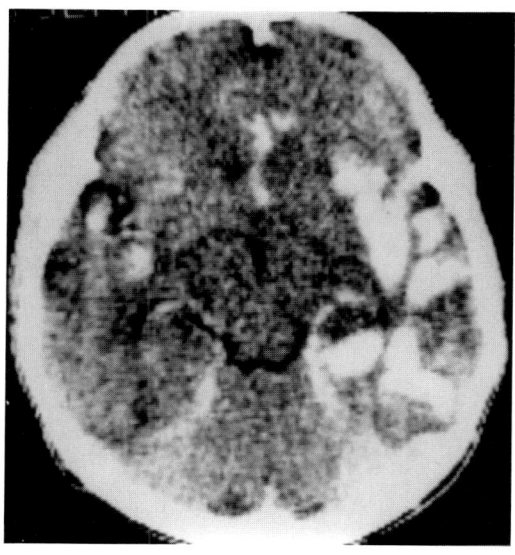

B

FIG SK20-13. Herpes simplex encephalitis. (A) Nonenhanced scan demonstrates a hypodense area deep in the left frontotemporal region (large black arrows) and a shift of midline structures. The putamen, with its well-defined lateral border (small white arrows), is unaffected by infection. (B) In another patient, there is dramatic gyral contrast enhancement that is most prominent on the left.[13]

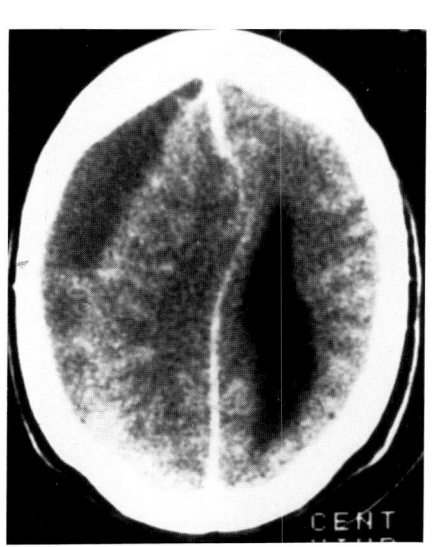

FIG SK20-14. Right subdural hematoma. Crescent-shaped, low-density region in the right frontoparietal area. Note the marginal contrast enhancement, dilated left ventricle, and evidence of subfalcine and transtentorial herniation.

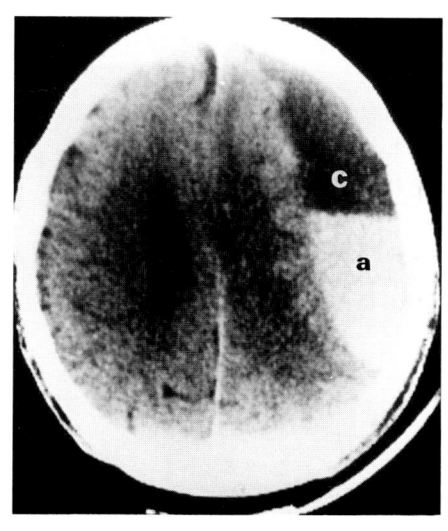

FIG SK20-15. Mixed acute and chronic left subdural hematoma. The high-density acute hemorrhage (a) is layered in the dependent portion of the hematoma, with the lower density chronic collection (c) situated anteriorly.

FIG SK20-16. Subdural empyema. Lens-shaped extra-axial hypodense collection (arrow) that complicated a severe sinus infection. Note the thin rim of peripheral contrast enhancement.

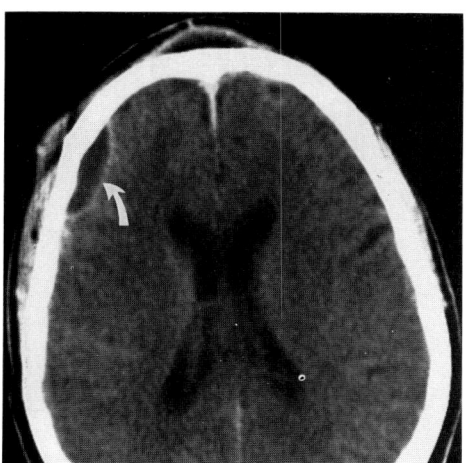

FIG SK20-17. Multiple sclerosis. Multiple discrete, homogeneous, and slightly irregular regions of diminished attenuation (arrows) adjacent to the slightly enlarged ventricles.[13]

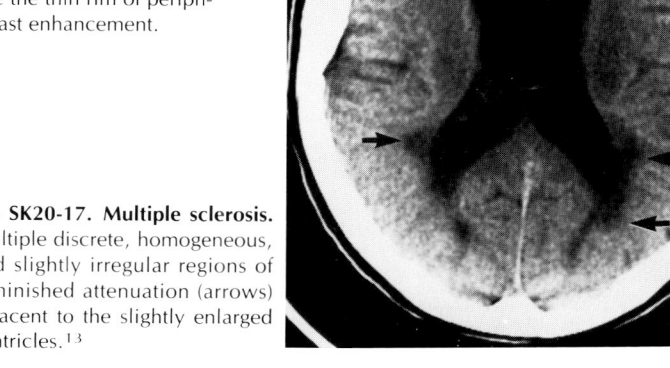

HIGH-ATTENUATION MASS IN A CEREBRAL HEMISPHERE ON COMPUTED TOMOGRAPHY

Condition	Imaging Findings	Comments
Meningioma (Figs SK21-1 and SK21-2)	Rounded, sharply delineated hyperdense mass in a juxtadural location. Often contains calcification and usually shows intense homogeneous contrast enhancement.	Benign tumor that arises from arachnoid lining cells and is attached to the dura. The hyperdense matrix of a meningioma is the result of diminished water content, tumor hypervascularity, and microscopic psammomatous calcification. The detection of hyperostosis is virtually pathognomonic.
Metastasis (Fig SK21-3)	Some dense metastases mimic meningiomas because of their superficial location and well-defined margins, though they are entirely intraparenchymal.	Metastatic colon carcinoma, which has a very dense cellular structure, and metastatic osteosarcoma, which contains osteoid and calcification, tend to be extremely dense. Melanoma and choriocarcinoma also tend to be hyperdense.
Primary lymphoma (Fig SK21-4)	Slightly hyperdense mass that enhances homogeneously and often intensely.	Rare malignant neoplasm derived from microglial cells (histologically similar to lymphocytes) that is often multifocal and has a markedly increased incidence in organ transplant recipients.
Acute intracerebral hemorrhage (Fig SK21-5)	Homogeneously dense, well-defined lesion with a round to oval configuration.	Causes include head trauma, surgery, hypertensive vascular disease, or rupture of a vascular malformation, mycotic aneurysm, or berry aneurysm.
Acute epidural hematoma (Figs SK21-6 and SK21-7)	Biconvex (lens-shaped), peripheral high-density lesion.	Caused by acute arterial bleeding; most commonly develops over the parietotemporal convexity.
Acute subdural hematoma (Fig SK21-8)	Peripheral zone of increased density that follows the surface of the brain and has a crescentic shape adjacent to the inner table of the skull.	Caused by venous bleeding, most commonly from ruptured veins between the dura and leptomeninges. Serial scans demonstrate a gradual decrease in the attenuation of a subdural lesion over several weeks.

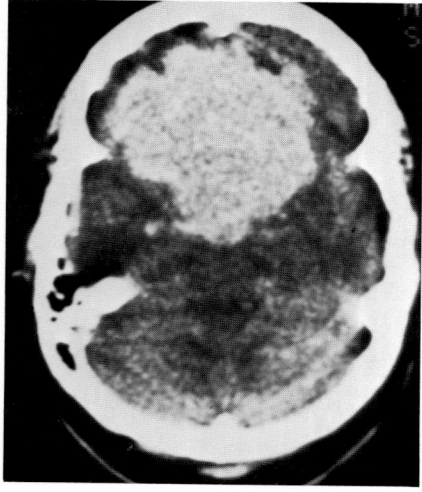

FIG SK21-1. **Meningioma.** Huge hyperdense mass in the frontal lobe.

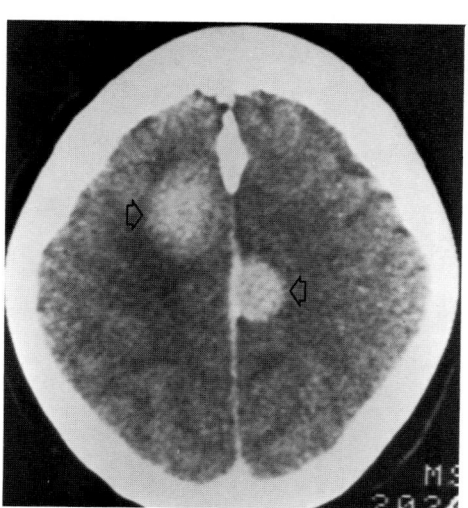

FIG SK21-2. **Meningioma.** Bilateral hyperdense masses (arrows) in juxtadural locations.

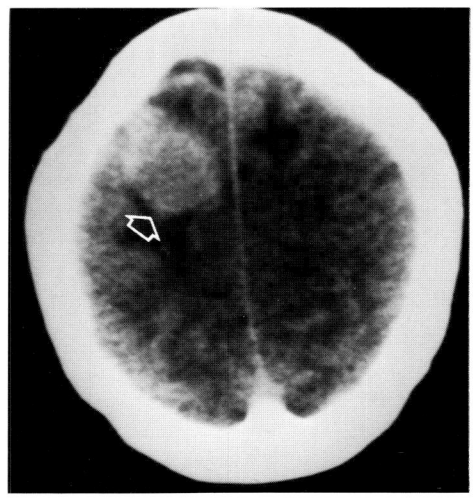

FIG SK21-3. Metastasis. Nonenhanced scan shows a hyperdense mass (arrow) in the right frontal region representing a metastasis from carcinoma of the lung.

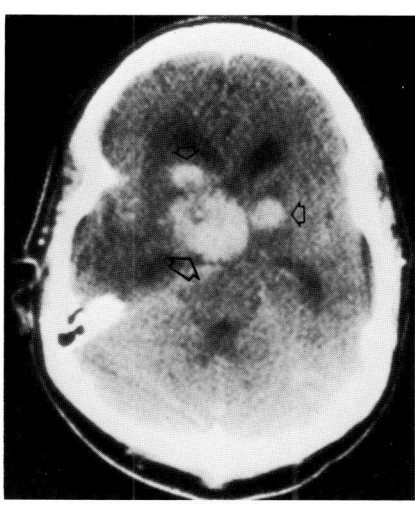

FIG SK21-4. Primary lymphoma. Multifocal hyperdense masses (arrows).

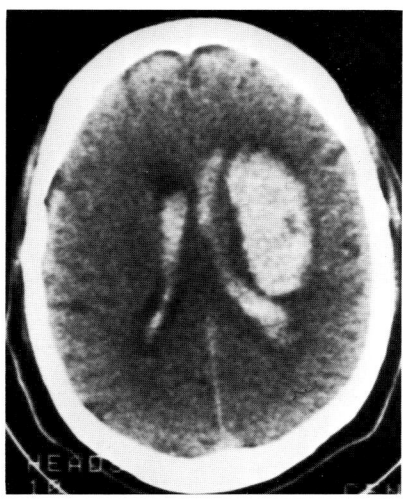

FIG SK21-5. Intracerebral hematoma. Large homogeneous high-density area with extensive acute bleeding into the lateral ventricles.

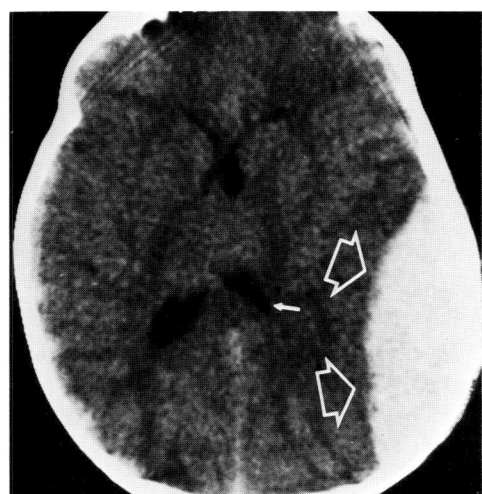

FIG SK21-6. Acute epidural hematoma. CT scan of a 4-year-old involved in a motor vehicle accident shows a characteristic lens-shaped epidural hematoma (open arrows). The substantial mass effect associated with the hematoma distorts the lateral ventricle (closed arrow).

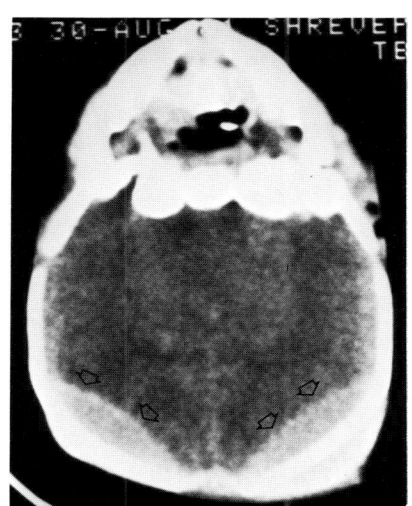

FIG SK21-7. Epidural hematoma. Bilaterally symmetric posterior high-density areas (arrows) with lens-shaped configurations.

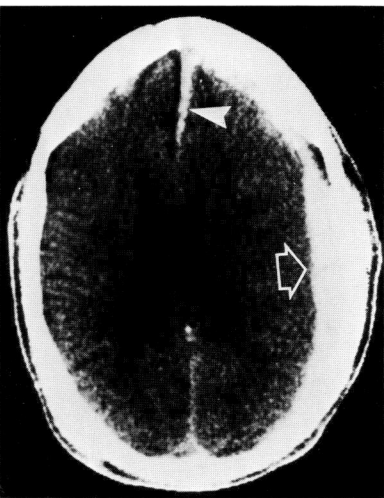

FIG SK21-8. Acute subdural hematoma. High-density, crescent-shaped lesion (open arrow) adjacent to the inner table of the skull. The hematoma extends into the interhemispheric fissure (closed arrowhead).

SUPRATENTORIAL MASSES ON MAGNETIC RESONANCE IMAGING

Condition	Imaging Findings	Comments
Astrocytoma **(Fig SK22-1)**	Hypointense lesion on T_1-weighted images. High-intensity signal on proton-density and T_2-weighted images.	Low-grade tumors tend to be homogeneous and lack central necrosis. They may contain large cystic components that have smooth walls and contain uniform-signal fluid, unlike the heterogeneous appearance of necrosis.
Glioblastoma multiforme **(Figs SK22-2 and SK22-3)**	Hypointense lesion on T_1-weighted images. Hyperintense signal on proton-density and T_2-weighted images.	These high-grade gliomas appear heterogeneous as a result of central necrosis with cellular debris, fluid, and hemorrhage. These tumors infiltrate along white matter fiber tracts. Deeper lesions frequently extend across the corpus callosum into the opposite hemisphere.
Oligodendroglioma **(Fig SK22-4)**	Hypointense lesion on T_1-weighted images. Hyperintense signal on proton-density and T_2-weighted images.	Although conventional spin-echo MRI is insensitive to the frequent calcification in these slow-growing tumors, it can demonstrate a heterogeneous appearance caused by cystic and hemorrhagic regions in the mass.

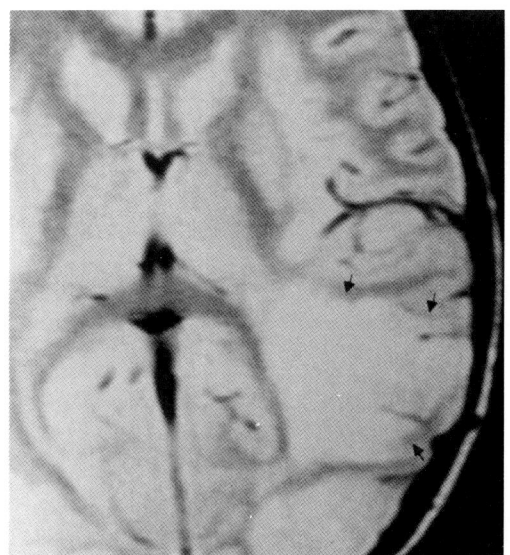

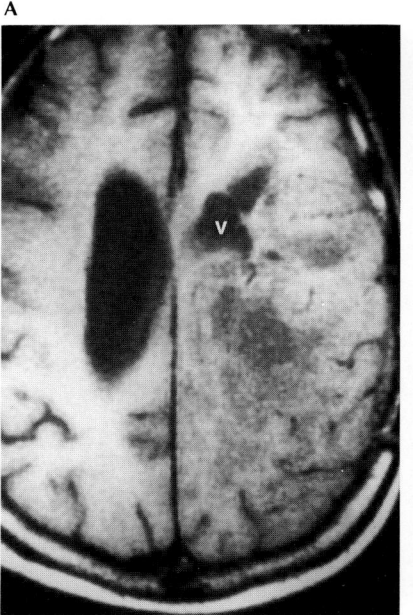
A

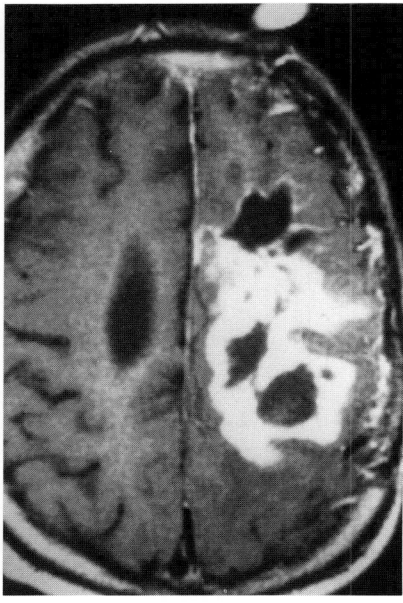
B

FIG SK22-1. Low-grade astrocytoma. Proton-density axial scan shows a high-intensity mass (arrows) involving the left posterior temporal-occipital cortex and subcortical white matter. The homogeneous appearance is typical of these slow-growing tumors.[20]

FIG SK22-2. Glioblastoma multiforme. (A) Axial T_1-weighted image shows a large mass of inhomogeneous low-intensity signal compressing the left lateral ventricle (v). (B) After the injection of gadolinium, there is striking enhancement of this complex necrotic mass.

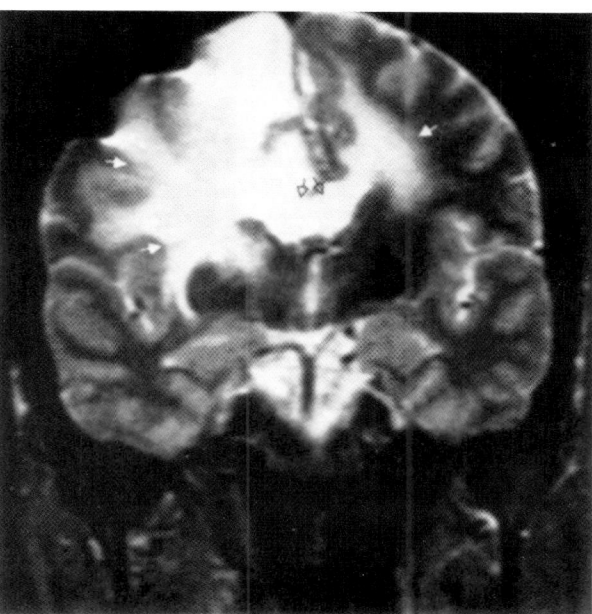

FIG **SK22-3.** **Glioblastoma** crossing the corpus callosum. Coronal T_2-weighted scan shows high signal intensity in the left and right centrum semiovale (white arrows) and extension of tumor across the corpus callosum (open arrows).[20]

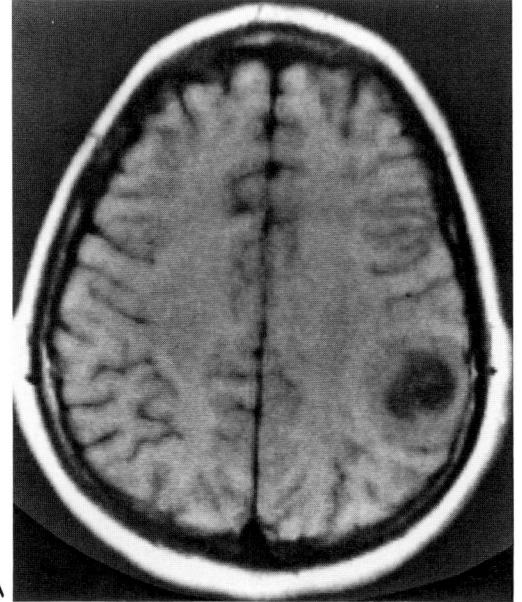 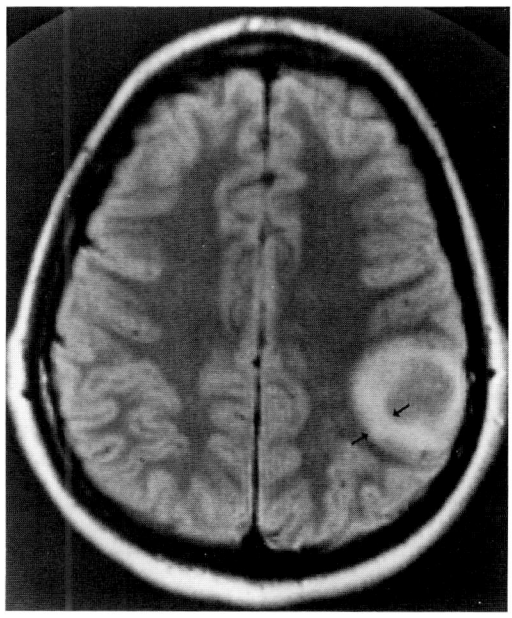

A   B

FIG **SK22-4.** **Oligodendroglioma.** (A) T_1-weighted and (B) proton-density images show a well-differentiated left parietal lobe mass containing a central cystic component. The arrows (B) point to the thickened wall of the enhancing lesion.[21]

Condition	Imaging Findings	Comments
Metastasis **(Fig SK22-5)**	Generally hypointense on T_1-weighted images and of increased signal intensity on proton-density and T_2-weighted images. Peritumoral edema is usually prominent, but unlike infiltrative gliomas, the edema accompanying a metastasis usually does not cross the corpus callosum or involve the cortex.	Areas of nonhemorrhagic cystic necrosis appear as irregular regions of intensity similar to that of cerebrospinal fluid (CSF) surrounded by the nonnecrotic portion of the lesion. Intratumoral hemorrhage occurs in about 15% to 20% of metastases, especially melanoma, choriocarcinoma, and renal cell, thyroid, and bronchogenic carcinoma. Melanotic melanoma metastases without hemorrhage typically are of high intensity on T_1-weighted images and are isointense or hypointense to cortex on T_2-weighted sequences.
Lymphoma **(Fig SK22-6)**	Hypointense or isointense mass on T_1-weighted images. Typically a homogeneous, slightly high-signal to isointense mass deep in the brain on T_2-weighted images.	The mild T_2 prolongation is probably related to dense cell packing in the tumor, leaving relatively little interstitial space for the accumulation of water. Like glioblastoma, lymphoma tends to extend across the corpus callosum into the opposite hemisphere. Central necrosis is uncommon, however, and there is usually only a mild or moderate amount of peritumoral edema.
Meningioma **(Fig SK22-7)**	Usually hypointense to white matter on T_1-weighted images. At 1.5 T, the lesion is hyperintense to white matter on T_2-weighted images.	At lower field strength, about half of meningiomas are isointense to cortex on T_1- and T_2-weighted images. The tumor usually has a mottled pattern resulting from a combination of flow void from vascularity, focal calcification, small cystic foci, and entrapped CSF spaces. An interface is often seen between the brain and the lesion, representing a CSF cleft, a vascular rim, or a dural margin.
Epidermoid **(see Fig SK30-4)**	Heterogeneous texture and variable signal intensity. Most epidermoids are of slightly higher signal than CSF on both T_1- and T_2-weighted images.	Some epidermoids appear bright on T_1-weighted images. The heterogeneous signal pattern is probably related to various concentrations of keratin, cholesterol, and water in the cyst as well as the proportion of cholesterol and keratin in crystalline form.
Dermoid	Heterogeneous texture as a result of the multiple cell types in it.	Fatty components are common and produce high signal on T_1-weighted images. A characteristic fat-fluid level may be seen.
Lipoma **(see Fig SK40-8B)**	High signal intensity on T_1-weighted images. Isointense or mildly hyperintense on proton-density images. Low intensity on T_2-weighted sequences.	Typically a midline lesion that is often associated with partial or complete agenesis of the corpus callosum.
Choroid plexus papilloma **(Fig SK22-8)**	Mildly hyperintense on T_2-weighted images.	Relatively homogeneous, although hypervascularity can result in areas of flow void. Intense, homogeneous contrast enhancement.

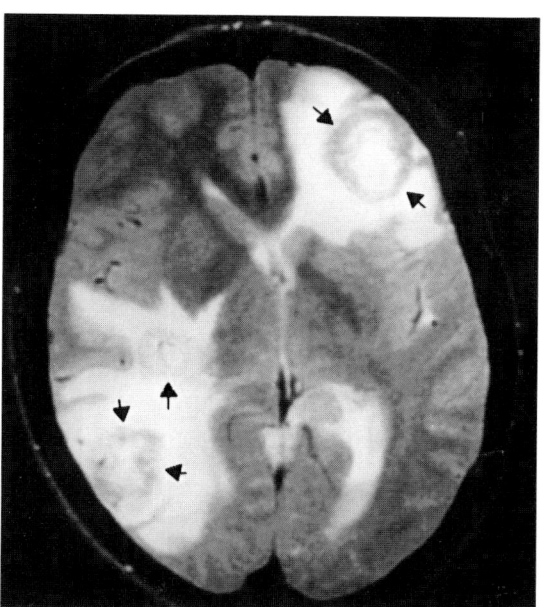

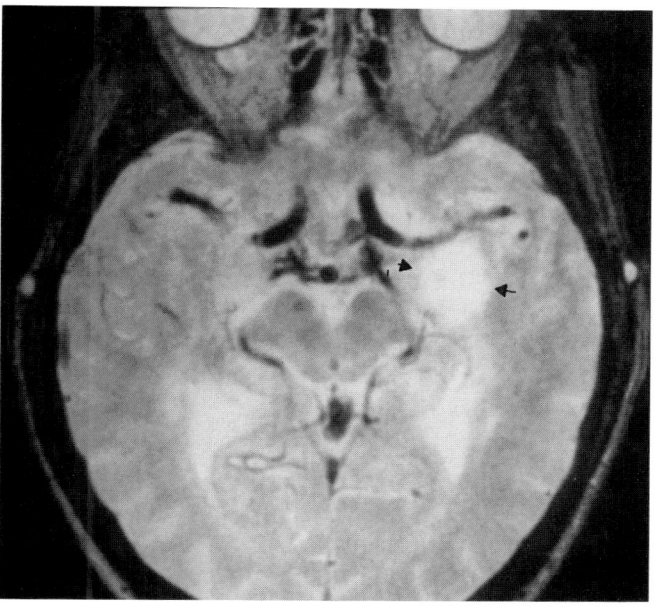

FIG SK22-5. Metastases. Axial T₂-weighted scan demonstrates three large masses (arrows) surrounded by extensive high-signal edema.

FIG SK22-6. Lymphoma. Homogeneous mass of increased signal intensity (arrows) extending to involve the uncus.

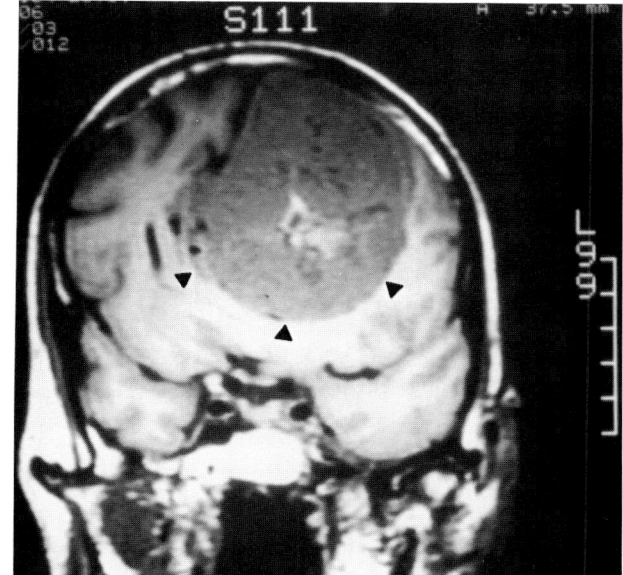

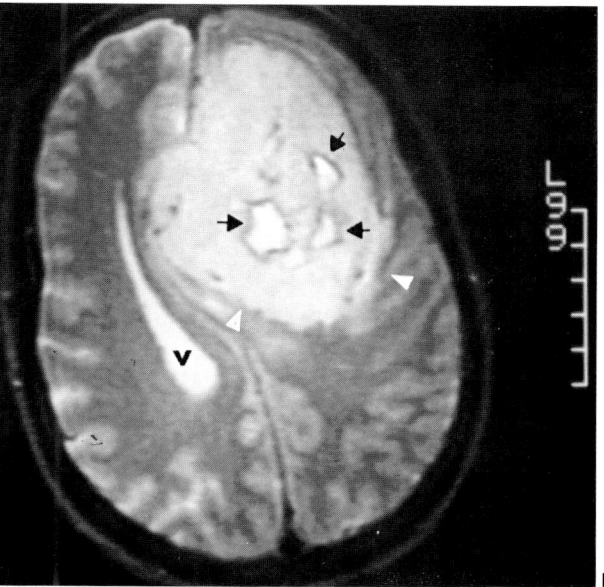

A

B

FIG SK22-7. Meningioma. Huge mass (black and white arrowheads) that appears hypointense on a T₁-weighted coronal scan (A) and hyperintense on a T₂-weighted image (B). Note the dramatic shift of the ventricle (v) caused by the mass effect of tumor. The arrows point to areas of hemorrhage in the neoplasm.

Condition	Imaging Findings	Comments
Colloid cyst (Fig SK22-9; see also Fig SK36-2)	Smoothly marginated spherical mass with two signal patterns: low density on CT, isointense on T_1-weighted MR images, and hyperintense on T_2-weighted MR images; and isodense or slightly hyperdense on CT with a high-signal capsule and a hypointense center on T_2-weighted MR images.	The first pattern corresponds to a fluid composition similar to CSF. In the second pattern, the hypointense center on MRI has been attributed to high concentrations of metal ions (sodium, calcium, magnesium, copper, and iron) or a high cholesterol content of the cyst fluid.
Cerebral abscess (Fig SK22-10)	Hypointense mass with isointense capsule surrounded by low-signal edema on T_1-weighted images. Hyperintense mass surrounded by a hypointense capsule and high-signal edema on T_2-weighted images.	In the cerebritis stage, there is high signal intensity on T_2-weighted images both centrally from inflammation and peripherally from edema. Areas of low signal are variably imaged on T_1-weighted scans. As this process develops into a discrete abscess, the capsule becomes highlighted as a relatively isointense structure containing and surrounded by low signal on T_1-weighted images and high signal on T_2-weighted images.
Herpes simplex encephalitis	Ill-defined areas of high signal intensity on T_2-weighted images. This process usually begins unilaterally but progresses to become bilateral.	MRI can demonstrate positive findings more quickly (as soon as 2 days) and more definitively than CT.
Intraparenchymal hematoma (Fig SK22-11)		Well-defined, although somewhat variable, progression of signal intensity changes primarily related to the paramagnetic effects of the breakdown products of hemoglobin.
Very acute (0–3 hours)	Isointense to slightly hyperintense on T_1-weighted images. Isointense to bright signal on T_2-weighted images.	Immediately after an intracerebral bleed, the liquefied mass in the brain substance contains oxyhemoglobin but no paramagnetic substances. Therefore, it looks like any other proteinaceous fluid collection.
Acute (3 hours–3 days)	Isointense or hypointense on T_1-weighted images. Markedly hypointense on T_2-weighted images.	Reduction in oxygen tension in the hematoma results in the formation of intracellular deoxyhemoglobin and methemoglobin in intact red cells. These substances have a paramagnetic effect that produces T_2 shortening. A thin rim of increased signal surrounding the hematoma on T_2-weighted images represents edema.
Subacute (3 days–3 weeks)	Bright rim of hyperintense signal on T_1-weighted images that extends inward to fill the entire lesion. Increased signal on T_2-weighted images, although to a lesser extent.	As red blood cells lyse, redistribution of methemoglobin into the extracellular space changes the effect of this paramagnetic substance to one of predominantly T_1 shortening. The longer T_2 results from a combination of (1) red blood cell lysis (T_2 shortening disappears), (2) osmotic effects that draw fluid into the hematoma, and (3) the repetition times (TR) that are in general use for T_2-weighted sequences, which are not sufficiently long to eliminate T_1 contrast effects in the image.
Chronic (3 weeks–3 months or more)	Variable appearance on T_1-weighted images. Pronounced hypointense rim or completely low-signal lesion on T_2-weighted images.	Phagocytic cells invade the hemorrhage (starting at the outer rim and working inward), metabolizing the hemoglobin breakdown products and storing the iron as superparamagnetic hemosiderin and ferritin.

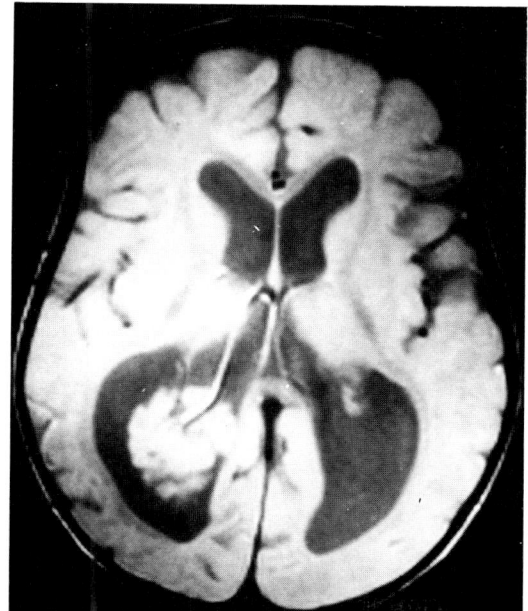

FIG SK22-8. **Choroid plexus papilloma.** Lobulated mass in the dilated occipital horn of the right lateral ventricle.

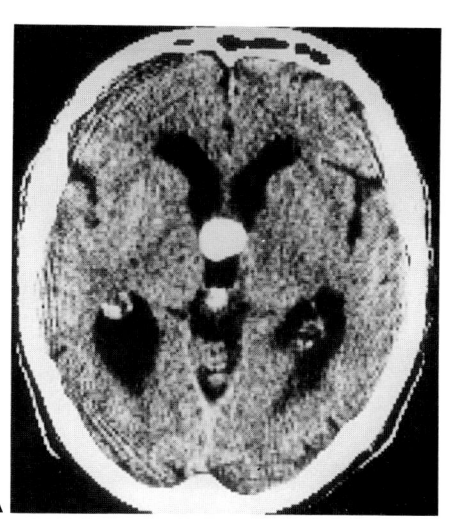

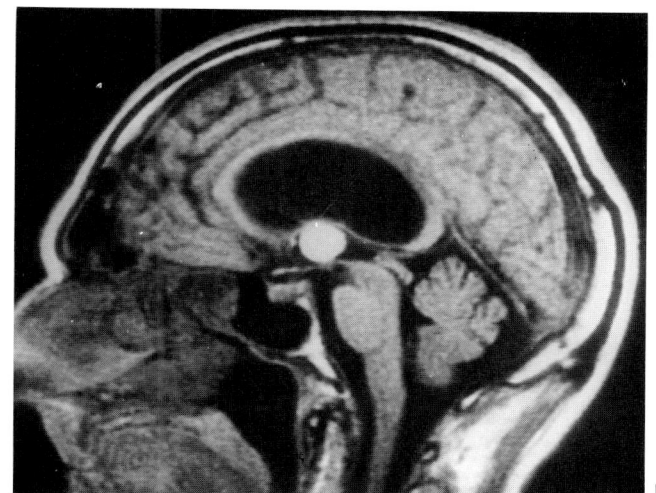

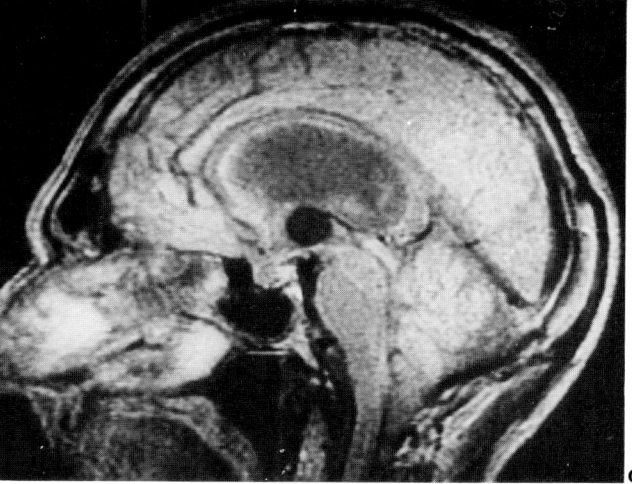

FIG SK22-9. **Colloid cyst.** (A) Unenhanced CT scan shows a very hyperdense mass in the anterosuperior portion of the third ventricle. (B) Midline sagittal T_1-weighted MR image shows a homogeneous intense mass in the anterosuperior third ventricle. (C) On a T_2-weighted image, the homogeneous mass has very low signal intensity.[22]

Condition	Imaging Findings	Comments
Vascular diseases		
Infarction **(Fig SK22-12)**	Hypointense on T_1-weighted images. Hyperintense on proton-density and T_2-weighted images. Old infarcts may have a more complex signal pattern that is related both to hemorrhagic components and to the evolution of infarcts, the latter resulting in areas of microcystic and macrocystic encephalomalacia and gliosis.	Classic pattern of cerebral infarction is a wedge-shaped abnormality that involves both the cortex and a variable amount of the subcortical tissue, in either a major vascular territory or a watershed area. Because MRI is extremely sensitive to edema, experimental infarcts have been detected as soon as 2 to 4 hours after vessel occlusion, at a time when CT has shown no abnormality.
Arteriovenous malformation (AVM) **(Fig SK22-13)**	Cluster of serpiginous flow voids (representing rapid blood flow) and areas of high signal (slow flow in draining veins).	The use of partial flip-angle techniques can distinguish hemosiderin or calcification associated with the lesion from vessels containing rapidly flowing blood.
"Cryptic" AVM **(Fig SK22-14)**	On T_2-weighted images, an island of bright signal (methemoglobin) is surrounded by an extensive region of very low signal (hemosiderin).	This lesion may be responsible for spontaneous hemorrhage but is angiographically occult.
Venous malformation	Solitary or stellate collection of flow voids (draining vein) that may be associated with increased signal in the body of the angioma.	Radiating or spokelike pattern of tributaries draining into a single large vein that courses perpendicular to the surface of the brain to enter a major vein or dural sinus.
Aneurysm **(Fig SK22-15)**	Flow void that may be surrounded by a heterogeneous signal intensity pattern representing turbulence or thrombus.	MRI may be unable to distinguish small aneurysms from normal vessels. Partial flip-angle imaging produces fairly consistent flow-related enhancement in the lumen and more clearly differentiates this from surrounding clot.

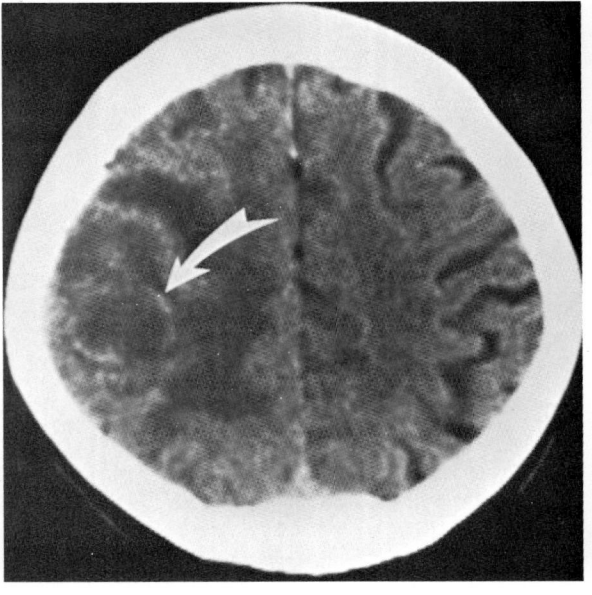
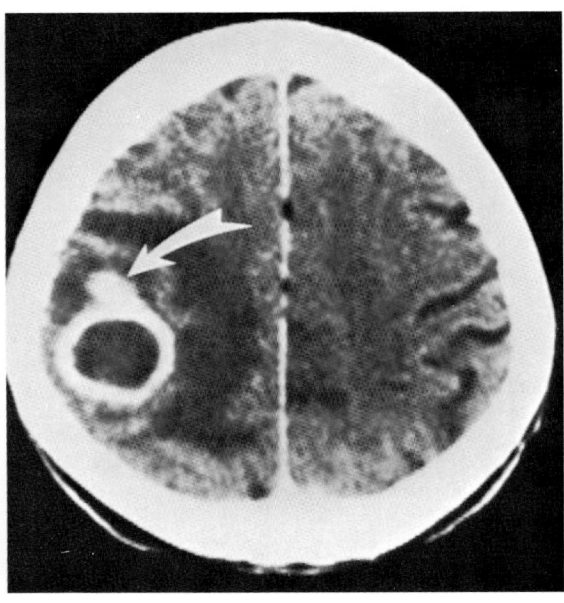

A   B

FIG SK22-10. Brain abscess. (A) Nonenhanced CT scan shows vasogenic edema in the right anterior parietal white matter. The isointense ring of the abscess capsule can be seen (white arrow). (B) Contrast-enhanced study shows a thick but uniformly enhancing capsule with the beginnings of a daughter abscess anteriorly (arrow). The enhancement of an abscess is typically circular and nearly uniform except along the medial surface.[23]

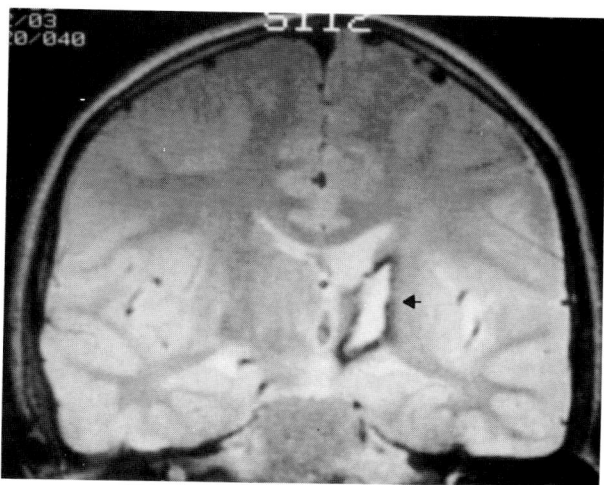

FIG SK22-11. **Intraparenchymal hematoma.** Coronal T_2-weighted scan shows a large hematoma in the left thalamic region (arrow). The hematoma consists of two portions: a central area of increased signal intensity representing methemoglobin, and a surrounding area of low signal intensity representing hemosiderin.

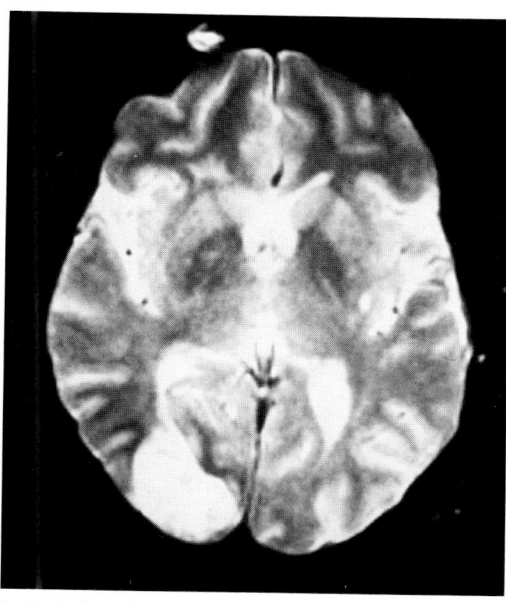

FIG SK22-12. **Infarction.** Axial T_2-weighted image shows a wedge-shaped area of increased signal intensity involving both cortex and sub-cortical tissue in the right occipital lobe.

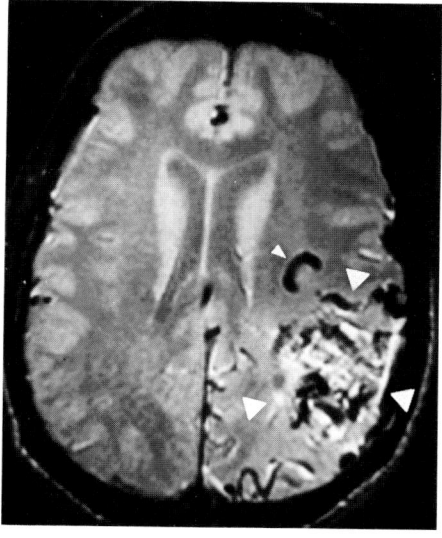

FIG SK22-13. **Arteriovenous malformation (AVM).** Axial proton-density scan shows a large left parietal mass (large arrowheads) consisting of vascular structures of various intensities, depending on whether there is rapid flow (black) or slow flow (white). Note the markedly dilated vessel (small arrowhead) that feeds the malformation.

FIG SK22-14. **Cryptic AVM.** Axial T_2-weighted scan shows the characteristic appearance of an island of bright signal (methemoglobin) surrounded by an extensive region of very low signal (hemosiderin).

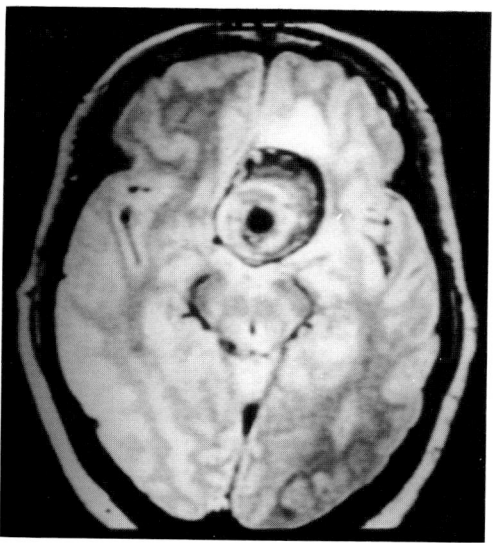

FIG SK22-15. **Aneurysm** of the supraclinoid portion of the internal carotid artery. The low-signal flow void representing the residual patent lumen is surrounded by a heterogeneous region of increased signal representing lamellar thrombus.

SELLAR AND JUXTASELLAR MASSES ON COMPUTED TOMOGRAPHY

Condition	Imaging Findings	Comments
Pituitary adenoma **(Figs SK23-1 and SK23-2)**	Typically a well-circumscribed tumor of slightly greater than brain density that shows homogeneous contrast enhancement. Regions of necrosis or cyst formation in the tumor produce internal areas of low density. Microadenomas (< 10 mm) are usually less dense than the normal pituitary gland.	Computed tomography can demonstrate adjacent bone erosion, extension of the tumor beyond the confines of the sella, and impression of nearby structures such as the third ventricle, optic nerves, or optic chiasm.
Craniopharyngioma **(Fig SK23-3)**	Typically a mixed-density lesion containing cystic and solid areas and dense globular or, less commonly, rim calcification. Variable contrast enhancement of the solid portion of the tumor.	Benign congenital, or rest-cell, tumor with cystic and solid components that usually originates above the sella turcica, depressing the optic chiasm and extending up into the third ventricle. Less commonly, a craniopharyngioma lies in the sella, where it compresses the pituitary gland and may erode adjacent bony walls.
Meningioma **(Fig SK23-4)**	Hyperdense mass that enhances intensely and homogeneously after intravenous administration of contrast material. May have associated hyperostosis of adjacent bone.	Suprasellar meningiomas arise from the tuberculum sellae, clinoid processes, optic nerve sheath, cerebellopontine angle cistern, cavernous sinus, or medial sphenoidal ridge.

Glioma
    Optic chiasm
    (Fig SK23-5)
	Suprasellar mass that is isodense on nonenhanced scans and shows moderate and variable enhancement after administration of contrast material.	Benign globular mass occupying the anterior aspect of the suprasellar cistern that most often occurs in adolescent girls, gradually produces bilateral visual abnormalities and optic atrophy, and is often associated with neurofibromatosis.

Hypothalamus	Usually a large, well-defined, irregularly contoured mass that is inhomogeneous with low-density and markedly enhancing regions.	Slow-growing astrocytoma that usually occurs in children and young adults. In infants, it typically produces a syndrome of failure to thrive despite adequate caloric intake, unusual alertness, and hyperactivity.
Chordoma **(Fig SK23-6)**	Well-defined mass with variable enhancement and homogeneity. Usually associated with destruction of the clivus and retrosellar calcification.	Locally invasive tumor that arises from remnants of the fetal notochord and most commonly occurs in patients 50 to 70 years of age.
Metastases **(Fig SK23-7)**	Smooth or irregular masses that usually enhance homogeneously and are associated with bone destruction.	Most metastases to the sellar and juxtasellar region originate from tumors of the lung, breast, kidney, or gastrointestinal tract or are due to direct spread from carcinomas of the nasopharynx or sphenoid sinus.
Germ cell tumor **(germinoma/teratoma)** **(Fig SK23-8)**	Various patterns of density and enhancement.	Occasionally involve the suprasellar region and frequently calcify (especially teratomas). May spread via cerebrospinal fluid pathways.

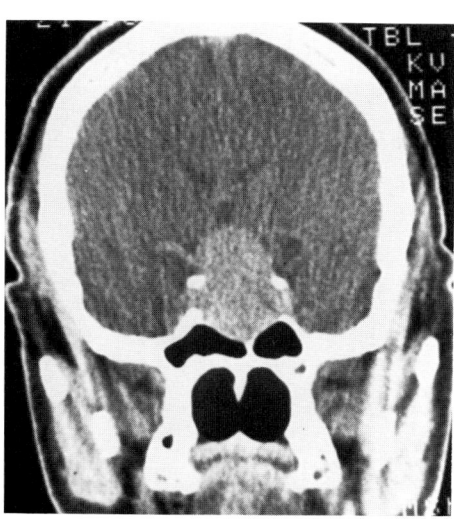

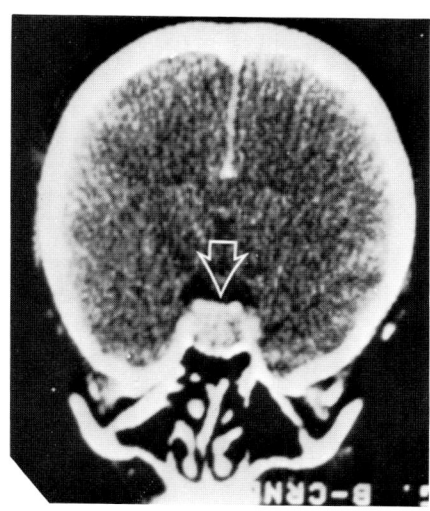

Fig SK23-1. Pituitary adenoma. Coronal scan shows an enhancing mass filling and extending out from the pituitary fossa. Note the remodeling of the base of the sella.

Fig SK23-2. Nelson's syndrome. Hyperdense tumor filling the enlarged sella (arrow) in a patient whose pituitary adenoma developed after adrenal surgery.

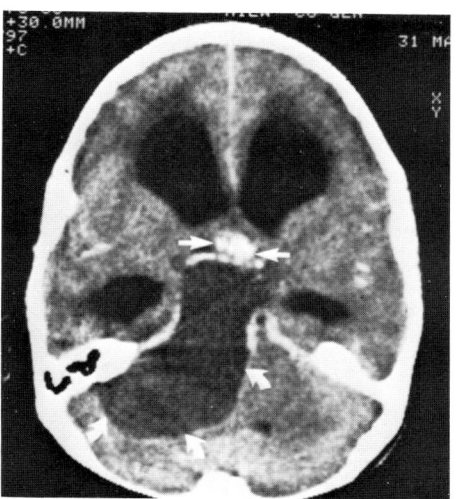

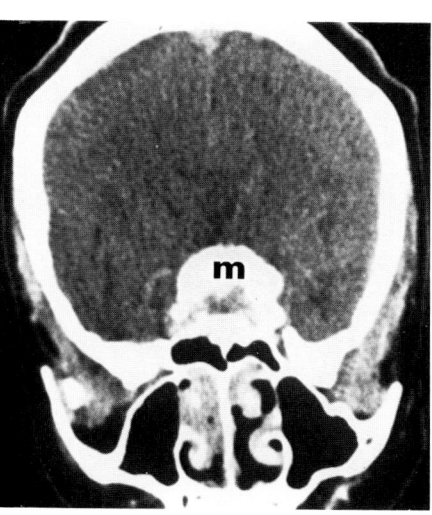

Fig SK23-3. Craniopharyngioma. The rim-enhancing tumor contains dense calcification (straight arrows) and a large cystic component (curved arrows) that extends into the posterior fossa. Note the associated hydrocephalus.[13]

Fig SK23-4. Meningioma. Coronal reconstruction shows the large calcified mass (m) and associated bone destruction.

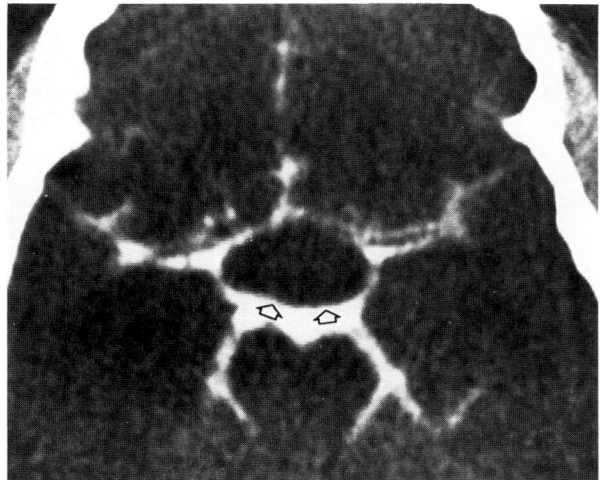

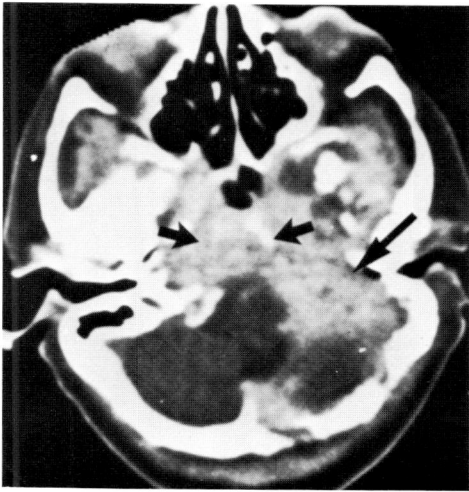

Fig SK23-5. Optic chiasm glioma. Axial suprasellar metrizamide cisternogram demonstrates a tumor filling the suprasellar cistern (arrows). Only faint enhancement was present on the standard contrast-enhanced CT scan.[24]

Fig SK23-6. Chordoma. Enlarging mass with destruction of the entire clivus (short arrows) and only small bone fragments remaining. The left petrous pyramid is also destroyed (long arrow).[17]

Condition	Imaging Findings	Comments
Epidermoid/dermoid **(Fig SK23-9)**	Smooth or lobulated suprasellar masses of low attenuation (usually of less than cerebrospinal fluid density). Usually nonenhancing (may have a thin peripheral rim of contrast enhancement).	Epidermoids are lined with squamous epithelium, while dermoids typically contain hair, dermal elements, calcification, and fat. Intrathecal contrast material may be required to find the margins of these lesions.
Neuroma	Inhomogeneously enhancing mass. A trigeminal tumor typically erodes the base of the skull (especially the foramen ovale and apex of the petrous pyramid).	Arises from cranial nerves III to VI. Gasserian ganglion neuroma appears as a large filling defect in the enhanced cavernous sinus.
Hamartoma of the tuber cinereum **(Fig SK23-10)**	Small, smooth, isodense and nonenhancing mass attached to the posterior aspect of the hypothalamus between the tuber cinereum and the pons.	Rare lesion of early childhood that usually presents with precocious puberty, seizures, and mental changes (behavioral disorders and intellectual deterioration).
Aneurysm **Intracavernous**	Well-defined, oval or teardrop-shaped, eccentric mass that is slightly denser than cerebral tissue on unenhanced scans and markedly and homogeneously enhanced after intravenous administration of contrast material.	Intracavernous internal carotid aneurysms are saccular, occasionally have an intrasellar component, and are bilateral in about 25% of cases. They may have rim calcification and contain a low-density area representing a thrombus. An aneurysm can erode bone and compress the cavernous sinus (causing cranial nerve palsy) or rupture and produce a carotid-cavernous fistula.
Suprasellar **(Fig SK23-11)**	Slightly hyperdense mass that enhances intensely and homogeneously. May have rim calcification and contain a low-density thrombus.	Usually most common in the fourth to sixth decades, congenital (berry aneurysm), and the result of maldevelopment of the media (especially at points of arterial bifurcation). The sudden onset of headache or neck stiffness suggests aneurysmal leakage or rupture.
Carotid-cavernous fistula	Focal or diffuse enlargement of one or both enhancing cavernous sinuses (most prominent on the side of the fistula) and enlargement of the superior ophthalmic vein (especially on the side of the fistula) and edematous extraocular muscles.	Arises from traumatic rupture of the internal carotid artery or spontaneous rupture of a carotid aneurysm. May occasionally produce a normal CT scan for a few days after head trauma because the fistula develops slowly or after a delay.
Arachnoid cyst **(Fig SK23-12)**	Well-defined, nonenhancing mass of cerebrospinal fluid density. Sharp, noncalcified margin.	A suprasellar cyst often causes hydrocephalus (most common in infancy), visual impairment, and endocrine dysfunction.
Inflammatory lesion	Various patterns.	Infrequent manifestation of sarcoidosis, tuberculosis, sphenoid mucocele, pituitary abscess, or lymphoid hypophysitis (an autoimmune disorder in which lymphocytes infiltrate the pituitary gland).
Histiocytosis X	Irregularly marginated, relatively well-defined enhancing suprasellar mass.	Involvement of the hypothalamus and sella turcica, which is most common in children, is usually associated with multiple destructive skeletal lesions.

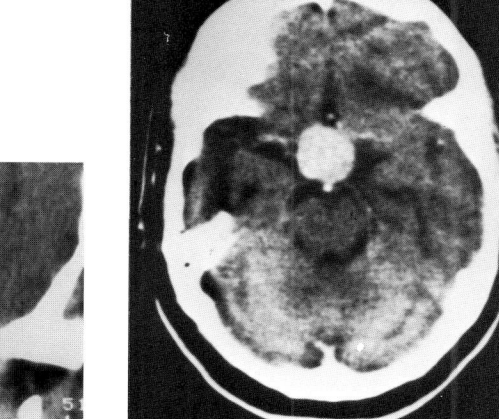

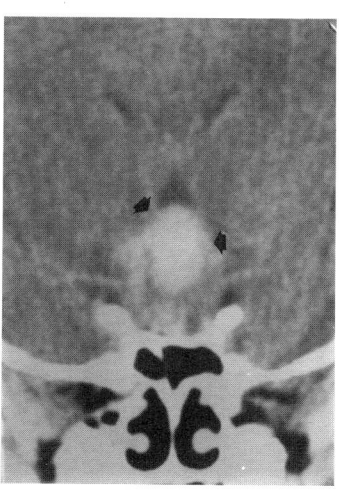

FIG SK23-7. Metastasis from oat cell carcinoma of the lung. (A) Noncontrast coronal scan shows a somewhat hyperdense mass filling the pituitary fossa and extending into the suprasellar region. (B) After intravenous injection of contrast material, there is dense enhancement of the metastasis.

FIG SK23-8. Ectopic pinealoma. Enhancing suprasellar mass (arrows).

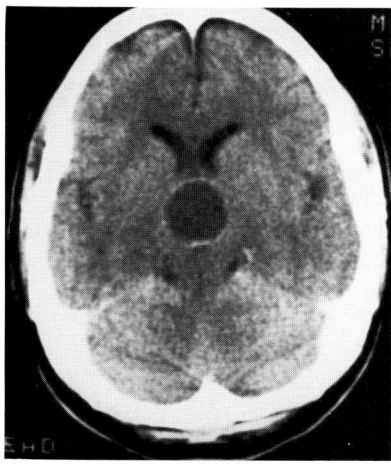

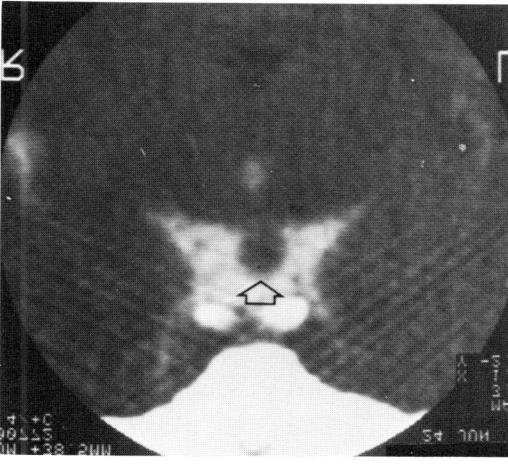

FIG SK23-9. Epidermoid. Smooth, low-attenuation suprasellar mass with a thin rim of contrast enhancement.

FIG SK23-10. Hamartoma of the tuber cinereum. Intrathecally enhanced coronal scan shows a small mass (arrow) that was isodense and nonenhancing on initial CT scans.

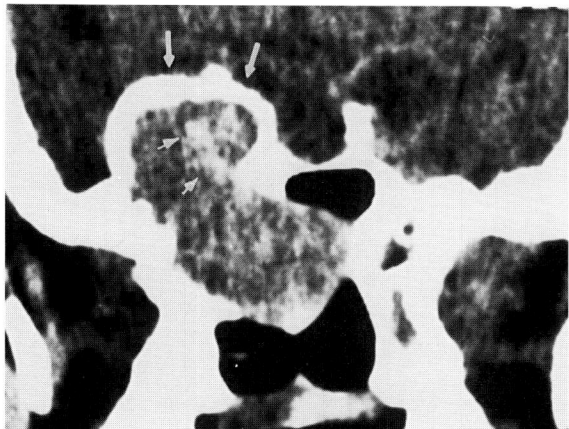

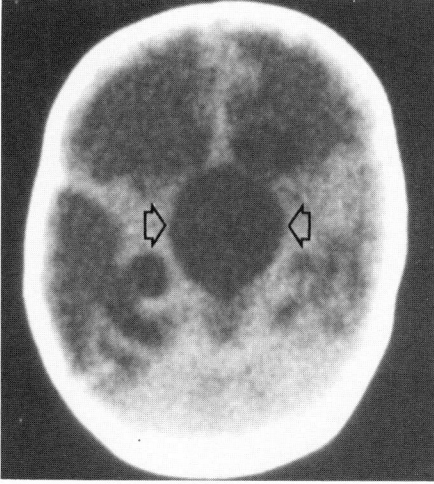

FIG SK23-11. Giant parasellar aneurysm. There is a rim of calcification (long arrows) along the superior margin of the aneurysm. Areas of enhancement in the aneurysm (short arrows) represent the patent lumen; the remainder of the aneurysm is filled with nonenhancing thrombus.

FIG SK23-12. Arachnoid cyst. Large, well-defined suprasellar mass of cerebrospinal fluid density (arrows). Note the prominent associated hydrocephalus.

SELLAR AND JUXTASELLAR MASSES ON MAGNETIC RESONANCE IMAGING

Condition	Imaging Findings	Comments
Pituitary adenoma **Microadenoma** **(Fig SK24-1)**	Usually hypointense compared with the normal gland on T_1-weighted images. After contrast injection, the tumor typically does not enhance to the same extent as the normal pituitary gland and thus stands out as an area of relative hypointensity.	Important secondary signs of microadenoma include asymmetric upward convexity of the gland surface, deviation of the infundibulum, and focal erosion of the sellar floor. The preferred imaging planes are coronal and sagittal.
Macroadenoma **(Fig SK24-2)**	Generally isointense to the normal gland and brain parenchyma unless there are cystic and hemorrhagic components. Homogeneous contrast enhancement permits clear demarcation of the tumor from normal suprasellar structures.	Adenoma larger than 10 mm. It may be hormone secreting (especially prolactin producing) and associated with amenorrhea and galactorrhea. MRI is ideal for demonstrating extension of tumor to involve the cavernous sinus, optic chiasm, inferior recesses of the third ventricle, and hypothalamus.
Craniopharyngioma **(Fig SK24-3)**	Variable appearance depending on the solid or cystic nature of the mass and the specific cyst contents. Solid lesions are hypointense on T_1-weighted images and hyperintense on T_2-weighted images. Cysts also have a long T_2 but show high signal intensity on T_1-weighted images if they have a high cholesterol content or methemoglobin.	The solid and wall portions of a craniopharyngioma show contrast enhancement. Truncation of the dorsum sellae and upward growth into the third ventricle may be seen. Calcification (seen well on CT) is not reliably detected by MRI.
Rathke's cleft cyst **(Fig SK24-4)**	Either a mass with CSF intensity on both T_1- and T_2-weighted images or a lesion that is markedly hyperintense on both sequences.	Remnant of an embryologic invagination cephalad up out of the pharynx that gives rise to the anterior and intermediate pituitary lobes. Bright signal on T_1-weighted images appears to reflect the high protein or starch content of the mucoid material in the cyst.
Meningioma **(Fig SK24-5)**	Isointense to hypointense mass on T_1-weighted images. Isointense or slightly hyperintense mass on T_2-weighted images. Marked homogeneous contrast enhancement.	Sagittal and coronal planes show the anatomic location of the mass as well as whether the internal carotid artery and its branches are encased by tumor and whether there is involvement of the optic nerve and chiasm. Unlike a pituitary adenoma, a suprasellar meningioma usually does not project into the intrasellar space.
Glioma **Optic chiasm** **(Fig SK24-6)**	Isointense or slightly hypointense on T_1-weighted images. Hyperintense on T_2-weighted images.	Posterior extension to the lateral geniculate body and beyond into the optic radiations appears as areas of increased signal on axial T_2-weighted images.
Hypothalamus	Isointense or slightly hypointense on T_1-weighted images. Hyperintense on T_2-weighted images.	Subtle deformity of the inferior recesses of the third ventricle can be visualized on coronal views. As with chiasmatic glioma, the tumor tends to have moderate contrast enhancement.

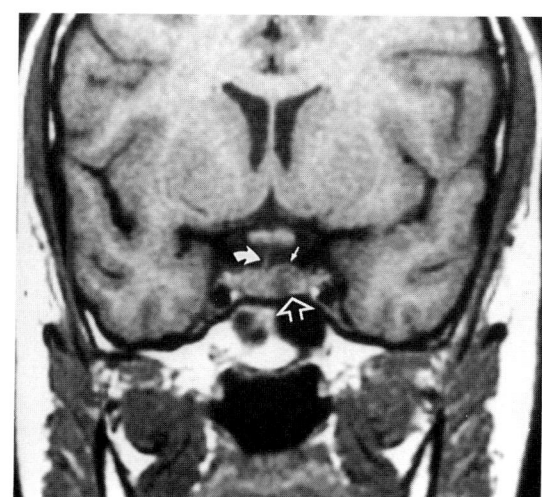

FIG SK24-1. Pituitary microadenoma. Coronal T$_1$-weighted image demonstrates a prolactin-secreting microadenoma (open arrow) as a focal area of decreased signal in the pituitary gland. Associated findings include displacement of the pituitary stalk contralaterally (curved arrow) and elevation of the upper border of the gland (straight solid arrow).[25]

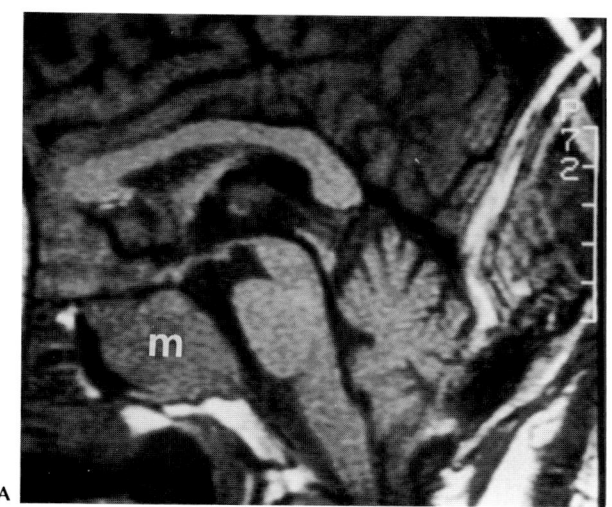

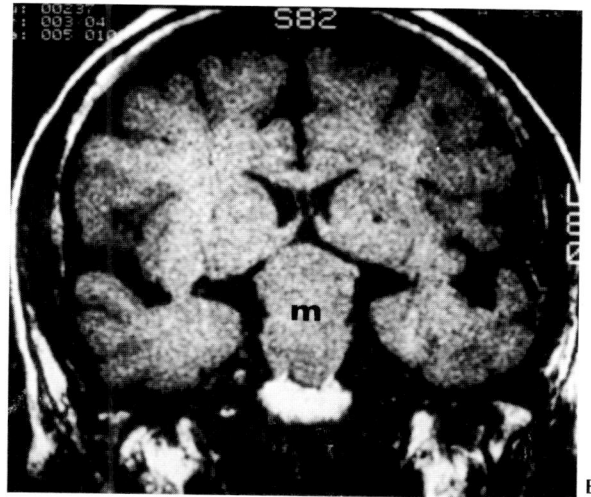

FIG SK24-2. Pituitary macroadenoma. (A) Sagittal and (B) coronal MR scans demonstrate a large mass (m) that arises from the sella turcica and extends upward to fill the suprasellar cistern. (C) In another patient, an axial scan shows tumor involvement of the right cavernous sinus with encasement of the ipsilateral carotid artery (arrow).

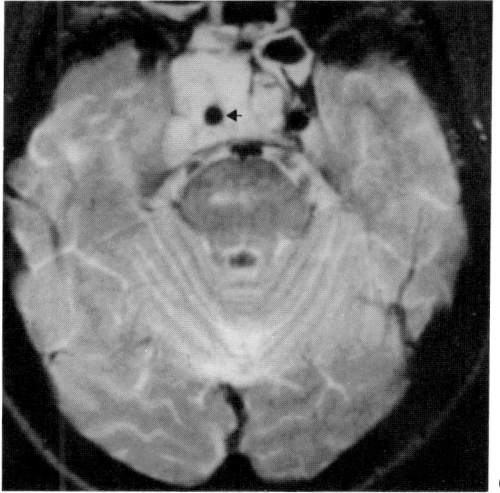

Condition	Imaging Findings	Comments
Chordoma (Fig SK24-7)	Hypointense lesion on T_1-weighted images. Hyperintense signal on T_2-weighted images.	Alteration of the normal high-signal fat in the clivus on T_1-weighted images is a sensitive indicator of disease.
Metastases (Fig SK24-8)	Hypointense lesion on T_1-weighted images. Hyperintense signal on T_2-weighted images.	Most metastases to the sellar and juxtasellar region originate from tumors of the lung, breast, kidney, or gastrointestinal tract or result from direct spread from carcinomas of the nasopharynx or sphenoid sinus.
Germ cell tumor (germinoma/teratoma)	Isointense to hypointense on T_1-weighted images. Slightly to moderately increased signal on T_2-weighted images.	Detection of a suprasellar germ cell tumor mandates close inspection of the pineal region because it may represent a forward extension of a pineal tumor or a multifocal process.
Epidermoid (Fig SK24-9)	Heterogeneous texture and variable signal intensity. Most are of slightly higher signal than CSF on both T_1- and T_2-weighted images.	Some epidermoids appear bright on T_1-weighted images.
Dermoid	Heterogeneous texture as a result of the multiple cell types in it.	Fatty components are common and produce high signal on T_1-weighted images.

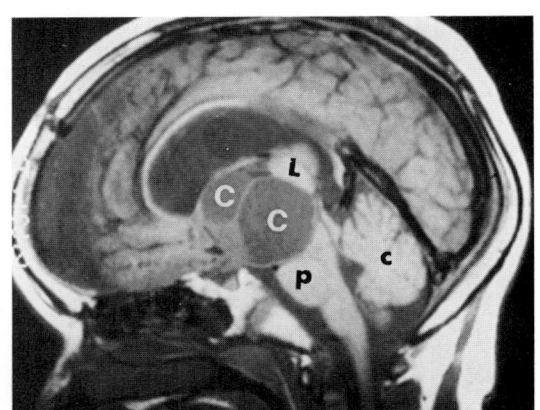

FIG SK24-3. **Craniopharyngioma.** Sagittal MR image demonstrates a large, multiloculated, suprasellar mass with cystic (C) and lipid (L) components. (p, Pons; c, cerebellum.)

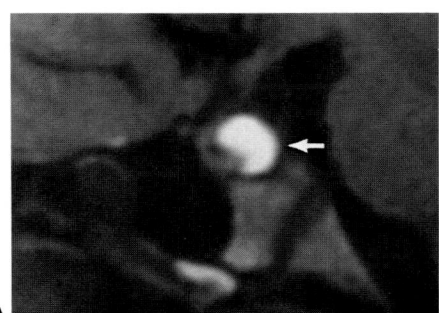

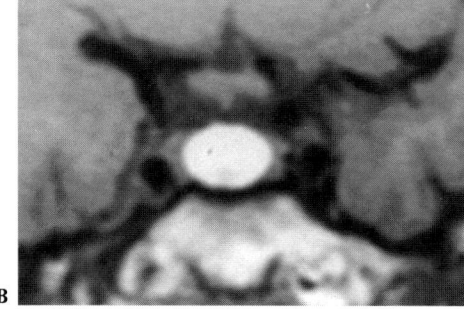

FIG SK24-4. **Rathke's cleft cyst.** (A) Sagittal and (B) coronal T_1-weighted images show an ovoid lesion of high signal intensity (arrow) in the middle to posterior portion of the pituitary fossa.[26]

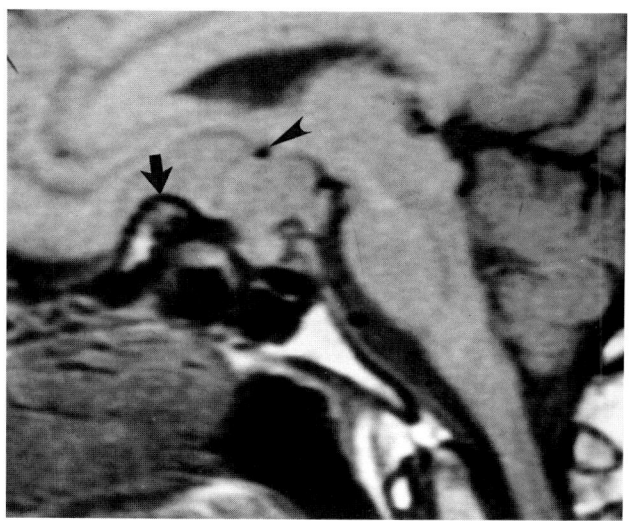

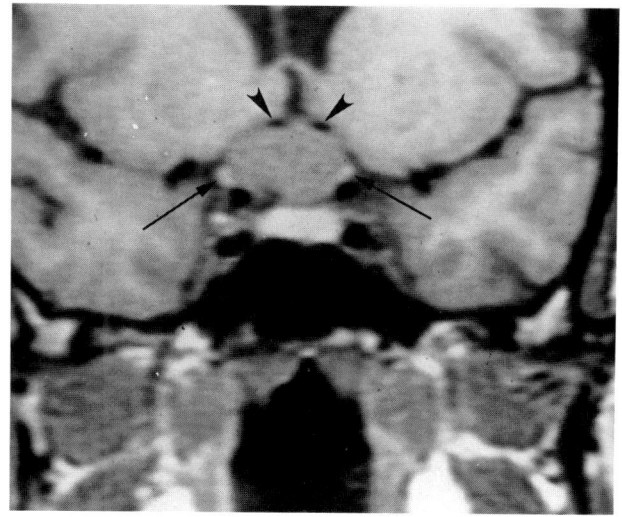

FIG SK24-5. **Planum sphenoidale meningioma** growing over the diaphragma sellae. (A) Sagittal T_1-weighted scan shows a soft-tissue mass isointense to brain that elevates the anterior cerebral artery (arrowhead) and produces hyperostosis of the planum sphenoidale (arrow). (B) Coronal T_1-weighted image shows a mass in the suprasellar space sitting on the diaphragma sellae, lying above the pituitary gland, elevating the two anterior cerebral arteries (arrowheads), and displacing both optic nerves (arrows).[26]

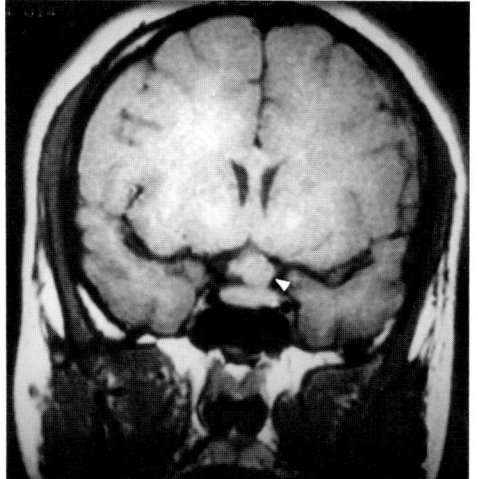

FIG SK24-6. **Optic chiasm glioma.** A suprasellar mass is seen on the left (arrowhead).

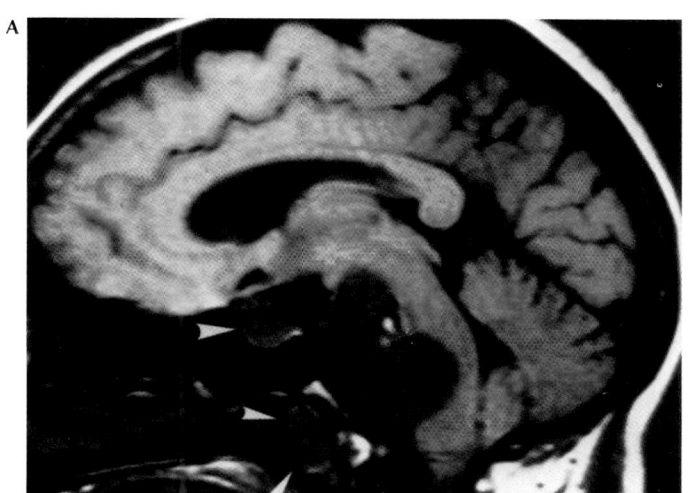

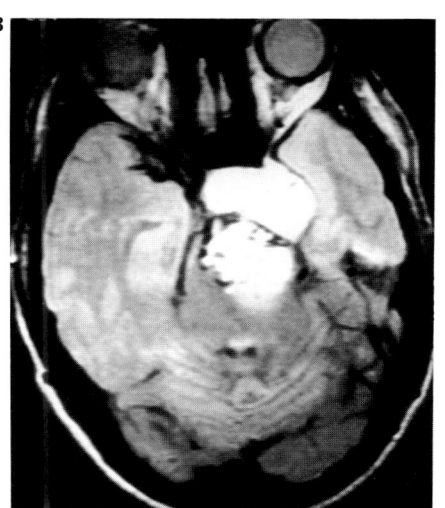

FIG SK24-7. **Clival chordoma.** (A) Sagittal MR scan shows a low-intensity multilobulated mass deforming and displacing the brainstem, destroying the clivus, and extending into the sella turcica (upper arrowhead) and nasopharynx (lower two arrowheads). (B) Axial T_2-weighted scan shows that the hyperintense mass with peripheral vessels invaginates into the brainstem and also occupies the region of the sella turcica and left cavernous sinus.[27]

Condition	Imaging Findings	Comments
Neuroma (Fig SK24-10)	Isointense or hypointense lesion on T_1-weighted images. Isointense to hyperintense lesion on T_2-weighted images.	Prominent homogeneous contrast enhancement. Coronal scans may show extension of a mandibular (V_3) neuroma downward through the foramen ovale.
Aneurysm (Fig SK24-11)	Flow void that may be surrounded by a pattern of heterogeneous signal intensity representing turbulence or thrombus.	Aneurysms in the suprasellar, intrasellar, and parasellar spaces can mimic a neoplasm by producing a mass lesion.
Arachnoid cyst	Smoothly marginated and homogeneous mass containing cyst fluid that is isointense to CSF on all pulse sequences.	The presence of mass effect and the lack of adjacent brain reaction are usually sufficient to differentiate an arachnoid cyst from atrophic encephalomalacia.
Ectopia of the posterior pituitary lobe (Fig SK24-12)	Posterior pituitary bright spot located cephalad in the median eminence of the hypothalamus rather than in its usual location.	Occurs most commonly in pituitary dwarfism (short stature), although it has been reported as being a normal variant. It also can be an acquired abnormality with traumatic stalk transection and compression or destruction of the neurohypophysis.
Lesion of the infundibular stalk	Various appearances.	True primary neoplasms (choristoma or pituicytoma) are extremely rare. More common neoplasms of the infundibulum are germinoma, lymphoma, leukemia, and other metastatic tumors. Nonneoplastic causes of infundibular enlargement include histiocytosis and sarcoidosis.

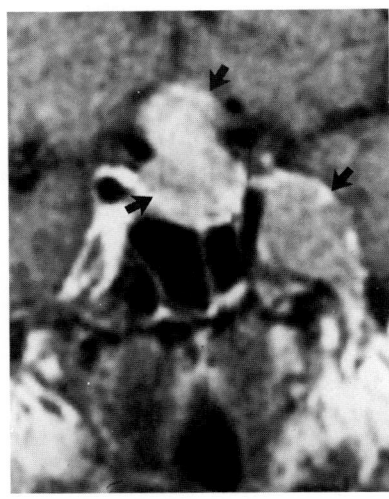

FIG SK24-8. Metastatic disease. Coronal T_1-weighted image shows an enhanced mass (arrows) in the sella, suprasellar space, and left parasellar cavernous sinus.[26]

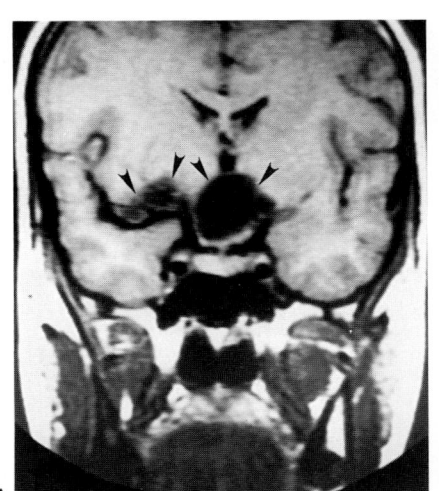

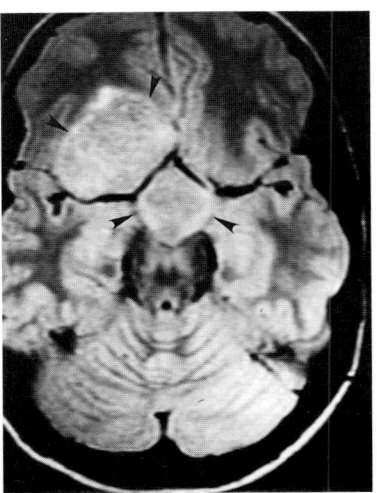

FIG SK24-9. Epidermoid tumor. (A) Coronal T_1-weighted image shows a hypointense suprasellar mass (arrowheads) that extends into the fissure of the right middle cerebral artery. (B) Axial proton-density image shows the suprasellar mass to have slightly increased signal intensity (arrowheads) and to extend into the inferior right frontal region.[26]

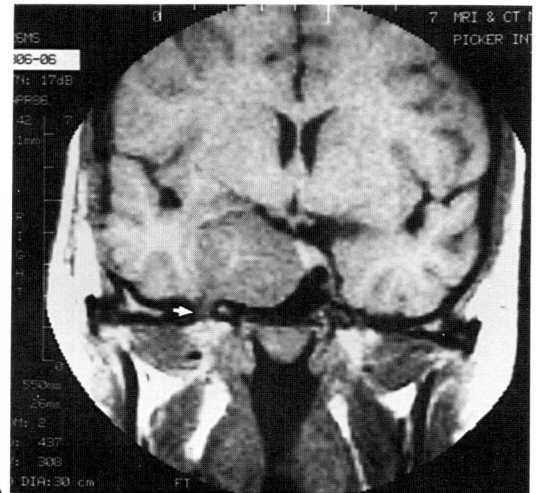

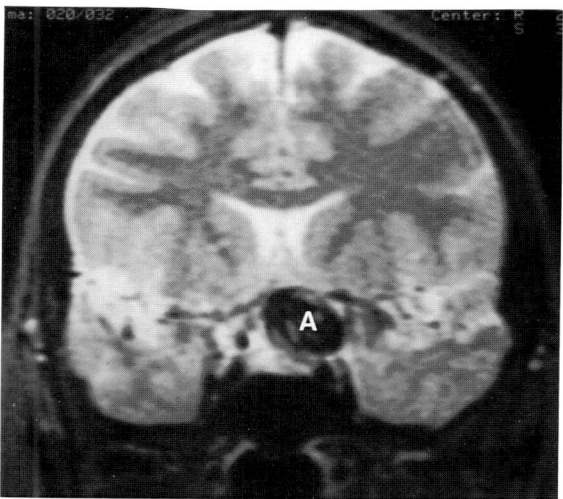

FIG SK24-11. **Distal left carotid artery aneurysm.** On this coronal T$_2$-weighted scan, the predominantly flow-void mass (A) extends into the suprasellar cistern and displaces the pituitary stalk.[25]

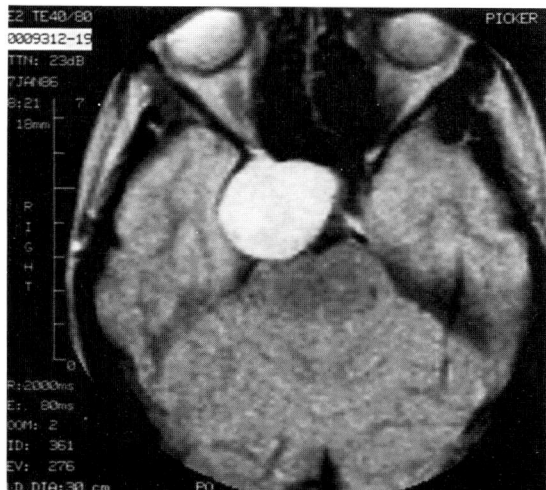

FIG SK24-10. **Trigeminal schwannoma** of the right gasserian ganglion. (A) T$_1$-weighted coronal image shows the mass to be of relatively low signal intensity and to involve the mandibular division (arrow). (B) On the T$_2$-weighted scan, the lesion has high homogeneous signal intensity.[28]

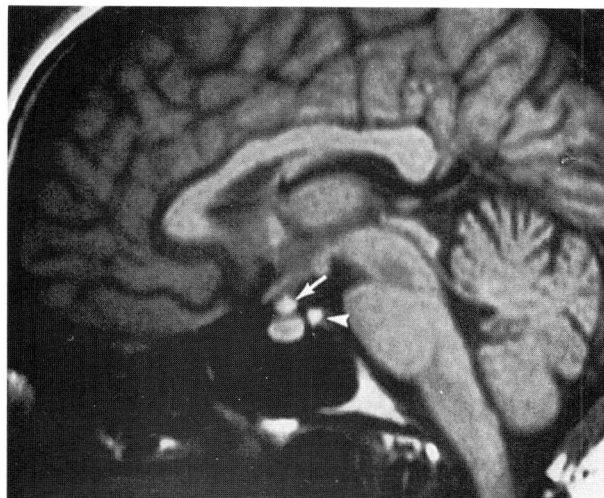

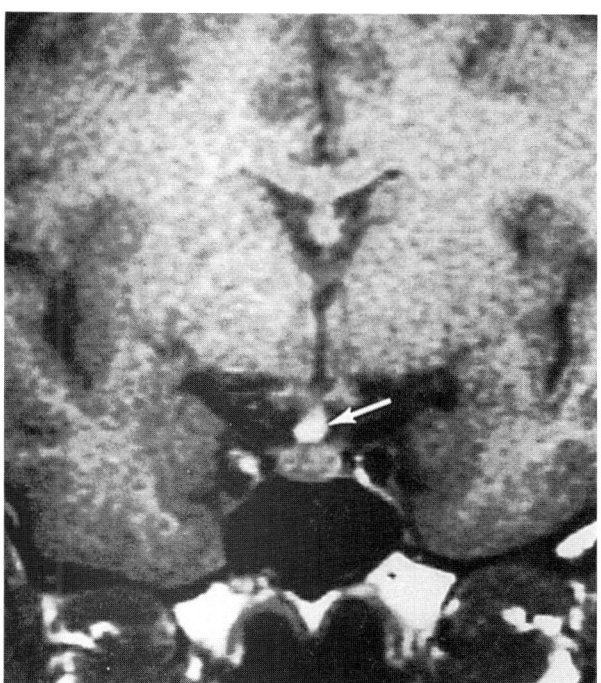

FIG SK24-12. **Ectopia of the posterior pituitary lobe.** (A) Sagittal and (B) coronal T$_1$-weighted images in a patient with diabetes insipidus that developed after an automobile accident. Hyperintensity in the region of the tuber cinereum (arrows) indicates transection of the pituitary stalk. Note the separate hyperintense area of fat in the dorsum sellae (arrowhead, A).[29]

MASSES IN THE PINEAL REGION

Condition	Imaging Findings	Comments
Pineal tumors **Germinoma ("atypical teratoma")** **(Figs SK25-1 and SK25-2)**	On CT, an isodense or hyperdense mass in the posterior third ventricle adjacent to or surrounding the pineal gland. Usually shows intense, homogeneous contrast enhancement. On MRI, usually isointense to brain on both T_1- and T_2-weighted images. A few lesions have long T_1 and T_2, which may correlate with embryonal cell elements.	Malignant primitive germ cell neoplasm that occurs almost exclusively in males, is usually radiosensitive, and is the most common tumor of the pineal region. May occur in association with a suprasellar germinoma. Because of their proximity to the aqueduct, these tumors frequently cause hydrocephalus. May produce ependymal or cisternal seeding.
Teratoma **(Figs SK25-3 and SK25-4)**	On CT, an inhomogeneous mass containing regions of low and high attenuation representing fat and calcification, respectively. On MRI, teratomas are of mixed signal intensity and often contain cystic components and fat.	Rare benign tumor that has a marked predominance in males and contains elements of all three germ layers. Usually shows minimal contrast enhancement (intense enhancement suggests malignant degeneration).
Teratocarcinoma	Irregularly marginated mass that varies in density and typically shows intense homogeneous contrast enhancement.	Malignant tumors (embryonal cell carcinoma; choriocarcinoma) that arise from primitive germ cells and are characterized by intratumoral hemorrhage, invasion of adjacent structures, and seeding via cerebrospinal fluid pathways.
Pineocytoma **(Fig SK25-5)**	On CT, a slightly hyperdense mass that often contains dense, focal calcification. Variable contrast enhancement. On MRI, a hypointense mass on T_1-weighted images that becomes hyperintense on T_2-weighted images.	Slow-growing tumor composed of mature pineal parenchymal cells and usually confined to the posterior third ventricle. Indistinct tumor margins suggest infiltration of adjacent structures. May spread via cerebrospinal fluid pathways.
Pineoblastoma **(Fig SK25-6)**	Poorly marginated, isodense or slightly hyperdense mass typically containing dense calcification. Homogeneous and intense contrast enhancement.	Highly malignant tumor of primitive pineal parenchymal cells that frequently spreads via cerebrospinal fluid pathways.
Metastasis **(Fig SK25-7)**	Indistinct hypodense or isodense mass that shows homogeneous enhancement. Occasionally hyperdense.	Infrequent manifestation that must be considered in older adults with known malignant disease.
Glioma of nonpineal origin	Low-density mass with poorly defined margins, minimal or moderate enhancement, and no calcification. May displace the normal calcified pineal gland.	Tumors arising from the thalamus, posterior hypothalamus, tectal plate of the mesencephalon, or splenium that extend into the quadrigeminal cistern. Usually occur in older patients.
Meningioma **(Fig SK25-8)**	On CT, a round, sharply delineated, isodense or hyperdense mass that is often calcified and shows intense homogeneous contrast enhancement. On MRI, generally a relatively isointense mass with intense enhancement.	Midline tumors arising from the edge of the tentorium may be difficult to distinguish from pineal tumors. However, they are usually eccentrically located and often have a flat border along the tentorium close to the dural margin.

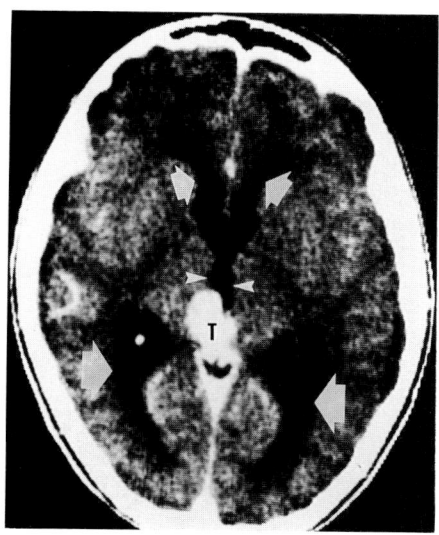

FIG SK25-1. **Germinoma.** Enhancing tumor (T) in the pineal region of a young girl with paralysis of upward gaze, headaches, and nausea (Perinaud's syndrome). The minimal dilatation of the third ventricle (arrowheads) and lateral ventricles (arrows) indicates mild hydrocephalus, which developed because of obstruction of the posterior portion of the third ventricle by the tumor.

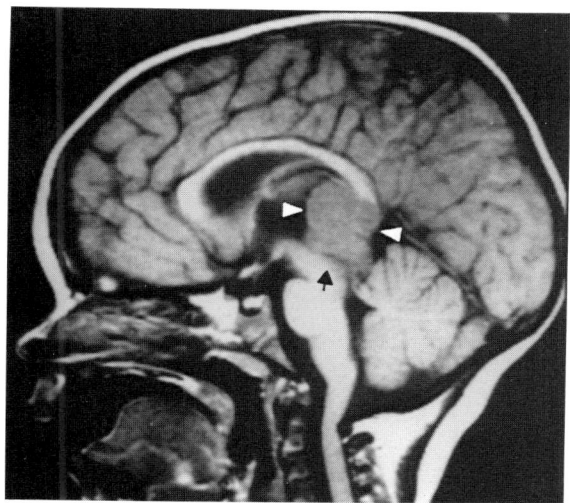

FIG SK25-2. **Germinoma.** Sagittal T₁-weighted MR image shows a large isointense mass (arrowheads) that compresses the midbrain (arrow) and elevates the splenium of the corpus callosum.

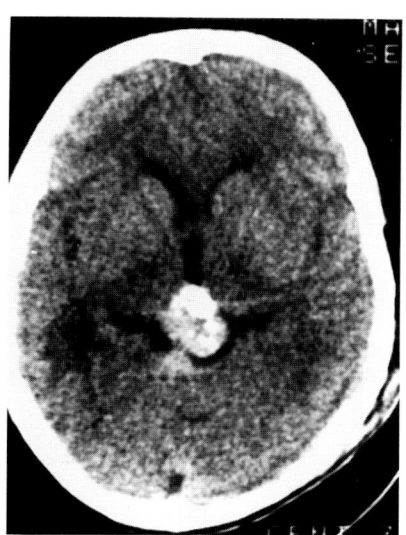

FIG SK25-3. **Teratoma.** Nonenhanced scan shows an inhomogeneous mass containing a large amount of calcification.

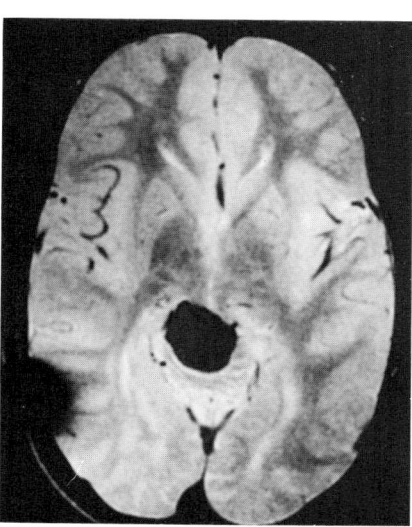

FIG SK25-4. **Teratoma.** Axial T₂-weighted MR image shows a pineal mass that is markedly hypointense because of high fat content and extensive calcification.

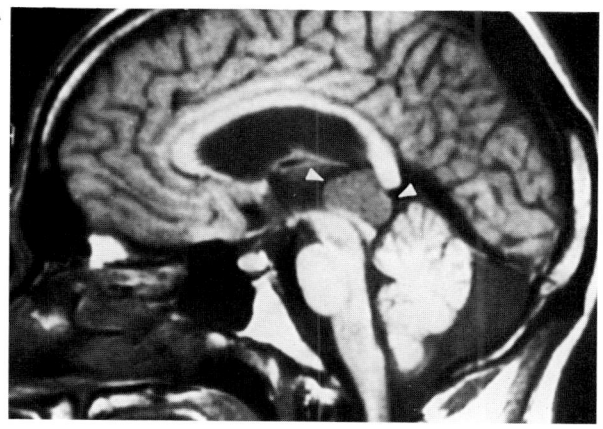

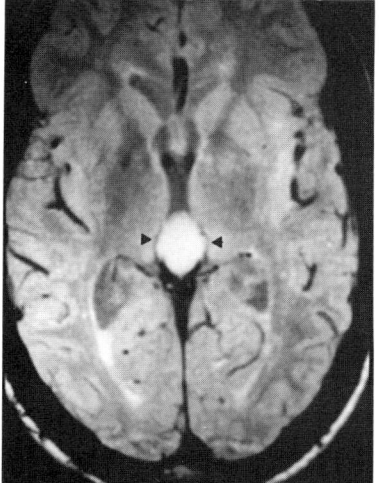

FIG SK25-5. **Pineocytoma.** Pineal mass that is hypointense (arrowheads) on a sagittal T₁-weighted image (A) and hyperintense (arrows) on an axial T₂-weighted image (B).

Condition	Imaging Findings	Comments
Vein of Galen aneurysm (Fig SK25-9)	Mass of uniform density and intense contrast enhancement that mimics a pineal tumor.	Arteriovenous malformation that often presents in childhood, produces high blood flow, and is an important cause of neonatal heart failure.
Pineal cyst (Fig SK25-10)	Sharply circumscribed mass that is best seen as a round area of high signal intensity on T_2-weighted images.	Benign lesion seen in 4% of normal patients in one series. They are not associated with hydrocephalus or a pineal mass and are of no clinical significance.

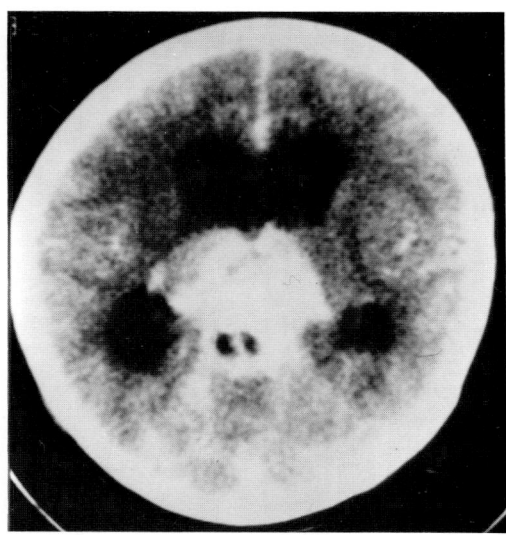

FIG SK25-6. Pineoblastoma. Huge densely calcified mass in the pineal region causing obstructive hydrocephalus.

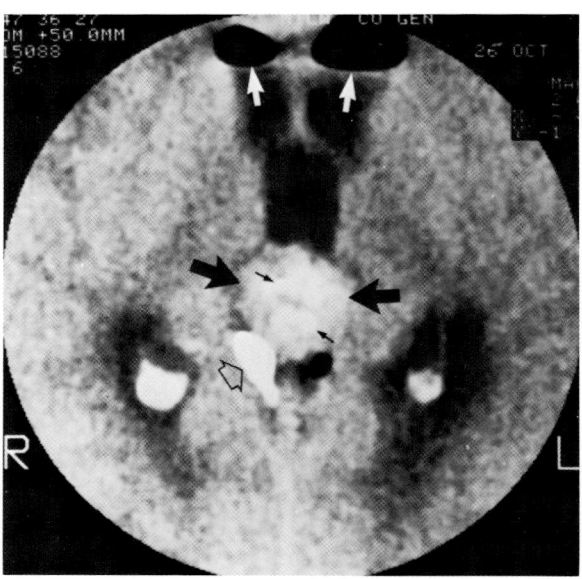

FIG SK25-7. Metastasis. In this patient with lung carcinoma, an unenhanced scan shows a well-circumscribed, hyperdense pineal mass (large arrows) containing dense punctate calcification (small arrows). Air in the frontal horns (white arrows) resulted from a recent ventricular shunting procedure. Note the tentorial calcification (open arrow) adjacent to the metastasis.[13]

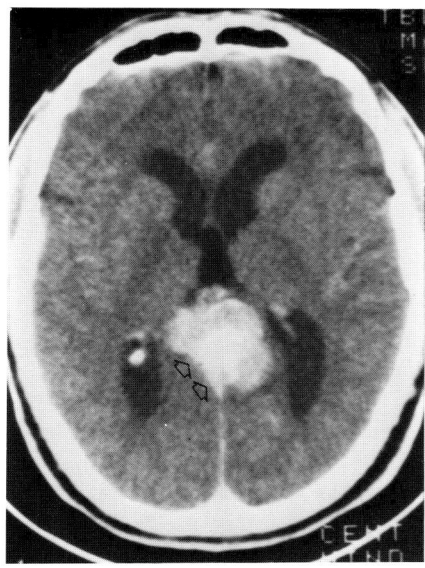

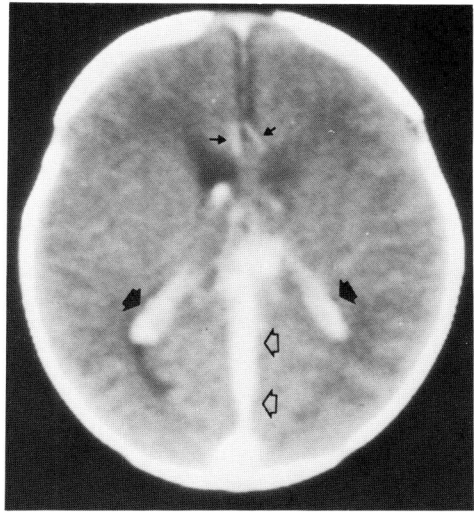

FIG **SK25-8. Meningioma.** Densely enhancing mass in the pineal region that arises from the incisura of the tentorium. Note the characteristic flat border (arrows) along the tentorium.

FIG **SK25-9. Vein of Galen aneurysm.** Contrast-enhanced scan shows dilatation of the vein of Galen and straight sinus (open arrows). Note the prominent feeding vessels of the choroid plexus (closed arrows) and the anterior cerebral arteries (thin arrows).

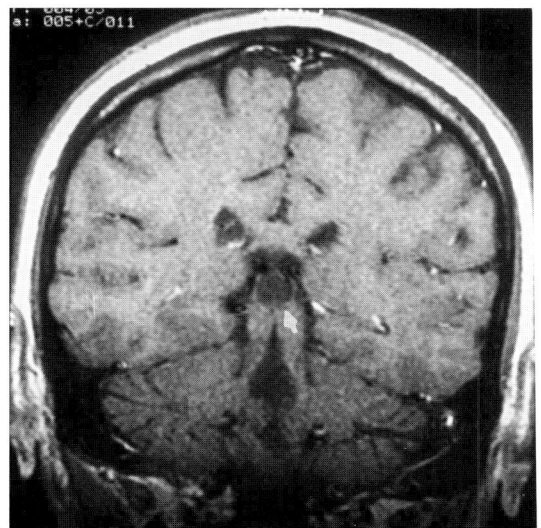

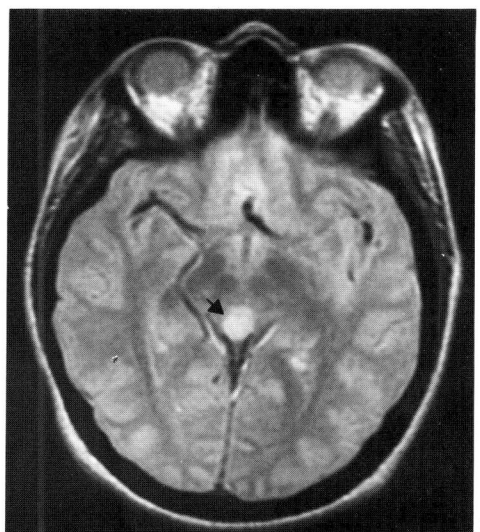

FIG **SK25-10. Pineal cyst.** Round pineal mass (arrows) that is markedly hypointense on a coronal T_1-weighted image (A) and hyperintense on an axial T_2-weighted image (B).

HYPOTHALAMIC LESIONS ON MAGNETIC RESONANCE IMAGING

Condition	Imaging Findings	Comments
Glioma (Fig SK26-1)	Suprasellar mass that is isointense or hypointense on T_1-weighted images and hyperintense on T_2-weighted images. Inhomogeneous contrast enhancement.	Hypothalamic gliomas frequently invade the optic chiasm and vice versa, so that the primary site of origin may be difficult to determine. The tumor is slow growing and usually occurs in children and young adults.
Germinoma (Fig SK26-2)	Usually mildly hypointense on T_1-weighted images and hyperintense on T_2-weighted images, though it may be isointense on both pulse sequences.	Second most frequent site (most common in the pineal region). Hypothalamic germinomas affect men and women equally, unlike the strong male predominance in pineal lesions. These low-grade malignant tumors are radiosensitive and may spread via CSF pathways.
Primary lymphoma (Fig SK26-3)	Slightly hypointense on T_1-weighted images. Variable appearance on T_2-weighted images. Usually shows contrast enhancement.	Prevalence of primary CNS lymphoma is increased in AIDS patients and other immunosuppressed individuals. Most common presentation is solitary or multicentric, well-defined enhancing masses in the deep gray nuclei, periventricular white matter, or corpus callosum.
Hamartoma (Fig SK26-4)	Mass in the region of the tuber cinereum that is isointense on T_1-weighted images and isointense or mildly hyperintense on T_2-weighted images. The lesion is stable over time and typically does not show contrast enhancement.	Rare lesion of early childhood that usually presents with precocious puberty, seizures, and mental changes (behavioral disorders and intellectual deterioration). It may be found incidentally in adults and mimic low-grade gliomas.

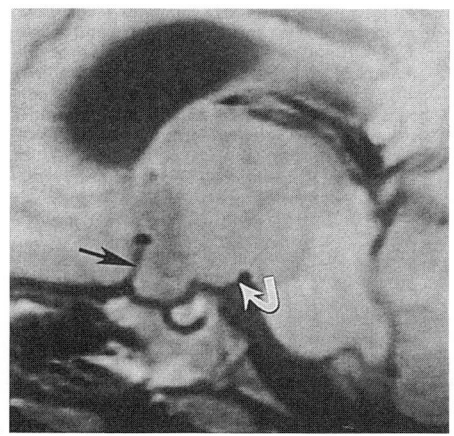

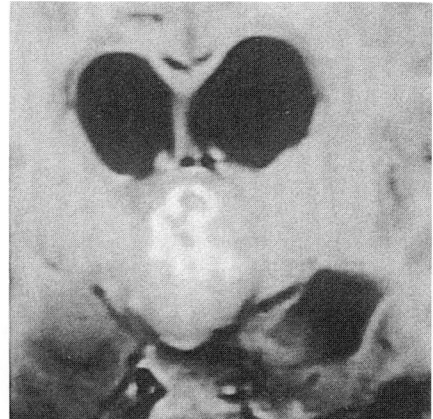

FIG SK26-1. Glioma. (A) Sagittal T_1-weighted image in a 2-year-old emaciated and hyperactive girl shows a large midline mass involving the optic chiasm (straight arrow) and hypothalamus (curved arrow). (B) Coronal contrast-enhanced T_1-weighted image shows non-uniform enhancement of the tumor, which extends superiorly to the foramen of Monro and causes obstructive hydrocephalus.[30]

A

B

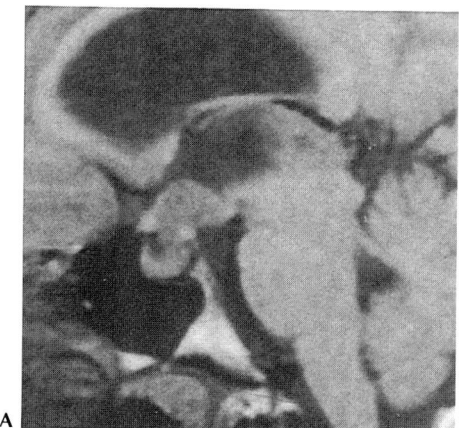
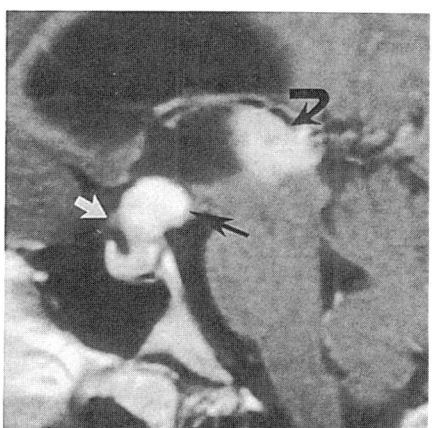

FIG SK26-2. Germinoma. Sagittal T_1-weighted scans before (A) and after (B) administration of contrast material in an 18-year-old man with diabetes insipidus show enhancing masses in the floor of the anterior third ventricle (straight black arrow) and pineal region (curved arrow). The optic chiasm (white arrow) is not involved. [30]

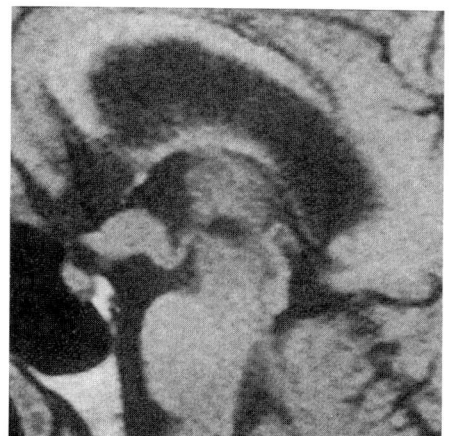
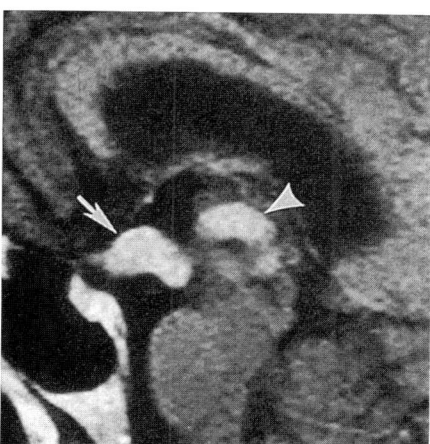

FIG SK26-3. Primary CNS lymphoma. (A) Sagittal and (B) axial T_1-weighted images after injection of contrast material show enhancing mass lesions in the hypothalamus (arrows) and left thalamus (arrowheads). [30]

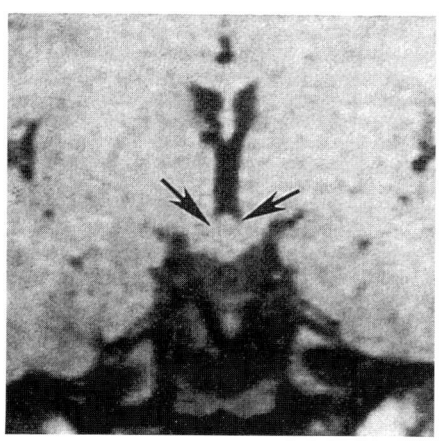
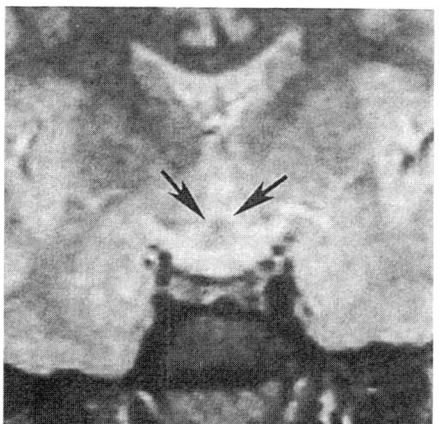

FIG SK26-4. Hamartoma. Coronal (A) T_1-weighted and (B) T_2-weighted scans in a 5-year-old girl with precocious puberty show a midline hypothalamic mass (arrows) bulging into the inferior floor of the third ventricle. The lesion is isointense on both images and is centered in the region of the tuber cinereum. [30]

Condition		Comments
Histiocytosis (Fig SK26-5)	Suprasellar mass involving the infundibulum and hypothalamus that is hypointense on T_1-weighted images and hyperintense on T_2-weighted images. The lesion enhances homogeneously with contrast material.	Multisystem disorder associated with proliferation of macrophages. Hypothalamic involvement, most common in children, is usually associated with multiple destructive skeletal lesions. Dramatic response to low-dose radiation strongly favors the diagnosis of histiocytosis over hypothalamic glioma.
Sarcoidosis (Fig SK26-6)	Leptomeningeal form, involving the infundibulum and hypothalamus, typically is isointense on T_1-weighted images and mildly hyperintense on T_2-weighted images. It shows homogeneous contrast enhancement.	Systemic noncaseating granulomatous disease that involves the central nervous system in about 5% of individuals. It is common in blacks and usually occurs in the third to fourth decades of life. There is usually a positive response to steroid therapy.
Ectopic posterior pituitary gland (Fig SK26-7)	Small midline mass within the tuber cinereum–infundibular region that has homogeneous high-signal intensity on T_1-weighted images and is isointense on T_2-weighted images. Characteristic absence of normal infundibulum and high-signal-intensity tissue within the posterior sella on T_1-weighted images.	May be caused by trauma or an adjacent mass or be of congenital origin. Often associated with dwarfism, though many patients are asymptomatic. Transection, compression, or absence of the infundibulum and its neurohypophyseal tract results in the proximal build up of neurosecretory granules within liposome vesicles before the point of interruption. The bright signal associated with the phospholipid membranes of these hormone-carrying vesicles is thus displaced proximally and cannot be seen in its normal location in the posterior lobe of the pituitary gland at the back of the sella.
Wernicke's encephalopathy (Fig SK26-8)	Nearly complete absence of the mamillary bodies, best seen on T_1-weighted images.	Atrophy of the mamillary bodies is a characteristic feature of this disorder. The disease is caused by thiamine deficiency and is most commonly seen in alcoholics. It is associated with the classic triad of oculomotor dysfunction, ataxia, and encephalopathy.

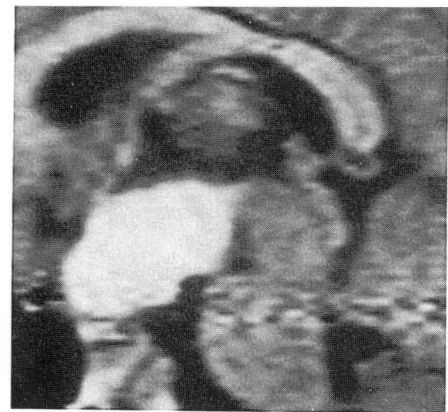
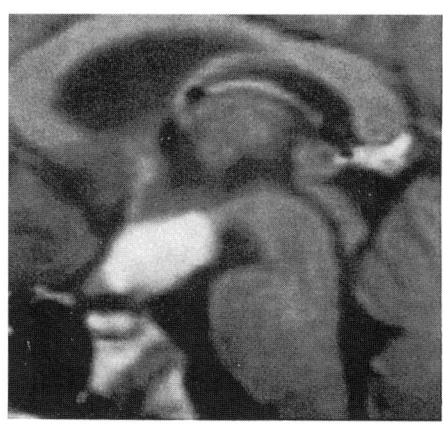

A   B

FIG SK26-5. **Histiocytosis.** (A) Initial sagittal T_1-weighted image after injection of contrast material in a 9-year-old boy with diabetes insipidus shows a large enhancing hypothalamic mass splaying the cerebral peduncles (arrows). (B) Corresponding image 3 weeks after low-dose radiation treatment shows a significant decrease in size of the lesion.[30]

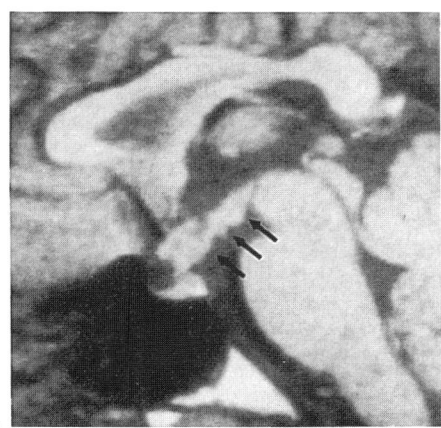

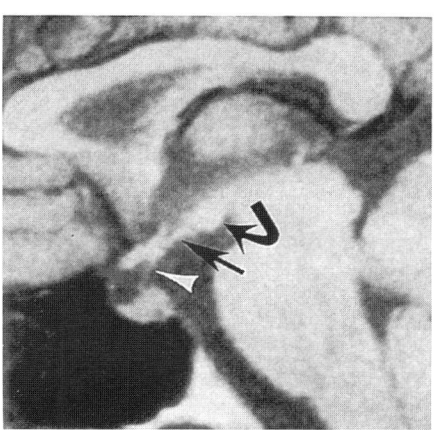

FIG SK26-6. Sarcoidosis. (A) Sagittal T$_1$-weighted image in a black woman with recent onset of visual difficulties shows abnormal thickening in the hypothalamic region (arrows) involving the tuber cinereum, mamillary bodies, and infundibulum. (B) After a 3-week course of steroids, a repeat sagittal scan shows dramatic resolution with a return to normal of hypothalamic region anatomy. Note the normal mamillary bodies (curved arrow), tuber cinereum (straight arrow), and infundibulum (arrowhead).[30]

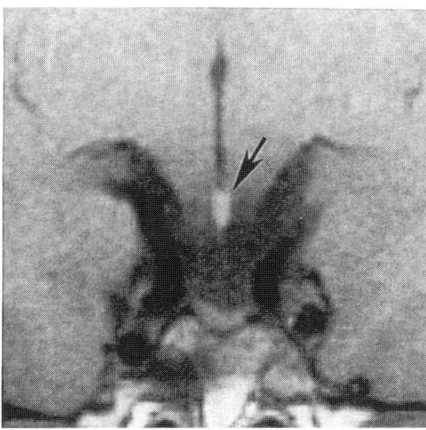

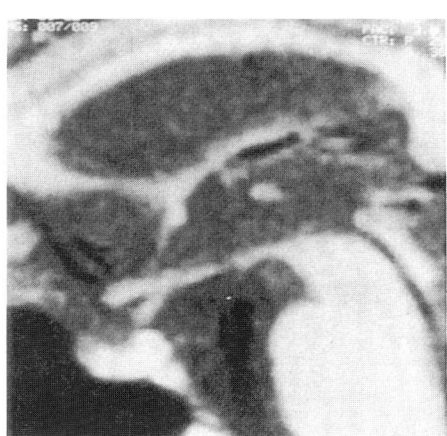

FIG SK26-7. Ectopic posterior pituitary gland. Coronal T$_1$-weighted image in a young boy with short stature shows a hyperintense, oblong nodule (arrow) in the inferior portion of the tuber cinereum. Pituitary tissue within the sella does not show high signal in its posterior portion, and there is no evidence of an infundibulum connecting the pituitary gland to the hypothalamus.[30]

FIG SK26-8. Wernicke's encephalopathy. Sagittal T$_1$-weighted image in an elderly alcoholic man shows striking atrophy of the mamillary bodies.[30]

CEREBELLAR MASSES ON COMPUTED TOMOGRAPHY

Condition	Imaging Findings	Comments
Astrocytoma **(Fig SK27-1)**	Cystic or hypodense solid mass. Variable contrast enhancement (cystic astrocytomas may display an enhancing rim of tissue surrounding the circumference of the cyst or an enhancing localized mural nodule along nonenhancing cyst margins).	Occurs more commonly in children (first or second most frequent tumor of the posterior fossa) than in adults. Affects the cerebellar hemispheres more commonly than the vermis, tonsils, or brainstem. About 20% of the tumors calcify. Malignant astrocytomas show edema and necrosis in addition to enhancement after the administration of contrast material.
Medulloblastoma **(Fig SK27-2)**	Sharply marginated, spherical midline mass that is hyperdense and shows uniform and intense contrast enhancement.	Embryonal tumor consisting of primitive and poorly differentiated cells that originate immediately above the fourth ventricle and migrate during gestation toward the surface of the cerebellum. One of the two most common posterior fossa tumors in children. May occur in the cerebellar hemispheres in older patients. Metastasizes along the cerebrospinal fluid pathways in about 10% of cases (abnormal contrast enhancement or irregular thickening of the lining of the subarachnoid spaces).
Ependymoma	Isodense or slightly hyperdense midline mass. Unlike medulloblastomas, ependymomas are often inhomogeneous with cystic or hemorrhagic areas and frequently calcify. The tumor margins are often irregular and poorly defined and the enhancement pattern is usually less homogeneous and intense than in medulloblastoma.	Fourth ventricular tumor that is more common in children than in adults. A characteristic finding is a thin, well-defined, low-attenuation halo that represents the distended and usually effaced fourth ventricle surrounding the tumor. The lesion frequently extends through the foramina of Luschka into the cerebellopontine angle or through the foramen of Magendie into the cisterna magna and typically causes hydrocephalus.
Hemangioblastoma **(Fig SK27-3)**	Most commonly a cystic hemispheric mass, typically with one or more small intensely enhancing mural nodules. May appear as a solid mass. Calcification is extremely rare.	Relatively uncommon tumor of the posterior fossa and spinal cord that is usually seen in adults. Hemangioblastomas tend to be smaller than hemispheric astrocytomas and almost never calcify. Characteristic intense tumor stain on angiography (more sensitive and specific than CT for this type of tumor).
Cerebellar sarcoma (lateral medulloblastoma) **(Fig SK27-4)**	Large, solid, lobulated mass that is hyperdense or heterogeneous.	Probably represents a variety of desmoplastic peripheral medulloblastoma that is never calcified or predominantly cystic (as may be a central medulloblastoma).
Metastases **(Fig SK27-5)**	Various appearances (densely enhancing nodules surrounded by edema; large, inhomogeneous, poorly enhancing mass; ring enhancement in tumors with central necrosis).	Most common cerebellar tumors of older patients. There is usually a history of an extracerebral tumor and evidence of other cerebral metastases.

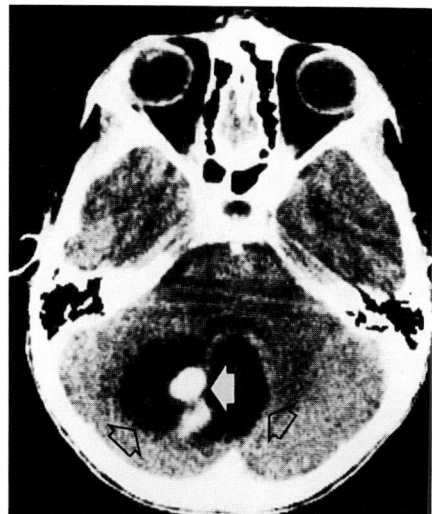

FIG SK27-1. Cystic astrocytoma. The cystic posterior fossa lesion (open arrows) contains a central nodular area of enhancement (closed arrow).

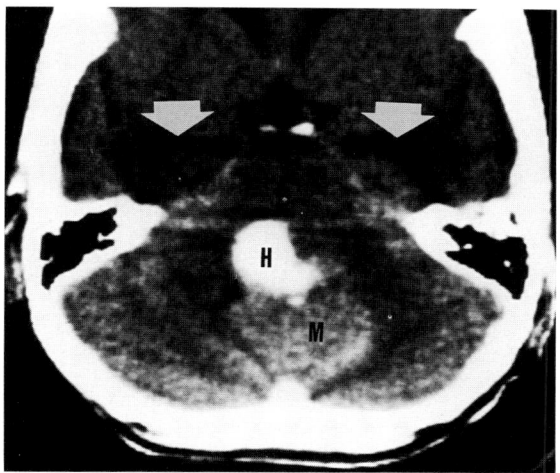
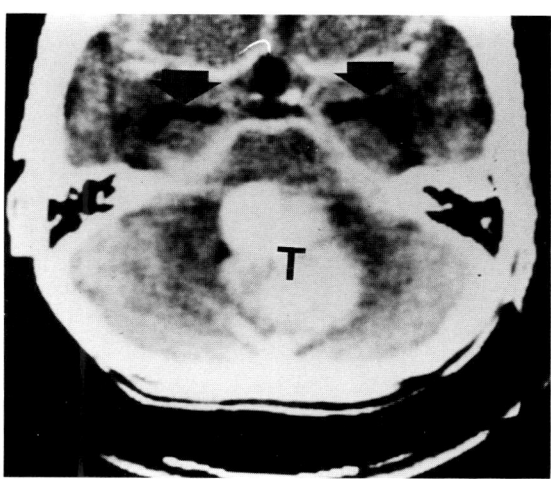

FIG SK27-2. Medulloblastoma. (A) Noncontrast scan in an 8-year-old girl shows the tumor as a mixed high-density (H) and medium-density (M) mass in the posterior fossa. (B) After the intravenous injection of contrast material, there was marked enhancement of the tumor (T). The arrows point to the dilated temporal horns representing hydrocephalus.

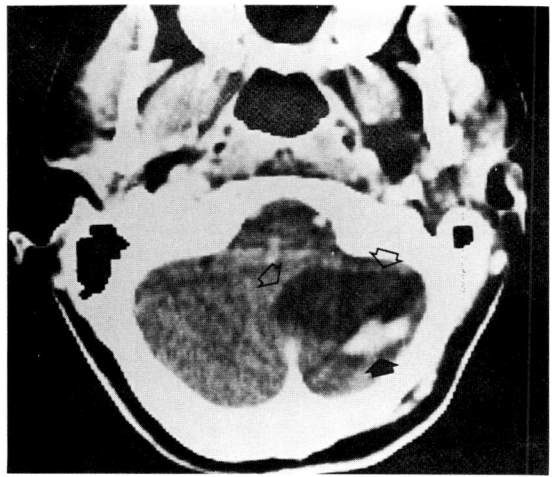
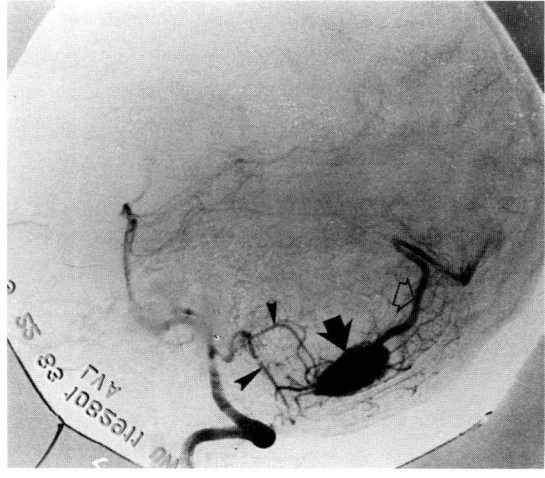

FIG SK27-3. Hemangioblastoma in von Hippel–Lindau syndrome. (A) CT scan shows a cystic lesion (open arrows) with an enhancing nodule (closed arrow) in the left cerebellar hemisphere. (B) Vertebral arteriogram shows the vascular nodule (solid arrow) of the tumor with multiple feeding arteries (black arrowheads) and a large draining vein (open arrow).

Condition	Imaging Findings	Comments
Lymphoma	Solid, hyperdense, densely enhancing mass that is located near the fourth ventricle or cerebellar surface and is usually associated with little or no edema.	Often multicentric with infiltration into adjoining tissue and across the midline (no respect for normal anatomic boundaries). Tumor margins are invariably poorly defined and irregular, probably because of the characteristic perivascular and vascular infiltration pattern of the tumor cells.
Epidermoid	Sharply marginated, nearly homogeneous, hypodense mass that may have an extremely low attenuation due to a high fat content.	Result of inclusion of ectodermal germ layer elements in the neural tube during its closure between the third and fifth weeks of gestation. Most commonly occurs in the cerebellopontine angle and suprasellar region, though it may develop in the fourth ventricle. Rupture into the ventricular system may produce a characteristic fat–cerebrospinal fluid level.
Choroid plexus papilloma	Homogeneous isodense or hyperdense intraventricular mass with smooth, well-defined, frequently lobulated margins. Intense homogeneous contrast enhancement.	Most commonly occurs in the first decade of life, usually in infancy. Typically develops in the lateral ventricles, though the fourth ventricle may be involved. In choroid plexus carcinoma, there are low-attenuation zones in the adjacent brain (representing edema or tumor invasion) and massive hydrocephalus.
Infarct (Fig SK27-6)	Well-defined, low-attenuation region in a cerebellar hemisphere.	Contrast enhancement in a subacute infarction may simulate a cerebellar tumor.
Hemorrhage (Fig SK27-7)	High-attenuation process that may appear round or irregular in shape and compress the fourth ventricle to cause hydrocephalus.	Hemorrhage into the cisterns usually produces a thin layer of higher-density tissue adjacent to the tentorium or in the pontine cistern.
Arteriovenous malformation (Fig SK27-8)	Large, tortuous, high-attenuation structures (representing serpiginous dilated vessels) that are seen after contrast enhancement.	An unruptured arteriovenous malformation may appear normal or only subtly abnormal on unenhanced CT studies, since the abnormal vessels are usually only slightly hyperdense with respect to the brain and are therefore difficult to identify. In some cases, calcification in the malformation or a low-density cyst or damaged cerebral tissue from previous hemorrhage suggests the presence of a malformation.
Abscess	Various patterns.	Pyogenic; tuberculous; fungal; parasitic.

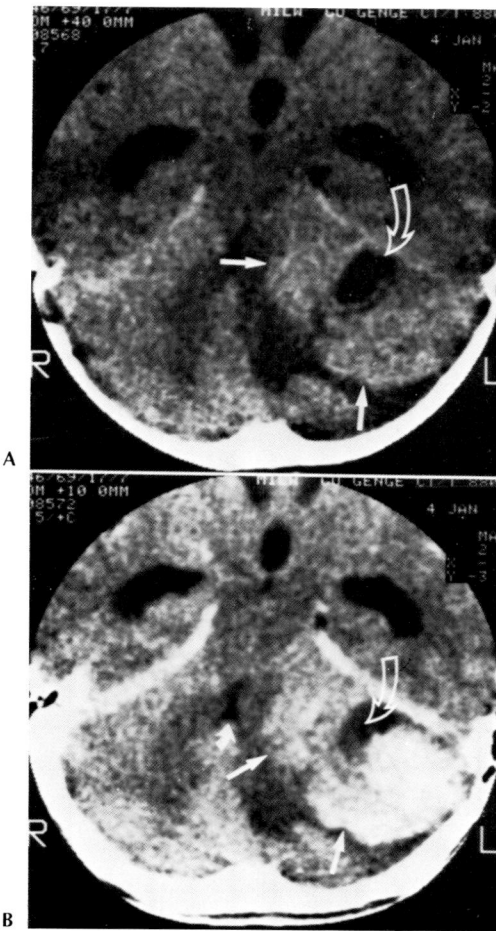

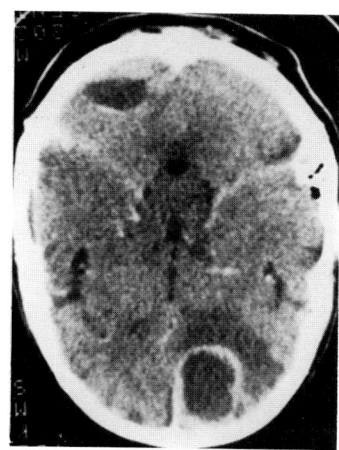

FIG SK27-4. **Cerebellar sarcoma.** (A) Noncontrast scan shows dense tumor (arrows) in the left cerebellar hemisphere. Note the cystic region (open curved arrow) within it. (B) After intravenous contrast infusion, the tumor is notably enhanced (arrows). The fourth ventricle is displaced severely from left to right (open curved arrow), causing noncommunicating hydrocephalus.[13]

FIG SK27-5. **Metastasis.** Ring-enhancing lesion with surrounding edema.

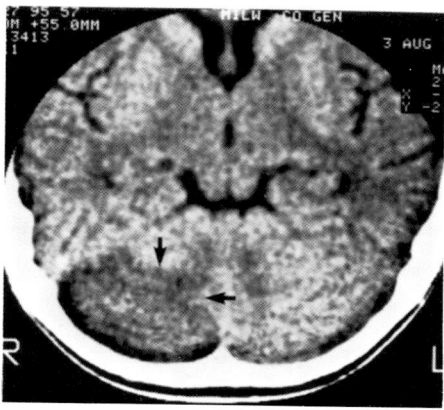

FIG SK27-6. **Right cerebellar infarction.** The low-attenuation process (arrows) has well-defined margins consistent with chronic infarction.[13]

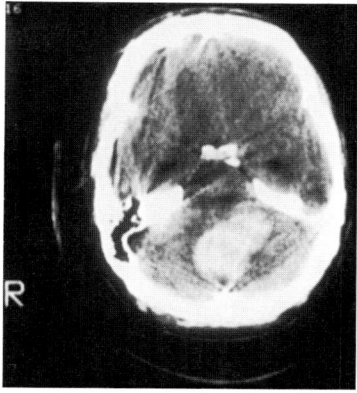

FIG SK27-7. **Cerebellar hemorrhage.** Well-circumscribed, high-attenuation mass.

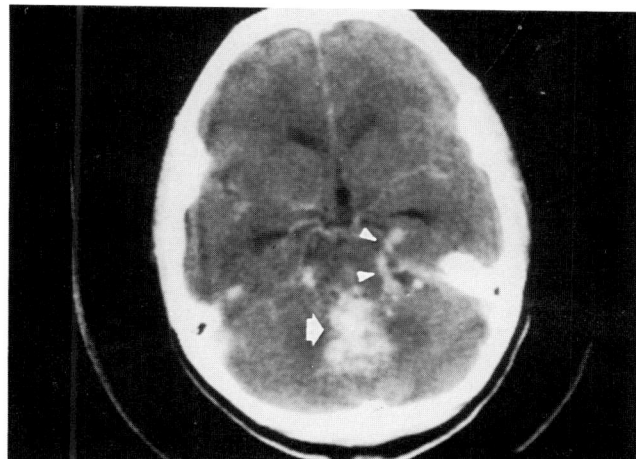

FIG SK27-8. **Arteriovenous malformation.** Irregular mass of increased attenuation in the vermis (arrow). Note the dilated vein (arrowheads) draining the lesion.

CEREBELLAR MASSES ON MAGNETIC RESONANCE IMAGING

Condition	Imaging Findings	Comments
Astrocytoma **(Fig SK28-1)**	Hypointense on T_1-weighted images. Increased signal intensity on T_2-weighted images.	More than 50% of these tumors are cystic with smooth margins and a relatively homogeneous appearance.
Medulloblastoma **(Fig SK28-2)**	Hypointense on T_1-weighted images. Increased signal intensity on T_2-weighted images.	Necrosis, hemorrhage, and cavitation are common and may produce a heterogeneous appearance (although to a lesser degree than with ependymoma). Dense cell packing with relatively little extracellular water may cause the tumor to appear only mildly hyperintense relative to brain on T_2-weighted images.
Ependymoma **(Fig SK28-3)**	Hypointense on T_1-weighted images. Increased signal intensity on T_2-weighted images.	Typically heterogeneous appearance because of frequent calcification and cystic and necrotic areas.
Hemangioblastoma **(Fig SK28-4)**	Cystic portion is hypointense on T_1-weighted images. The solid tumor nodules are isointense to or of slightly lower intensity than gray matter. Generalized increased signal intensity on T_2-weighted images.	Classic MR appearance is a cystic mass with a brightly enhancing nodule. The hypervascular tumor often shows areas of signal void, representing enlarged tumor vessels either in the mass or on its periphery.
Metastases **(Fig SK28-5)**	Hypointense on T_1-weighted images. Increased signal intensity on T_2-weighted images.	Contrast-enhanced MRI is the most sensitive technique for the evaluation of posterior fossa metastases. Hemorrhagic tumors (eg, melanoma, choriocarcinoma, and lung, thyroid, and renal carcinoma) produce various patterns depending on the chronicity of the bleeding.
Lymphoma	Hypointense or isointense mass on T_1-weighted images. Typically homogeneous, slightly high-signal to isointense mass on T_2-weighted images.	The mild T_2 prolongation is probably related to dense cell packing in the tumor, leaving relatively little interstitial space for the accumulation of water. The mass may be multicentric and exhibit infiltration into adjoining tissue and across the midline (no respect for normal anatomic boundaries).
Epidermoid	Heterogeneous texture and variable signal intensity. Most are of slightly higher signal than CSF on both T_1- and T_2-weighted images.	Some epidermoids appear bright on T_1-weighted images because of their high fat content.
Infarct **(Figs SK28-6 and SK28-7)**	Well-defined lesion that is hypointense on T_1-weighted images and hyperintense on T_2-weighted images. Old infarcts may have a more complex signal pattern that is related both to hemorrhagic components and to the evolution of infarcts, the latter resulting in areas of microcystic and macrocystic encephalomalacia and gliosis.	Involvement of both the cortex and a variable amount of subcortical tissue in a defined vascular territory. Contrast enhancement in a subacute infarction may simulate the appearance of a cerebellar tumor.
Hemorrhage **(Fig SK28-8)**	Variable pattern of signal intensity depending on the chronicity of the process.	The lesion may appear round or irregular in shape and may compress the fourth ventricle to cause hydrocephalus.

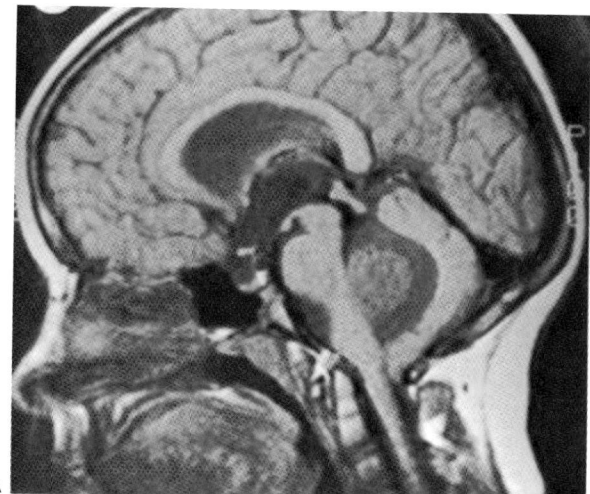

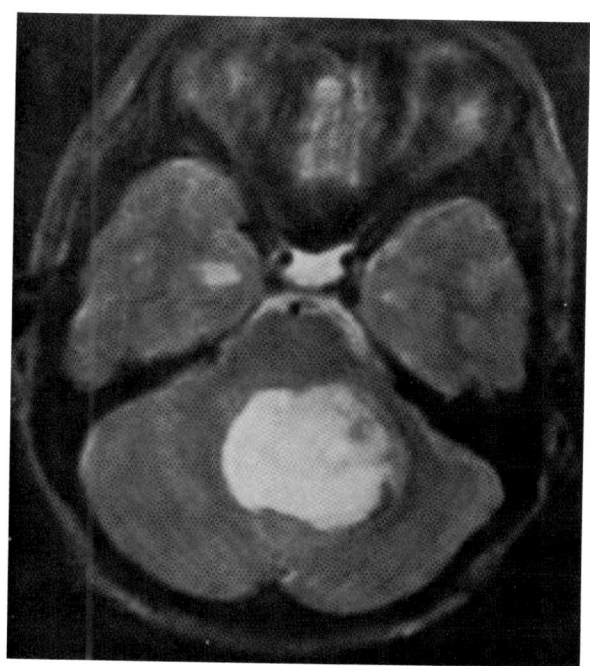

FIG SK28-1. Cystic astrocytoma. (A) Sagittal T$_1$-weighted image shows a large cerebellar vermian cyst containing fluid that is more intense than the dilated third ventricle. There is a central nodule of decreased intensity relative to the cerebellum. (B) On the axial T$_2$-weighted image, the cyst fluid is markedly hyperintense. The central nodule has a somewhat lesser signal intensity.[36]

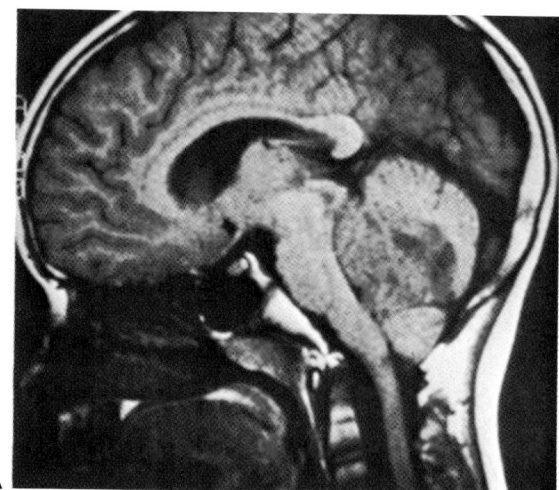

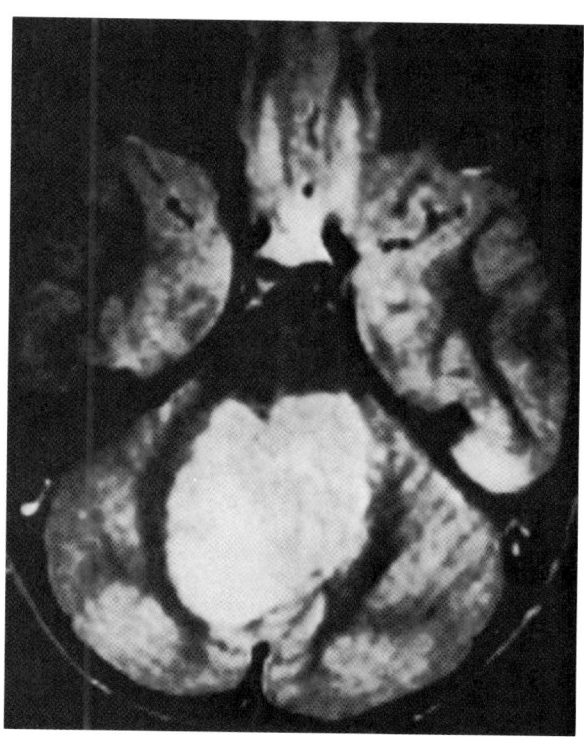

FIG SK28-2. Cystic medulloblastoma. (A) Sagittal T$_1$-weighted image demonstrates a mottled but predominantly hypointense cerebellar vermian lesion compressing the roof of the fourth ventricle. (B) Axial T$_2$-weighted image shows the solid portion of the tumor to be hyperintense, while the cystic-necrotic component has an even more marked hyperintensity.[36]

Condition	Imaging Findings	Comments
Arteriovenous malformation	Cluster of serpiginous flow voids (representing rapid blood flow) and areas of high signal (slow flow in draining veins).	The use of partial flip-angle techniques can distinguish hemosiderin or calcification associated with the lesion from vessels containing rapidly flowing blood.
Abscess	Hypointense mass with an isointense capsule surrounded by low-signal edema on T_1-weighted images. Hyperintense mass surrounded by a hypointense capsule and high-signal edema on T_2-weighted images.	Pyogenic; tuberculous; fungal; parasitic.

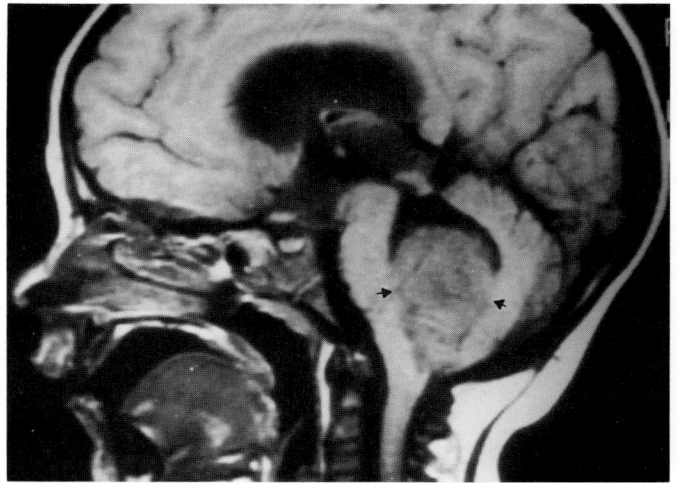

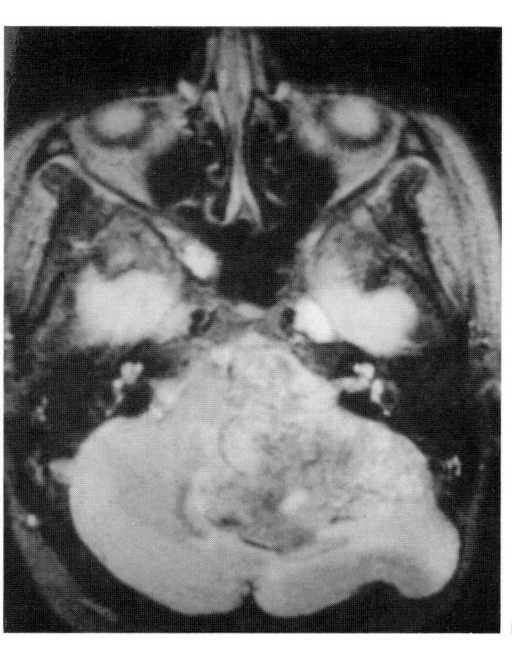

FIG SK28-3. Ependymoma. (A) Sagittal T_1-weighted image shows a large hypointense mass (arrows) in an expanded fourth ventricle. (B) Axial T_2-weighted image shows the markedly heterogeneous quality of the mass. Note the extension of peritumoral edema into the adjacent cerebellar hemisphere.

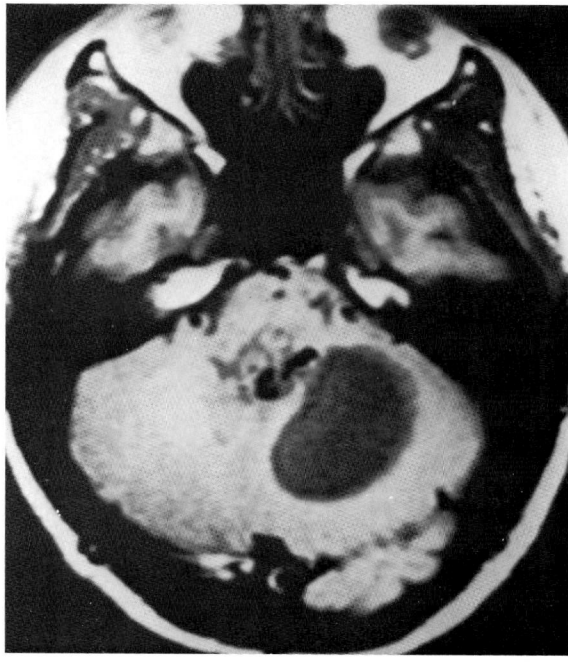

FIG SK28-4. Cystic hemangioblastoma. Axial T_1-weighted scan demonstrates a large cystic mass within the left cerebellar hemisphere. The cyst is markedly hypointense and well marginated and has a nodular component along its medial aspect. Note the virtually pathognomonic appearance of large arteries feeding the solid component of this cystic lesion.[36]

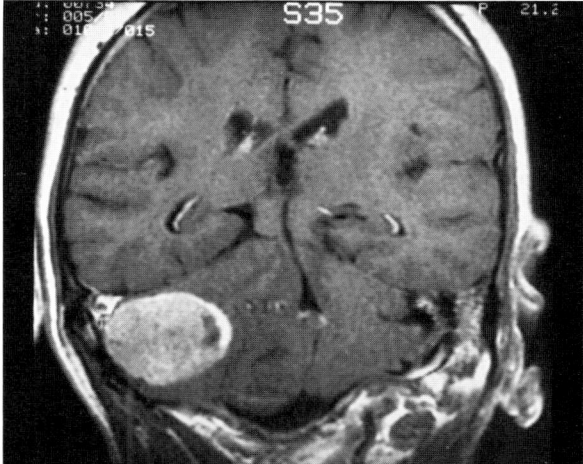

Fig SK28-5. **Metastasis.** Coronal MR scan after gadolinium administration shows an enhancing right cerebellar lesion with a pronounced mass effect on midline structures.

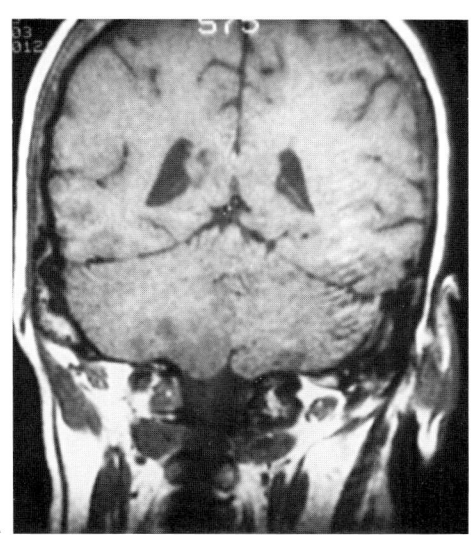

A

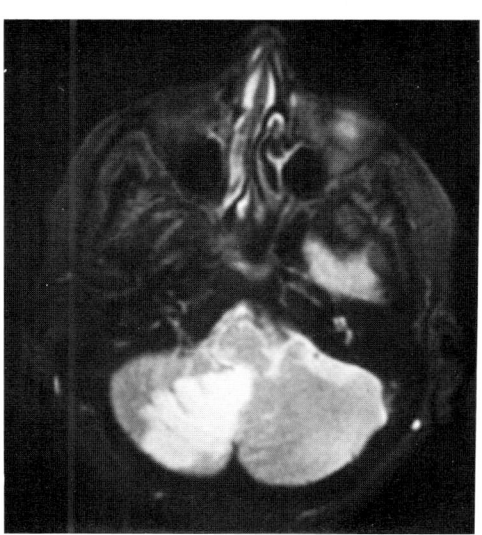

B

Fig SK28-6. **Infarction** in the territory of the right posterior inferior cerebellar artery. The well-defined lesion is hypointense on the coronal T_1-weighted image (A) and hyperintense on the axial T_2-weighted scan (B).

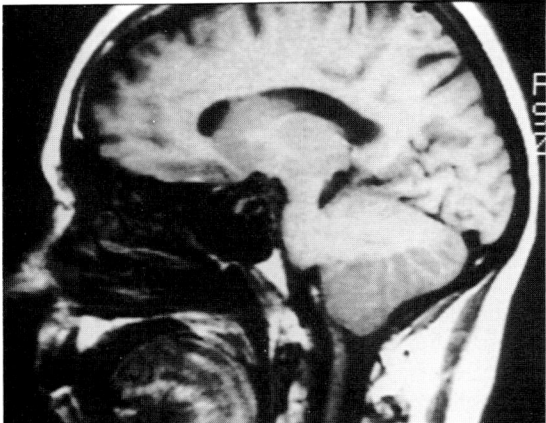

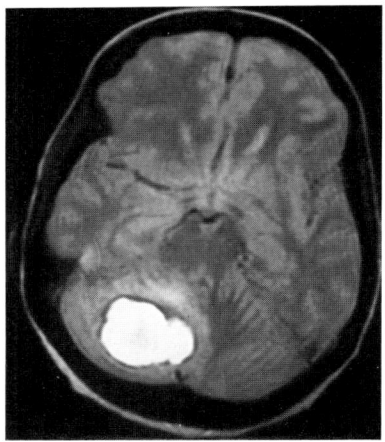

Fig SK28-7. **Infarction** in the territory of the left posterior inferior cerebellar artery. Parasagittal T_1-weighted image shows hypointensity of the entire lower half of the cerebellar hemisphere on that side.

Fig SK28-8. **Resolving hemorrhage.** The right cerebellar mass consists of hyperintense methemoglobin surrounded by a thin, hypointense rim of hemosiderin.

CEREBELLOPONTINE ANGLE MASSES
ON COMPUTED TOMOGRAPHY

Condition	Imaging Findings	Comments
Acoustic neuroma (Figs SK29-1 to SK29-3)	Well-defined, uniformly enhancing tumor with smooth, rounded margins. Typically there is enlargement and erosion of the internal auditory canal. May contain low-attenuation cystic areas and simulate an epidermoid. Bilateral acoustic neuromas suggest neurofibromatosis.	Represents about 10% of primary intracranial tumors and accounts for most masses in the cerebellopontine angle. Small intracanalicular tumors confined to the internal auditory canal may cause bony changes or clinical findings suggesting an acoustic neuroma in the absence of CT evidence of a discrete mass. In such cases (if MRI not available), repeat CT examination is required after the intrathecal administration of contrast material (metrizamide or air).
Meningioma (Fig SK29-4)	Hyperdense mass on noncontrast scans that shows dense enhancement after the intravenous injection of contrast material. Unlike acoustic neuromas, meningiomas commonly show calcification and cystic changes. Typically they are larger and more broadly based along the petrous bone than neuromas.	Second most common cerebellopontine angle mass. Usually centered above or below the internal auditory meatus and infrequently associated with widening of the internal auditory canal (or hearing loss).
Epidermoid (Fig SK29-5)	Low-density mass on both pre- and postcontrast scans (though occasional high-density and enhancing lesions have been recorded). Infrequently has a calcified margin.	Most common location for this fat-containing tumor. Because the tumor tends not to stretch or distort the brainstem or cranial nerves but to surround them, an extensive neoplasm may be present before symptoms occur.
Metastasis (Fig SK29-6)	Enhancing mass with bone erosion (often without distinct margins) and sometimes edema in the adjacent cerebellum.	Usually a history of a primary neoplasm elsewhere.
Arachnoid cyst (Fig SK29-7)	Cystic structure with a density equal to that of cerebrospinal fluid. With positive contrast cisternography, there is enhancement of the adjacent cisterns without enhancement of the cyst (some intrathecal contrast eventually penetrates the cyst).	Typically displaces adjacent brainstem and cerebellar structures to a much greater degree than a cystic epidermoid tumor. Arachnoid cysts do not calcify, unlike epidermoids.
Aneurysm of basilar or vertebral artery (Fig SK29-8)	Usually has greater than brain density on precontrast scans.	The amount of contrast enhancement depends on the degree of luminal thrombosis. A characteristic appearance is concentric or eccentric circles representing the enhanced lumen, the less dense thrombus, and the dense wall of the aneurysm.
Arterial ectasia	Curvilinear, homogeneously enhancing structure that may simulate a cerebellopontine angle tumor.	Elongation and ectasia of the vertebral, basilar, or inferior cerebellar artery. Digital or conventional arteriography or dynamic CT can show the true nature of the process.

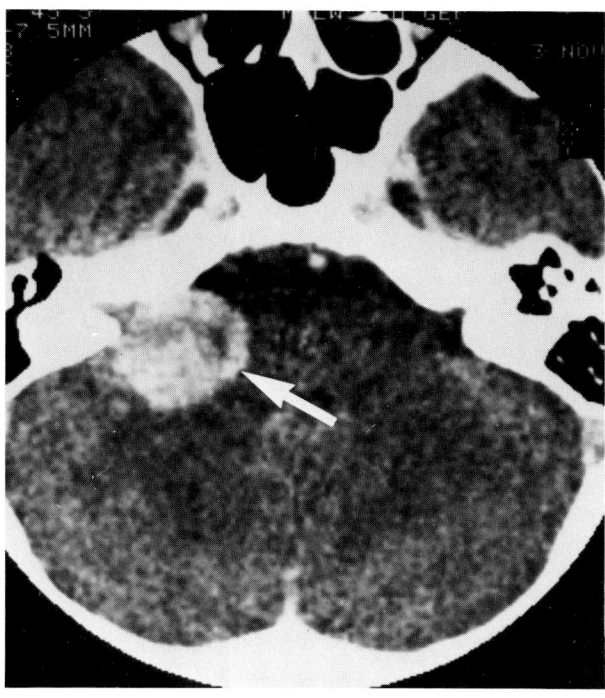

FIG SK29-1. Acoustic neuroma. Contrast-enhancing mass (arrow) in the right internal auditory canal and cerebellopontine angle cistern.[13]

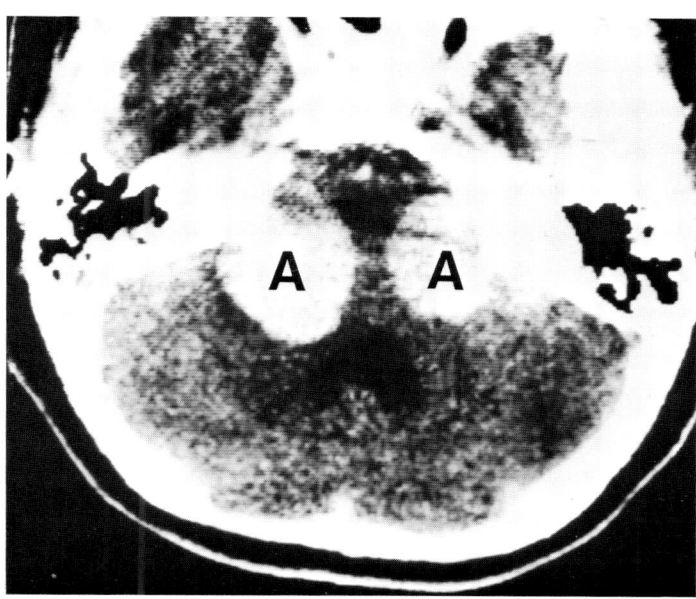

FIG SK29-2. Neurofibromatosis. Bilateral acoustic neuromas (A) in a young girl with progressive bilateral sensorineural hearing loss.

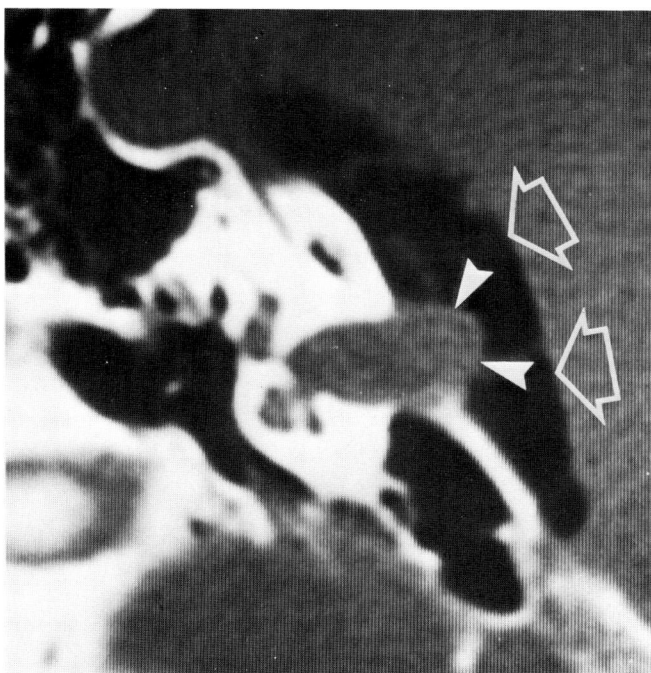

FIG SK29-3. Intracanalicular acoustic neuroma. Air injected into the subarachnoid space shows the cerebellopontine angle cistern (open arrows) and outlines the small tumor (arrowheads).

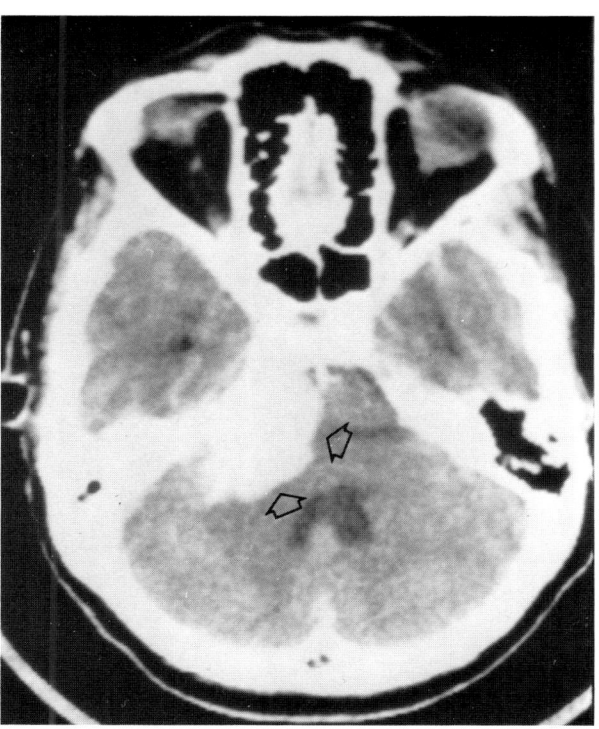

FIG SK29-4. Meningioma. Dense enhancing lesion (arrows) that is more broadly based along the petrous bone than a typical acoustic neuroma.

Condition	Imaging Findings	Comments
Glomus jugulare tumor (Fig SK29-9)	Lobulated, uniformly dense, and densely enhancing mass. Although the highly vascular mass may simulate other enhancing extra-axial lesions at this site, associated erosion of the jugular foramen usually permits the diagnosis.	The tumor arises in the middle ear and produces a blue or red polypoid mass, which can be visualized otoscopically, or a mass in the jugular foramen. Although most of these tumors are histologically benign, they may be locally invasive and cause irregular and poorly defined bone erosion suggesting malignancy.
Extension of adjacent tumor	Various patterns.	May be secondary to brainstem or cerebellar glioma, chordoma, pituitary adenoma, craniopharyngioma, fourth ventricular tumor, choroid plexus papilloma, or neuroma of one of the lowest four cranial nerves.

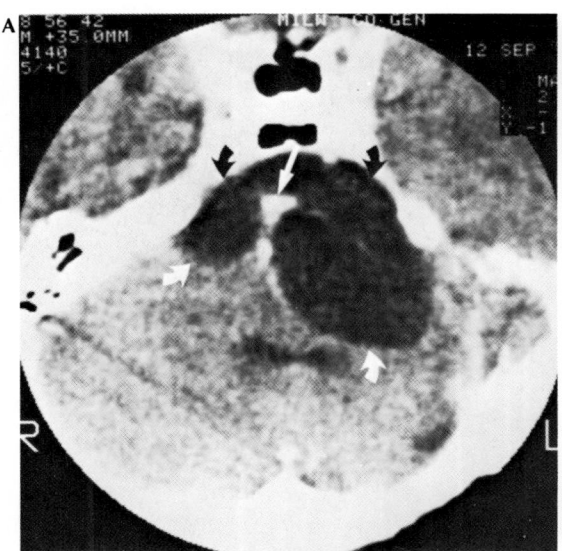
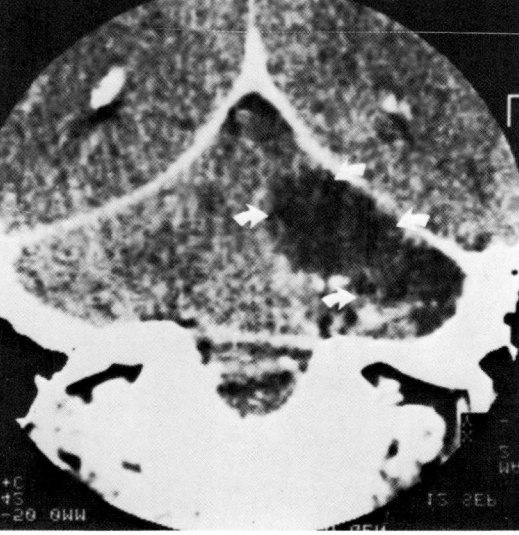

FIG SK29-5. **Epidermoid.** Irregularly shaped, low-density mass (curved arrows) in front of the basilar artery (arrow) and brainstem on (A) axial and (B) coronal images.[13]

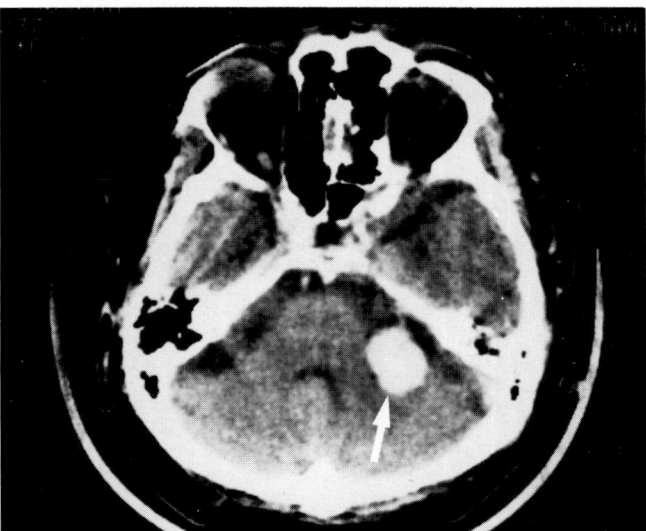

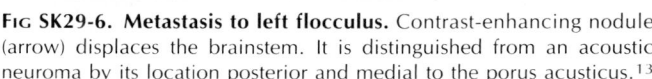

FIG SK29-6. **Metastasis to left flocculus.** Contrast-enhancing nodule (arrow) displaces the brainstem. It is distinguished from an acoustic neuroma by its location posterior and medial to the porus acusticus.[13]

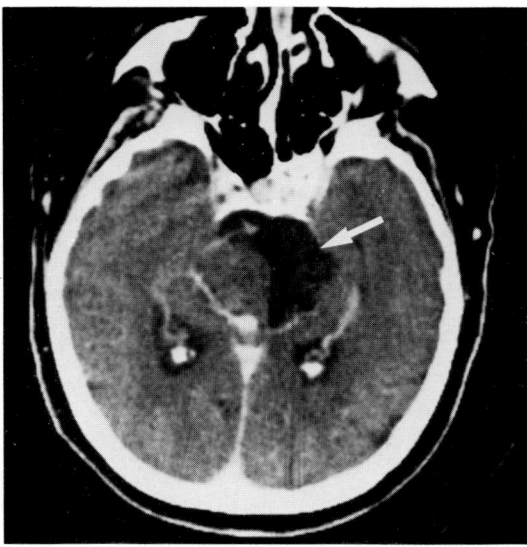

FIG SK29-7. **Arachnoid cyst.** Slightly irregular cystic mass (arrow) of cerebrospinal fluid density that displaces the brainstem and basilar artery to the right.[13]

Condition	Imaging Findings	Comments
Normal flocculus	Nodule along the lateral surface of the cerebellum near the internal auditory canal.	The flocculus is located posterior to the internal auditory canal, does not enhance as prominently as the usual acoustic neuroma, and is not associated with widening of the internal auditory canal.

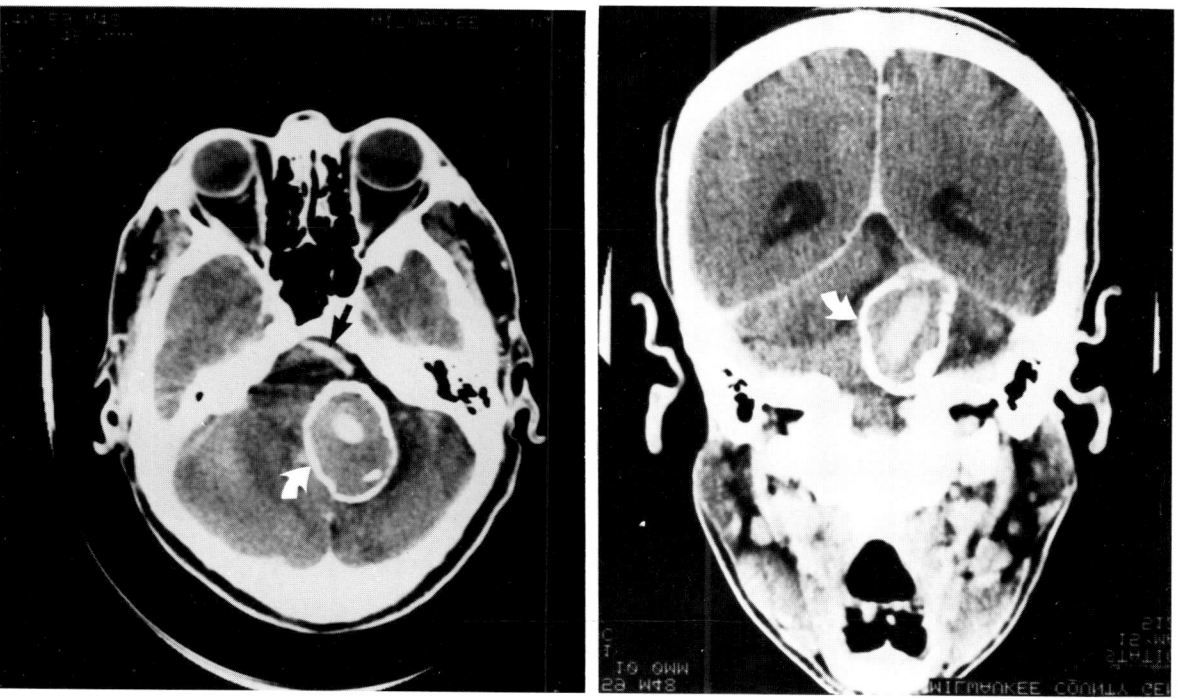

FIG SK29-8. Giant aneurysm with thrombus simulating meningioma. (A) Axial and (B) coronal images show the mass (curved arrow) with calcific rim and high density within it displacing the pons and cerebellum. The aneurysm fails to enhance as densely as the basilar artery (arrow).[13]

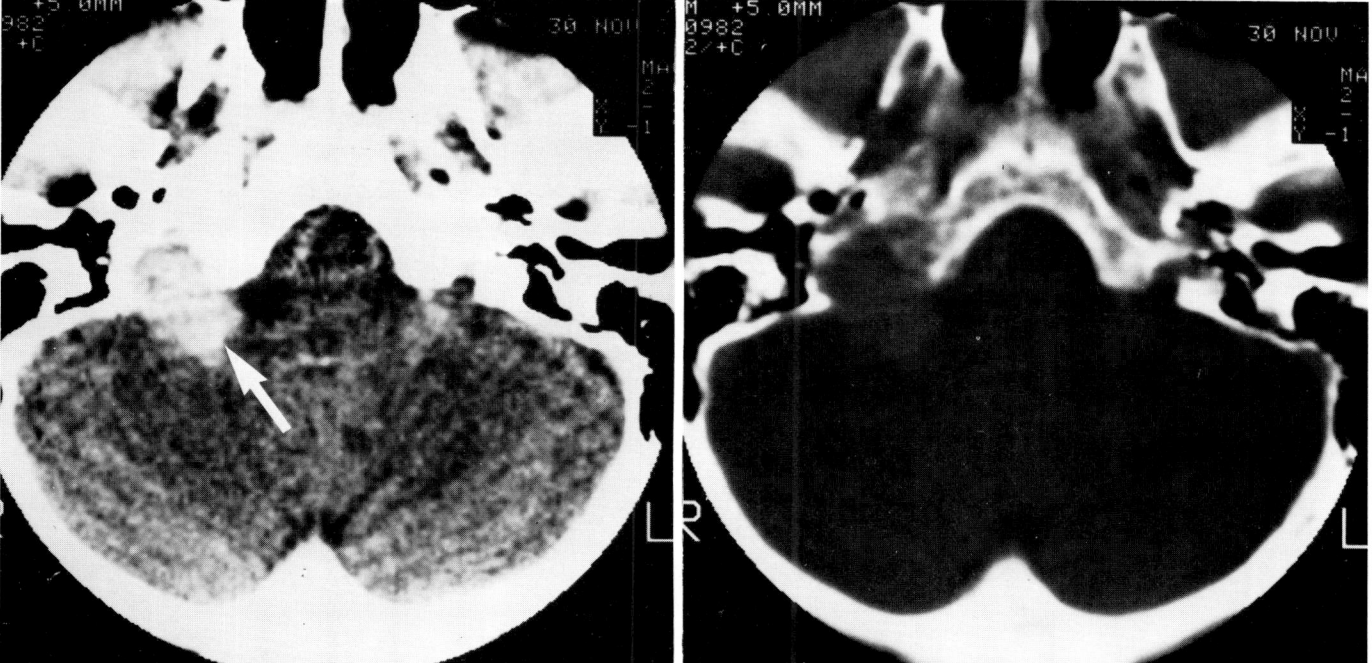

FIG SK29-9. Glomus jugulare tumor. Densely enhancing mass (arrow) that has eroded the osseous margins adjacent to the right jugular foramen.[13]

CEREBELLOPONTINE ANGLE MASSES ON MAGNETIC RESONANCE IMAGING

Condition	Imaging Findings	Comments
Acoustic neuroma (Figs SK30-1 and SK30-2)	Isointense or slightly hypointense lesion on T_1-weighted images. Hyperintense signal on T_2-weighted images.	Prominent contrast enhancement permits demonstration of even small intracanalicular masses on coronal or axial images.
Meningioma (Fig SK30-3)	Usually hypointense to white matter on T_1-weighted images. At 1.5 T, the lesion is hyperintense to white matter on T_2-weighted images.	Prominent and homogeneous contrast enhancement. Typically larger and more broadly based along the petrous bone than an acoustic neuroma.
Epidermoid (Fig SK30-4)	Heterogeneous texture and variable signal intensity. Most are of slightly higher signal than CSF on both T_1- and T_2-weighted images.	Some epidermoids appear bright on T_1-weighted images.
Metastasis	Generally hypointense on T_1-weighted images and of increased signal intensity on T_2-weighted images.	Intratumoral hemorrhage and cystic necrosis may occur. There is usually a history of a primary neoplasm elsewhere.
Arachnoid cyst	Smoothly marginated and homogeneous lesion containing cyst fluid that is isointense to CSF on all pulse sequences.	Typically displaces adjacent brainstem and cerebellar structures to a much greater degree than a cystic epidermoid tumor.
Aneurysm of basilar or vertebral artery	Flow void that may be surrounded by a pattern of heterogeneous signal intensity representing turbulence or thrombus.	Partial flip-angle imaging produces fairly consistent flow-related enhancement in the lumen and more clearly differentiates it from surrounding clot.

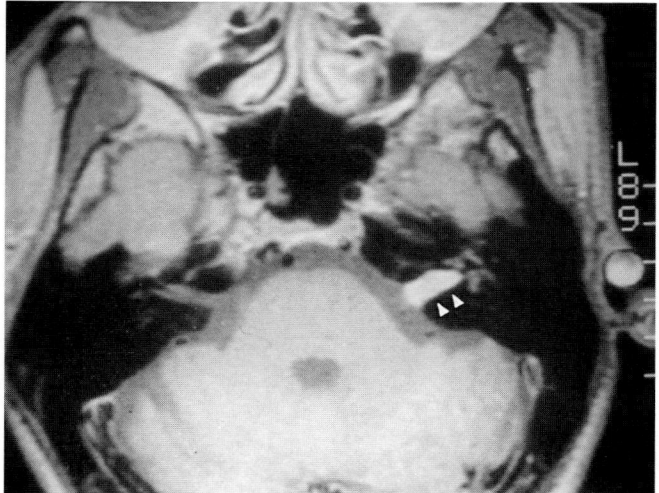

FIG SK30-1. Acoustic neuroma. Marked contrast enhancement of the left-sided lesion (arrowheads). Note the normal neural structures on the right.

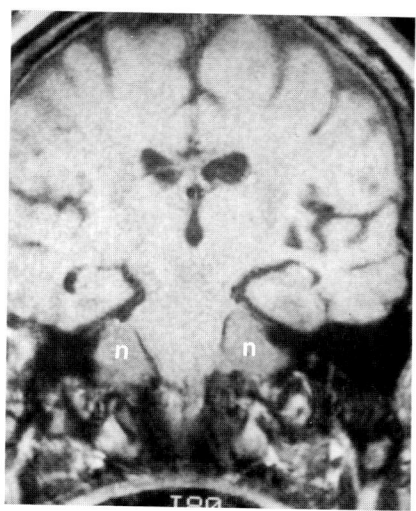

FIG SK30-2. Acoustic neuroma. Bilateral tumors (n) are seen in this coronal scan of a patient with neurofibromatosis.

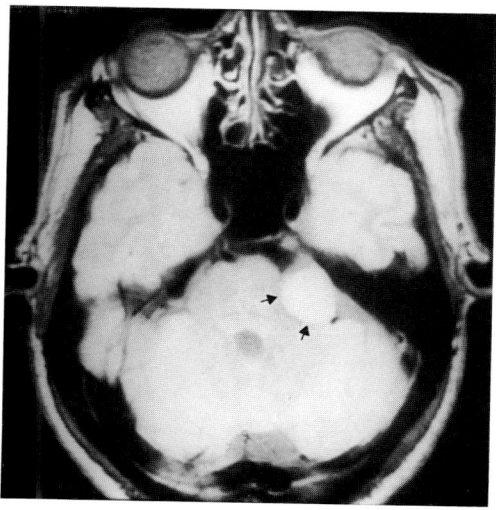

FIG SK30-3. Meningioma. Note that the mass (arrows) has a relatively broad base along the petrous bone.

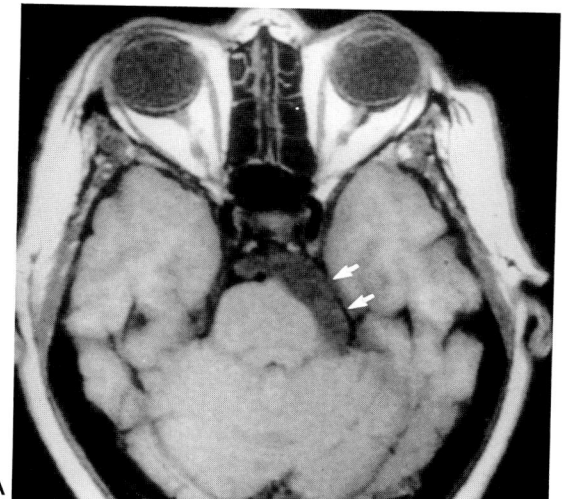

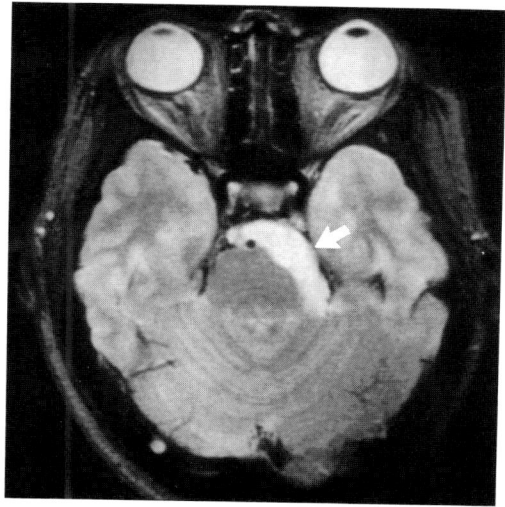

FIG SK30-4. Epidermoid. (A) Axial T_1-weighted and (B) axial T_2-weighted scans show an oblong mass (arrowheads) of slightly higher signal than CSF enveloping the basilar artery and extending around the pons.

Condition	Imaging Findings	Comments
Arterial ectasia	Curvilinear flow void that may simulate a cerebellopontine angle tumor.	Elongation and ectasia of the vertebral, basilar, or superior cerebellar artery.
Glomus jugulare tumor (Fig SK30-5)	Isointense lesion on T_1-weighted images. Hyperintense signal on T_2-weighted images.	This highly vascular tumor contains multiple signal voids representing enlarged vessels. There is marked contrast enhancement.
Extension of adjacent tumor (Fig SK30-6)	Generally a hypointense lesion on T_1-weighted images. Hyperintense signal on T_2-weighted images.	May be secondary to brainstem or cerebellar glioma, chordoma, pituitary adenoma, craniopharyngioma, fourth ventricular tumor, choroid plexus papilloma, or neuroma of the 5th or 9th through 12th cranial nerves.

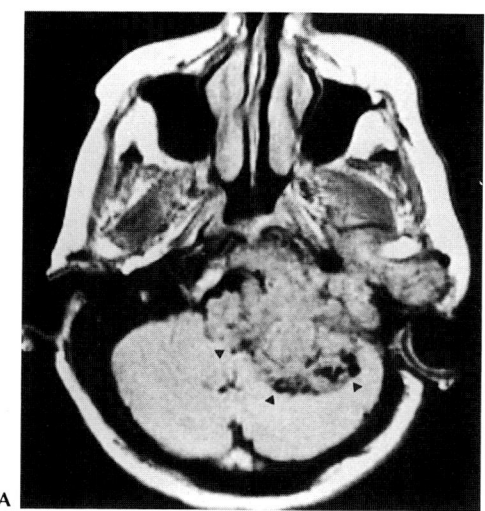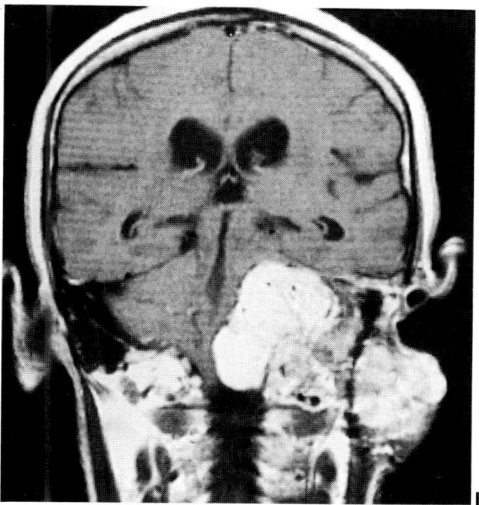

Fig SK30-5. Glomus jugulare tumor with intracranial involvement and bony erosion. (A) Axial T$_1$-weighted image shows the mass (arrowheads) in the left temporal bone and posterior fossa extending across the midline. Note the large veins on the surface of the tumor. (B) Coronal contrast-enhanced image shows displacement of the brainstem, bony erosion from the large enhanced mass, and parotid involvement.[31]

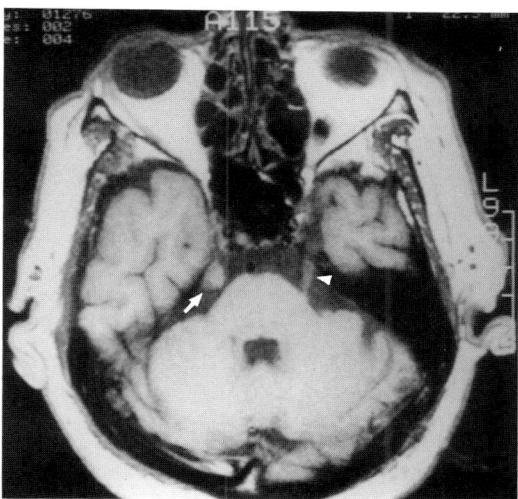

Fig SK30-6. Trigeminal neuroma. Isointense mass on the right (arrow). Note the normal 5th cranial nerve on the left (arrowhead).

LOW-DENSITY MASS IN THE BRAINSTEM ON COMPUTED TOMOGRAPHY

Condition	Imaging Findings	Comments
Glioma **(Fig SK31-1)**	Typically a low-attenuation area with indistinct margins in an asymmetrically expanded brainstem. The tumor may be relatively isodense (and be difficult to detect) or occasionally show increased attenuation or even gross calcification.	The mass effect depends on tumor size and may be generalized or focal. Contrast enhancement may be obvious, minimal, or absent. Cysts may occur, allowing palliative decompression.
Metastasis **(Fig SK31-2)**	Mass of inhomogeneous density with expansion of the brainstem and variable contrast enhancement (typically better defined than with gliomas).	More likely than primary glioma in a patient over 50 years of age with progressive brainstem signs. Usually there is evidence of other intracranial lesions (isolated metastasis to the brainstem is unusual).
Other tumors	Various patterns.	Hamartoma; teratoma; epidermoid; lymphoma.
Infarction **(Fig SK31-3)**	Combination of low attenuation, mass effect, and vague contrast enhancement may resemble a tumor.	Clinical information or follow-up scans can usually establish the diagnosis.
Multiple sclerosis	Combination of low attenuation, mass effect, and vague contrast enhancement may resemble a tumor.	Clinical information or follow-up scans can usually establish the diagnosis.
Central pontine myelinolysis **(Fig SK31-4)**	Central region of diminished attenuation in the pons and medulla without marked contrast enhancement.	Although initial reports were largely confined to chronic alcoholics, the condition is also seen in patients with electrolyte disturbances (particularly hyponatremia) that have been corrected rapidly.
Syringobulbia **(Fig SK31-5)**	Central mass of cerebrospinal fluid density within and usually enlarging the medulla. Sharply defined margins. Does not show contrast enhancement (unlike cystic neoplasm).	Cystic process in the medulla that is most frequently found in conjunction with syringomyelia (an Arnold-Chiari malformation) and less often with a tumor or degeneration in the brain.
Granuloma/abscess	Appearance mimicking that of a neoplasm.	Rare manifestation of tuberculosis, sarcoidosis, or infection. Diagnosis may require biopsy.

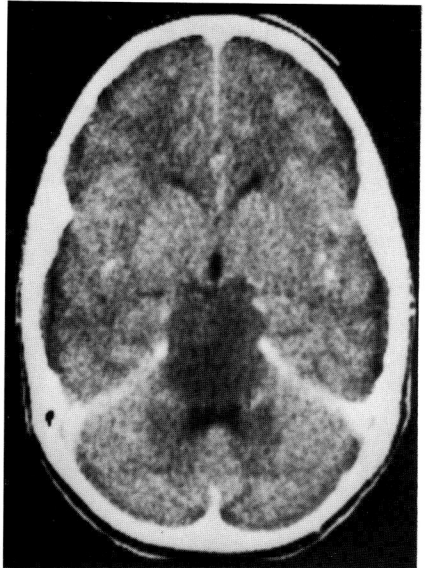

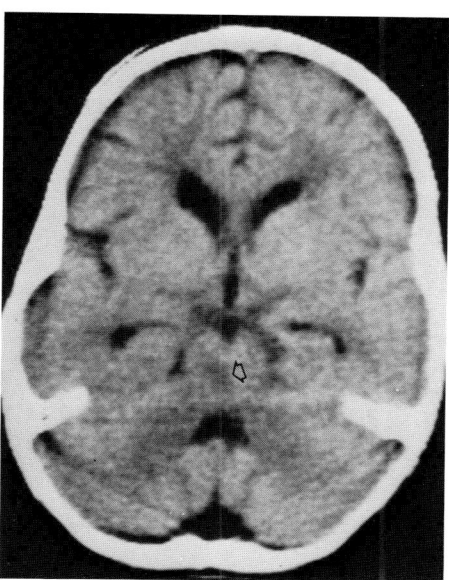

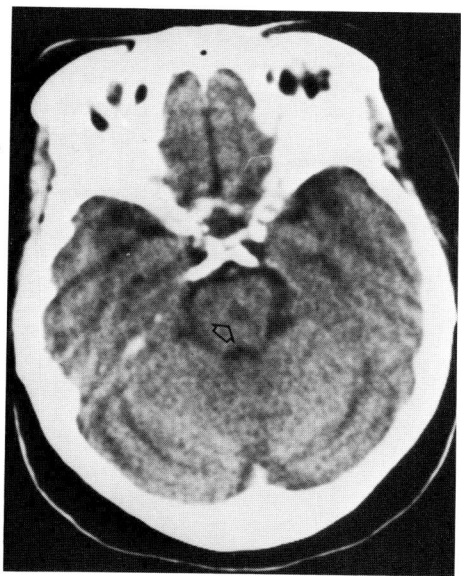

FIG SK31-1. Glioma. Poorly defined low-attenuation mass causing irregular expansion of the brainstem and compression of the fourth ventricle.

FIG SK31-2. Metastasis. Subtle, ill-defined area of low density (arrow).

FIG SK31-3. Infarction. Central low-attenuation region (arrow).

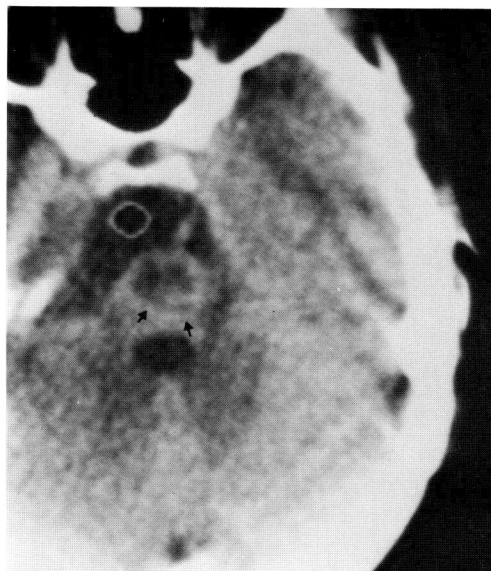

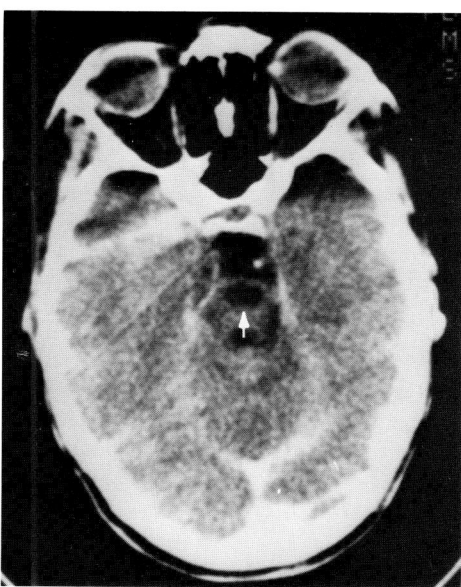

FIG SK31-4. Central pontine myelinolysis. Low-attenuation region (arrows) in the center of the pons in a comatose alcoholic patient. Note the widening of the prepontine subarachnoid space, indicating loss of brainstem volume due to atrophy.

FIG SK31-5. Syringobulbia. Well-demarcated mass of cerebrospinal fluid density (arrow) in the center of the brainstem.

BRAINSTEM LESIONS ON MAGNETIC RESONANCE IMAGING

Condition	Imaging Findings	Comments
Glioma (Fig SK32-1)	Hypointense mass on T_1-weighted images. High-intensity signal on proton-density and T_2-weighted images.	The mass effect depends on tumor size and may be generalized or focal. Low-grade tumors tend to be homogeneous; high-grade gliomas may be heterogeneous as a result of central necrosis with cellular debris, fluid, and hemorrhage.
Metastasis (Fig SK32-2)	Generally hypointense on T_1-weighted images and of increased signal intensity on proton-density and T_2-weighted images.	More likely than primary glioma to be seen in a patient older than 50 years of age with progressive brainstem signs. Usually there is evidence of other intracranial lesions (isolated metastasis to the brainstem is unusual).
Other tumors	Various patterns.	Hamartoma; teratoma; epidermoid; lymphoma.
Infarction	Hypointense on T_1-weighted images. Hyperintense on proton-density and T_2-weighted images.	Associated mass effect and vague contrast enhancement may resemble features of a neoplasm.
Multiple sclerosis	Hypointense on T_1-weighted images. Hyperintense on proton-density and T_2-weighted images.	Usually associated with similar areas of demyelination elsewhere in the brain.
Central pontine myelinolysis (Fig SK32-3)	Central region of hypointensity on T_1-weighted images and hyperintensity on T_2-weighted images in the pons and medulla.	Although initially reported in chronic alcoholics, this condition also presents in patients with electrolyte disturbances (especially hyponatremia) that have been corrected rapidly. In extreme cases, there may be extension to the tegmentum, midbrain, thalamus, internal capsule, and cerebral cortex.

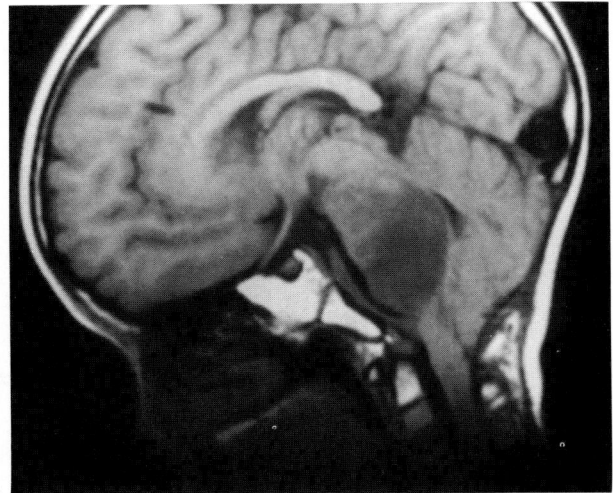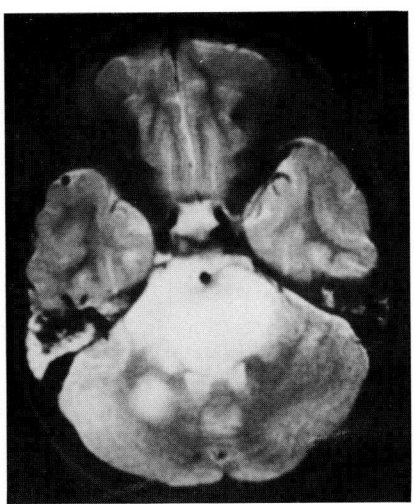

FIG SK32-1. Brainstem glioma. (A) Sagittal scan shows a huge low-intensity mass involving most of the pons and medulla and compressing the fourth ventricle. (B) On an axial scan, the mass is hyperintense, encases the basilar artery, and extends to affect the cerebellar peduncles and right cerebellar hemisphere.

Condition	Imaging Findings	Comments
Syringobulbia	Central mass of CSF density (hypointense on T_1-weighted images; hyperintense on T_2-weighted images) lying in and usually enlarging the medulla. Sharply defined margins, and no contrast enhancement (unlike cystic neoplasm).	Cystic process in the medulla that is more frequently found in conjunction with syringomyelia and less often with a tumor or degenerative process.
Granuloma/abscess	Appearance mimicking that of a neoplasm.	Rare manifestation of tuberculosis, sarcoidosis, or infection. Diagnosis may require biopsy.

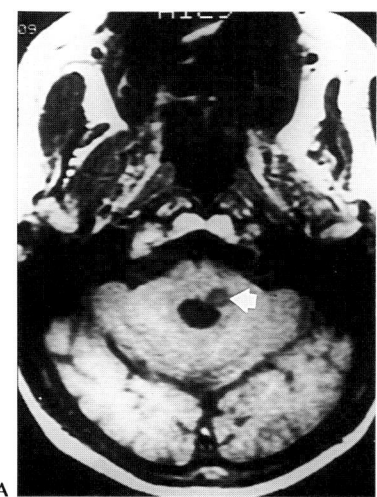 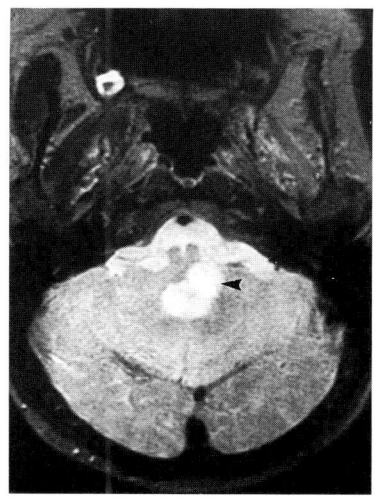

FIG SK32-2. **Metastasis.** Pontine mass (arrow) that appears hypointense on a T_1-weighted image (A) and hyperintense on a T_2-weighted scan (B).

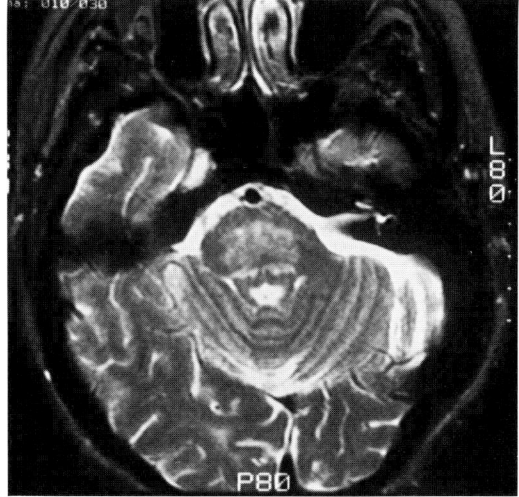 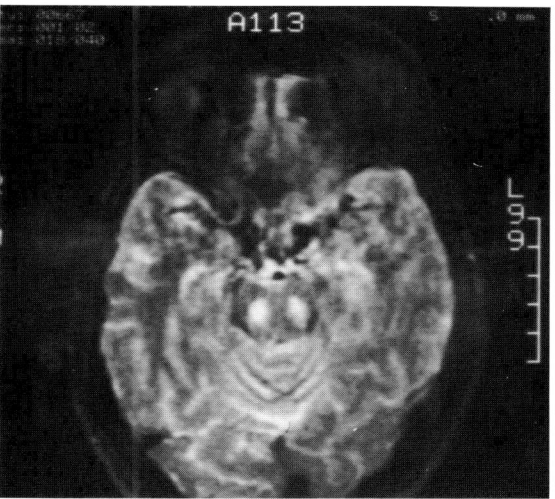

FIG SK32-3. **Central pontine myelinolysis.** (A) T_2-weighted axial image shows a hyperintense lesion in the central portion of the midpons. (B) More rostral scan shows symmetric lesions in the cerebral peduncles.

MASSES INVOLVING THE JUGULAR FORAMEN ON MAGNETIC RESONANCE IMAGING

Condition	Imaging Findings	Comments
Glomus jugulare tumor **(Fig SK33-1)**	Large, irregular mass that obscures the contents of the jugular foramen. It is nearly isointense with the brainstem on T_1-weighted images and usually has high signal intensity on T_2-weighted images. Intense contrast enhancement.	A characteristic finding is the appearance of prominent blood vessels within the mass. These vessels show negligible signal on T_1-weighted images and high-signal intensity on gradient echo images. Computed tomography (CT) better shows the ill-defined osseous erosion at the margins of a glomus tumor.
Neurofibroma/schwannoma **(Fig SK33-2)**	Smooth or irregular mass that is nearly isointense with the brainstem on T_1-weighted images and generally shows high signal intensity on T_2-weighted images. Intense contrast enhancement.	Typically no prominent vessels can be identified within the tumor. CT better shows adjacent bony erosion.
Meningioma **(Fig SK33-3)**	Mass with a signal intensity that is usually the same as the brainstem on T_1-weighted images and variable on T_2-weighted images. Intense contrast enhancement.	Extension of tumor along the posteromedial edge of the petrous bone into a jugular foramen can be demonstrated by MRI even when no bony erosion can be detected by CT. Calcification may produce areas of low signal intensity within the tumor. No prominent vessels are typically seen within the lesion.
Other tumors **(Fig SK33-4)**	Various patterns. Some tumors may contain areas of hemorrhage that produce high signal intensity on both T_1- and T_2-weighted images. Prominent blood vessels may sometimes be demonstrated.	Rare aggressive tumors (carcinoma, metastases, non-Hodgkin's lymphoma, childhood rhabdomyosarcoma, minor salivary gland malignancy, chondrosarcoma) may be difficult to differentiate from the more common lesions.

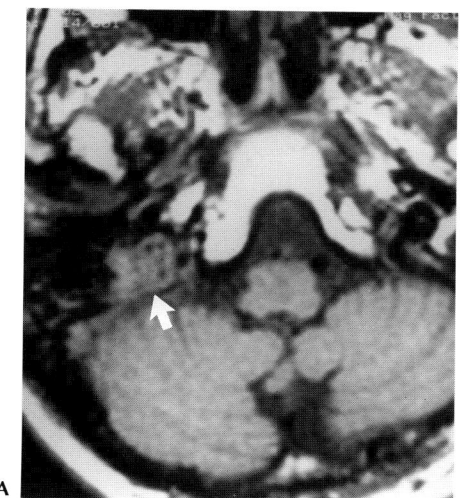

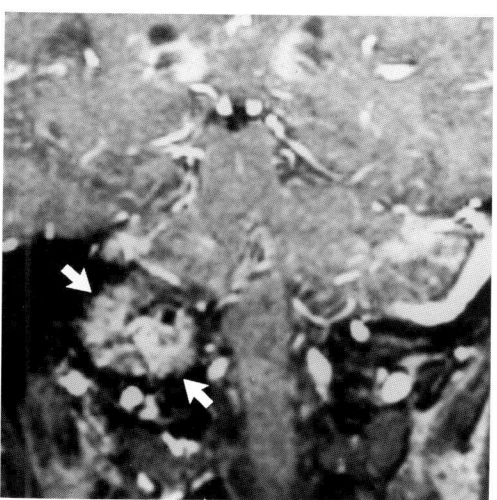

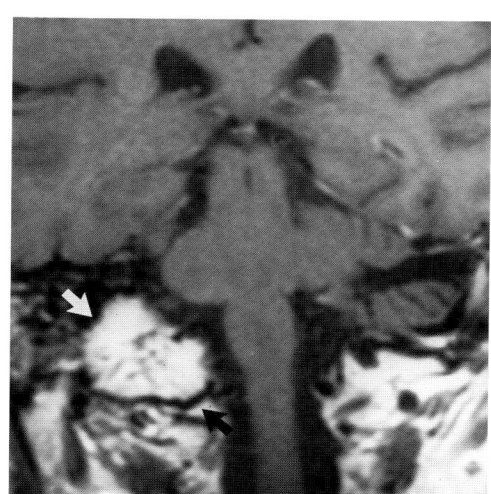

Fig SK33-1. Glomus jugulare tumor. T_1-weighted (A) axial, (B) coronal, and (C) contrast-enhanced coronal images show the tumor (arrows). The tumor contains small blood vessels, which demonstrate negligible signal intensity in A and C and high signal intensity in B. The tumor occludes the ipsilateral jugular bulb.[32]

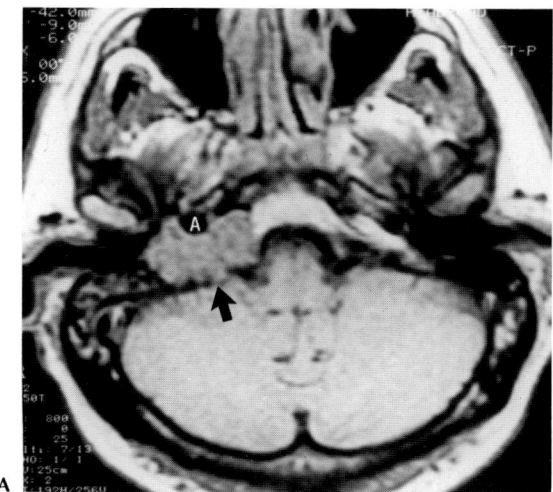

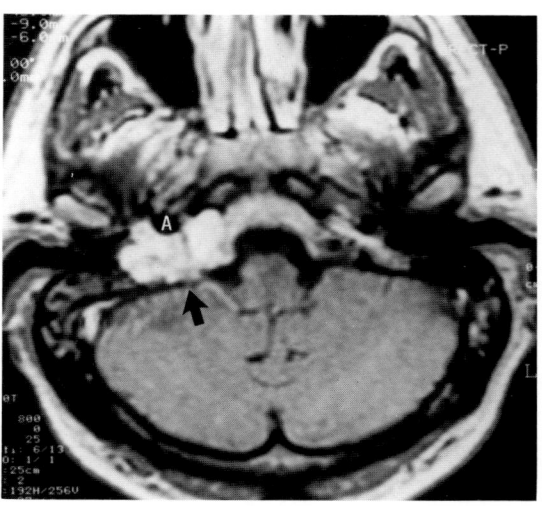

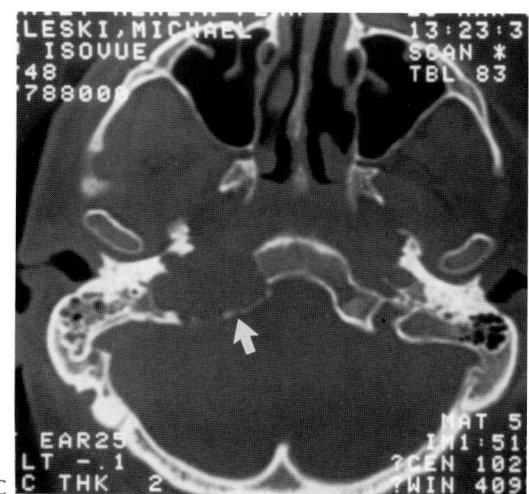

FIG SK33-2. **Schwannoma of 10th cranial nerve.** (A) Initial and (B) postcontrast T$_1$-weighted axial images show intense enhancement of the tumor (arrows). Note the anterior displacement of the internal carotid artery (A). (C) Axial CT scan with bone-window technique shows irregular erosion of the right jugular foramen area by the tumor (arrow).[32]

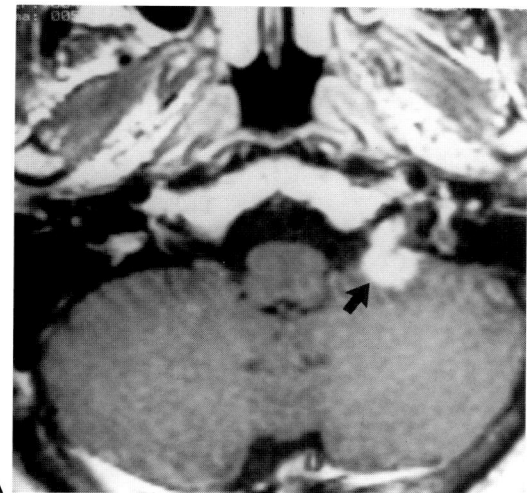
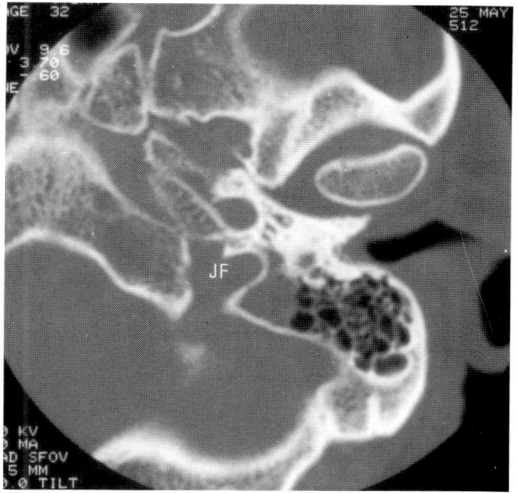

FIG SK33-3. Meningioma. (A) Axial T$_1$-weighted scan after administration of contrast material shows the enhancing tumor (arrow) extending into the jugular foramen. (B) Axial CT scan with bone-window technique demonstrates that the tumor has not eroded the margins of the jugular foramen (JF).[32]

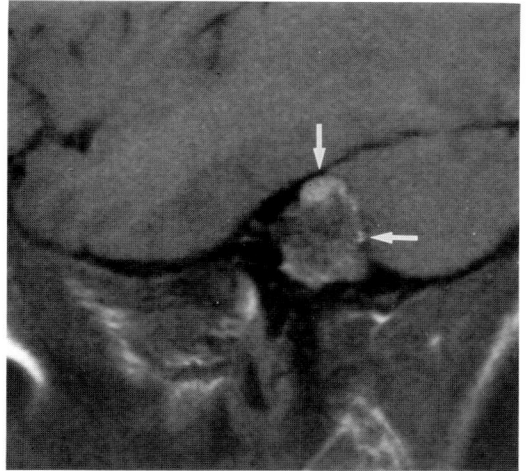
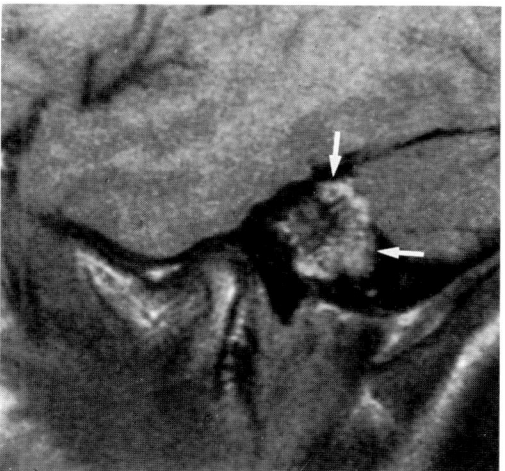

FIG SK33-4. Adenocarcinoma. (A) T$_1$-weighted and (B) T$_2$-weighted parasagittal images of the tumor (arrows) in the jugular foramen. Note regions of high signal intensity from chronic hemorrhage, and small blood vessels with negligible signal.[32]

PERIVENTRICULAR WHITE MATTER ABNORMALITIES ON MAGNETIC RESONANCE IMAGING

Condition	Imaging Findings	Comments
Virchow-Robin spaces (Fig SK34-1)	CSF spaces that appear as punctate (1–2 mm) areas of high signal intensity on T_2-weighted images but isointense or of low intensity on proton-density images.	Small subarachnoid spaces that follow the pia mater that is carried along with nutrient vessels as they penetrate the brain substance. Commonly seen in superficial white matter on higher axial sections through the cerebral hemispheres, where nutrient arteries for the deep white matter enter the brain. Other common locations include the lower basal ganglia and the lateral aspects of the anterior commissure, where the lenticulostriate arteries enter the anterior perforated substance.
Deep white matter ischemia (Fig SK34-2)	Multiple high-intensity foci on both T_2-weighted and proton-density images. Individual lesions have well-defined but irregular margins, tend to become confluent, and are usually relatively symmetric. No contrast enhancement is seen unless there is superimposed subacute infarction.	Most frequently detected in patients with ischemic cerebrovascular disease, hypertension, and aging, although in general there is poor correlation between the MR findings and neurologic function. The most common locations are the periventricular white matter, optic radiations, basal ganglia, centrum semiovale, and brainstem, in decreasing order of frequency.
Multiple sclerosis (Fig SK34-3)	Periventricular high-intensity foci best shown on proton-density scans (high-signal plaques may be obscured by CSF on T_2-weighted images). Typically found in a periventricular distribution, particularly along the lateral aspects of the atria and occipital horns. Usually there are discrete foci with well-defined margins. Contrast enhancement can be detected for up to 8 weeks after acute demyelination.	Chronic inflammatory disease of myelin that produces a relapsing and remitting course and is characterized by disseminated lesions in central nervous system white matter. In addition to involving periventricular sites, multiple sclerosis commonly involves the corona radiata, internal capsule, centrum semiovale, brainstem, and spinal cord. In contrast to deep white matter ischemia, multiple sclerosis is a disease of young adults and frequently involves the subcortical U fibers and the corpus callosum, where plaques often have a characteristic horizontal orientation.
Radiation injury (Fig SK34-4)	Symmetric high-signal foci in the periventricular white matter on both T_2-weighted and proton-density images. As the process extends outward to involve the peripheral arcuate fibers of the white matter, the margins become scalloped.	Effects of radiation injury to the brain are first detected on imaging studies about 6 to 8 months after the initial therapy. Imaging findings may continue to progress for 2 years or more after radiation therapy. With high-dose therapy, radiation necrosis may lead to profound edema, focal mass effect, and contrast enhancement. In such cases, it may be extremely difficult if not impossible to distinguish radiation change from recurrent tumor.

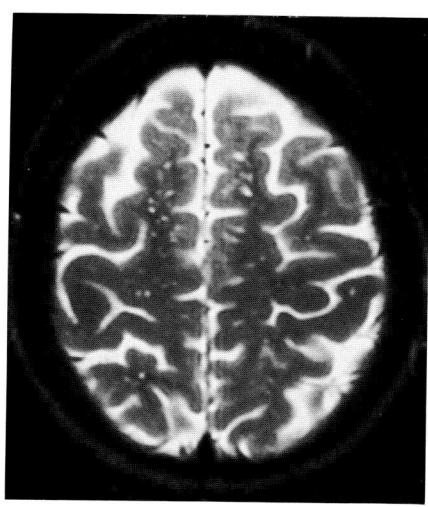

FIG SK34-1. **Prominent Virchow-Robin spaces.**

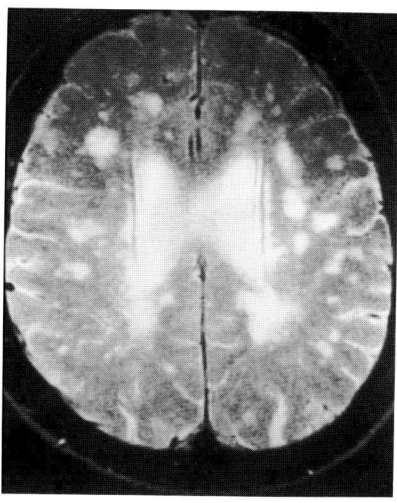

FIG SK34-2. **Deep white matter ischemia.** Multiple areas of increased signal intensity around the ventricles and in the deep white matter.

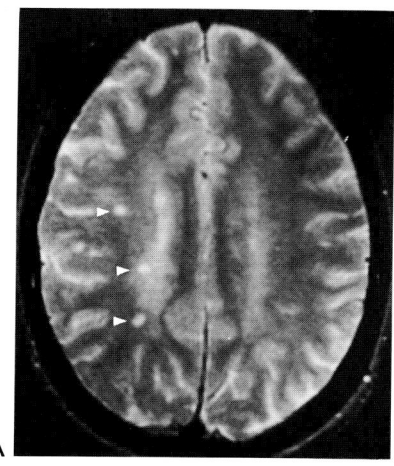

A

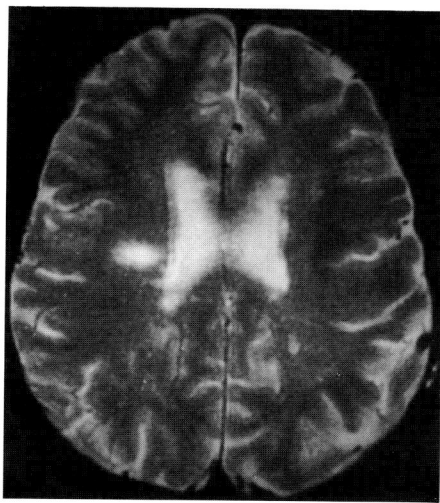

B

FIG SK34-3. **Multiple sclerosis.** (A) Characteristic areas of increased signal intensity (arrowheads) in the deep white matter of this 35-year-old woman. (B) In another patient, note the characteristic horizontal orientation of the right periventricular plaque.

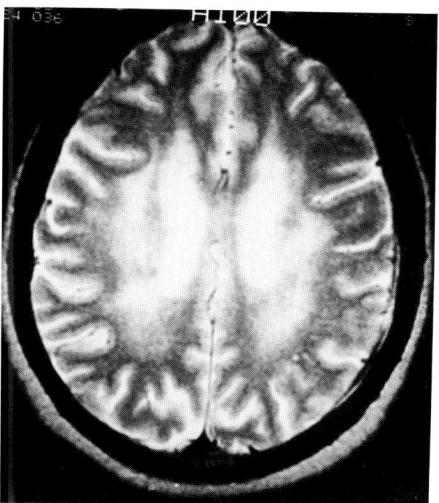

FIG SK34-4. **Radiation injury.** Symmetric foci of high signal intensity in the periventricular white matter on this T_2-weighted image.

Condition	Imaging Findings	Comments
Hydrocephalus with transependymal CSF flow	Smooth high-signal halo of relatively even thickness along the lateral ventricles, which are dilated out of proportion to the cortical sulci.	Must be distinguished from the normal appearance on axial T_2-weighted images of a cap of high signal around the frontal horns of the lateral ventricles ("ependymitis granularis"), which represents a normal accumulation of fluid in this subependymal area containing a loose network of axons with low myelin content.
Leukodystrophy	Symmetric, diffuse, and confluent pattern of involvement.	Genetic disorders of children (adrenoleukodystrophy, metachromatic leukodystrophy, globoid cell leukodystrophy, Canavan's disease, Krabbe's disease, Alexander's disease, Pelizaeus-Merzbacher disease) that result in abnormal accumulation of specific metabolites in brain tissue and lead to progressive visual failure, mental deterioration, and spastic paralysis early in life.
Subacute white matter encephalitis (Fig SK34-5)	Bilateral, diffuse, patchy to confluent areas of increased signal intensity with poorly defined margins.	Inflammatory process involving the white matter of the cerebrum, cerebellum, and brainstem. It is occurring with increasing frequency in patients with acquired immunodeficiency syndrome (AIDS) secondary to human immunodeficiency virus (HIV) or cytomegalovirus infection.
Progressive multifocal leukoencephalopathy (PML) (see Fig SK42-7)	Patchy, round or oval foci of increased signal intensity that eventually become large and confluent. The process is often distinctly asymmetric and initially involves the peripheral white matter, following the contours of the gray matter–white matter interface to give outer scalloped margins. Although PML is not primarily a periventricular process, the deeper white matter is also affected as the disease progresses.	Demyelinating disease resulting from reactivation of latent papovavirus in an immunocompromised individual. In the past, most cases occurred in patients with Hodgkin's disease or chronic lymphocytic leukemia or in those treated with steroids or immunosuppressive drugs. PML is occurring with increasing frequency in persons with AIDS.
Vasculitis	Multifocal periventricular high-intensity foci.	Seen in systemic lupus erythematosus and Behçet's disease. These conditions occur in young adults and can produce a neurologic picture similar to that of multiple sclerosis. Factors suggesting vasculitis include associated systemic features and the presence of cortical infarcts in addition to the periventricular lesions.
Migraine (Fig SK34-6)	Periventricular hyperintense foci.	Lesions resembling those of multiple sclerosis and deep white matter ischemia have been reported in about half the patients with migraine. The classic pattern of headaches should suggest the correct diagnosis.

Condition		Comments
Mucopolysaccharidoses	Multifocal periventricular high-intensity foci. Dural thickening and hydrocephalus may be noted.	Group of inherited metabolic diseases in which an enzyme deficiency leads to the deposition of mucopolysaccharides in various body tissues. Punctate white matter lesions reflect perivascular involvement with the disease, in which there is a large accumulation of vacuolated cells distended with mucopolysaccharide. As the disease progresses, the lesions become more widespread and larger, reflecting the development of infarcts and demyelination.

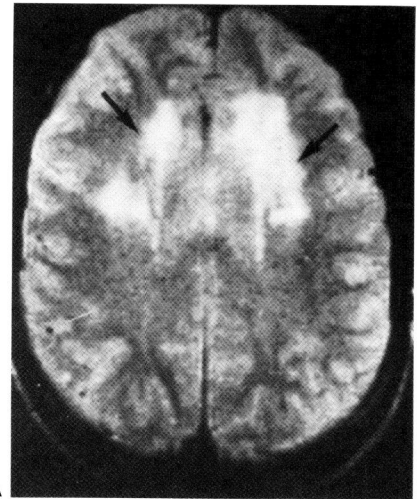
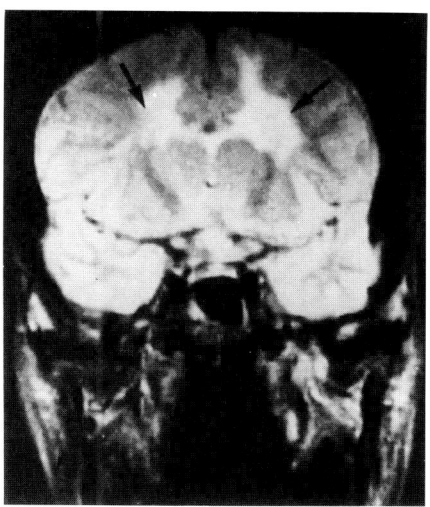

A   B

Fɪɢ SK34-5. HIV encephalitis. (A) Axial and (B) coronal T$_2$-weighted images show extensive white matter lesions (arrows) around the ventricles and in the centrum semiovale without evidence of mass effect.[33]

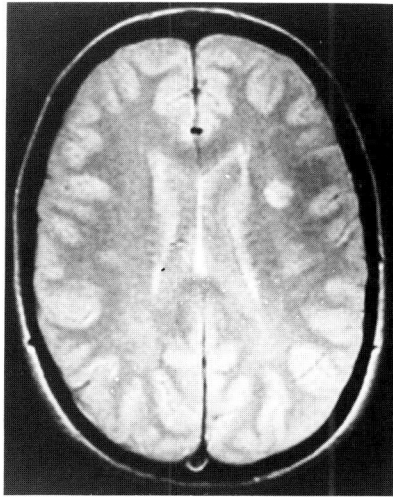

Fɪɢ SK34-6. Migraine. Focal area of hyperintensity in the left frontal white matter in a 47-year-old woman with classic migraine headaches.[34]

DEGENERATIVE AND METABOLIC DISORDERS OF THE BRAIN ON MAGNETIC RESONANCE IMAGING

Condition	Imaging Findings	Comments
Degenerative disorders **Parkinsonism** **(Fig SK35-1)**	Generalized atrophy with prominent sulci and arachnoid spaces. Described findings include (1) areas of hypointensity (correlating with sites of iron deposition) in the putamen, (2) return to normal signal intensity rather than the usual low signal of the dorsolateral aspect of the substantia nigra; and (3) narrowing of the pars compacta, a band of relatively increased signal between the hypointense red nucleus and the pars reticularis of the substantia nigra.	Extrapyramidal disorder that characteristically presents with slowness of movement, poverty of facial expression, flexed posture, immobility, and resting tremor. Pathologically, there is a loss of pigmented cells in the pars compacta of the substantia nigra.
Parkinsonism-plus syndromes	Various patterns in addition to generalized atrophy and enlarged cortical sulci and arachnoid spaces.	A term that refers to the approximately 25% of patients with Parkinsonian features who have more severe symptoms and respond poorly to dopamine replacement therapy.
Striatonigral degeneration **(Fig SK35-2)**	Striking hypointensity of the putamen, particularly along its posterolateral margin, on T_2-weighted images.	Degree of hypointense putaminal signal (representing pigment accumulation) has a significant correlation with the severity of rigidity.
Shy-Drager syndrome	Various patterns, depending on associated degenerative processes.	Pontocerebellar atrophy and neuronal degeneration in the sympathetic and vegetative nuclei causing orthostatic hypotension, urinary incontinence, and an inability to sweat.
Olivopontocerebellar atrophy **(Fig SK35-3)**	Atrophy and abnormal signal in the pons, middle cerebellar peduncles, cerebellum (hemispheric greater than vermian), and inferior olives.	Atrophic changes with prominent demyelination. Degenerative neuronal abnormalities in the substantia nigra, putamen, globus pallidus, dentate nuclei, and subthalamic nucleus of Luys.
Progressive supranuclear palsy **(Fig SK35-4)**	Focal atrophy or signal changes (or both) of midbrain structures.	In addition to the neuronal degeneration and gliosis in the areas noted above, there are symptoms of supranuclear ocular palsies, nuchal dystonia, generalized hypotonia, and disturbances of wakefulness.
Alzheimer's disease **(Fig SK35-5)**	In addition to generalized cortical and central atrophy, there is typical focal enlargement of the temporal horns (correlating with hippocampal atrophy) best seen on coronal scans.	Characterized by disorders of memory followed by language disturbances and visuospatial disorientation. Although there are few specific findings, the absence of white matter abnormality, hydrocephalus, mass lesion, or metabolic disorder in a demented patient strongly indicates Alzheimer's (or Parkinson's) disease.

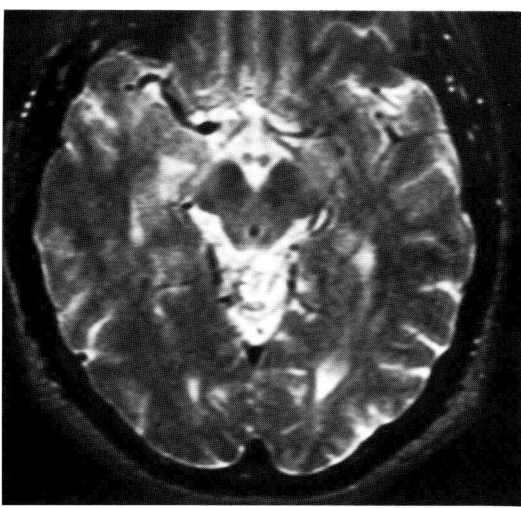

FIG SK35-1. Parkinson's disease. Complete loss bilaterally of the normal hyperintense band between the red nuclei and the pars reticularis of the substantia nigra.[35]

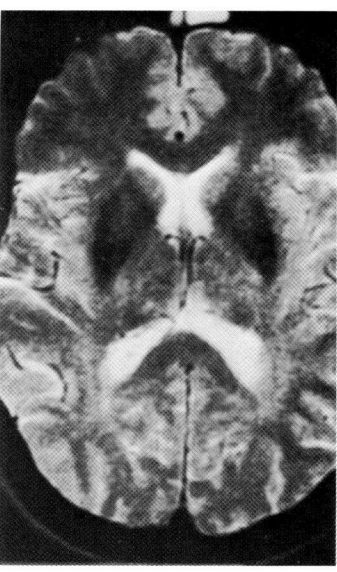

FIG SK35-2. Striatonigral degeneration. Axial T_2-weighted image shows striking hypointensity in the putamen.[36]

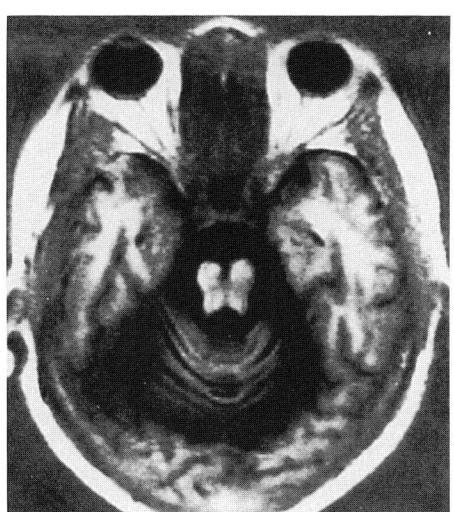

FIG SK35-3. Olivopontocerebellar atrophy.[37]

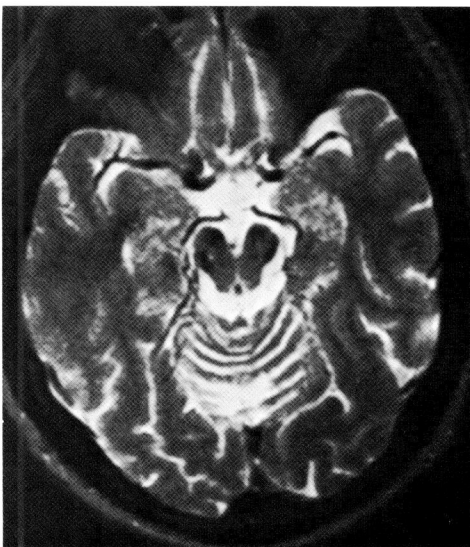

FIG SK35-4. Progressive supranuclear palsy. Axial T_2-weighted scan shows atrophy of the midbrain with prominence of the perimesencephalic cisterns.[38]

Condition	Imaging Findings	Comments
Pick's disease (Fig SK35-6)	Striking focal atrophy of both gray and white matter, typically involving the inferior frontal and temporal lobes, with severe reduction of affected gyri to a paper-thin edge ("knife-blade atrophy").	Much less common disorder in which the symptoms are largely indistinguishable from those of Alzheimer's disease, although abnormal behavior and difficulty with language occur more frequently than memory disturbances.
Huntington's chorea (Fig SK35-7)	Atrophy of the head of the caudate nucleus and putamen bilaterally and moderate frontotemporal atrophy.	Inherited disorder (autosomal dominant) characterized by dementia and choreoathetosis that progresses relentlessly.
Creutzfeldt-Jakob disease (**spongiform encephalopathy**) (Fig SK35-8)	Rapid progression of central and peripheral atrophy. On T_2-weighted images there is increased signal intensity of gray matter affecting the corpus striatum, thalamus, and cerebral cortex.	Caused by a virus-like infectious agent with a long incubation period of up to several years. Unremitting and fatal course characterized by severe dementia, ataxia, visual disturbances, and myoclonus. Relatively few white matter abnormalities, unlike dementia related to vascular disorders.
Wernicke's encephalopathy	Atrophic changes in the superior vermis and mamillary bodies with generalized sulcal enlargement. On T_2-weighted images there may be increased signal in multiple subcortical areas.	Disorder due to alcoholism or nutritional deficiency (or both) that is associated with confusion, apathy, truncal ataxia, and ophthalmoparesis.
Metabolic disorders **Central pontine myelinolysis** (see Fig SK32-3)	Central region in the pons and medulla that is hypointense on T_1-weighted images and hyperintense on T_2-weighted images.	Although initially reported in chronic alcoholics, this condition also presents in patients with electrolyte disturbances (especially hyponatremia) that have been corrected rapidly. In extreme cases, there may be extension to the tegmentum, midbrain, thalamus, internal capsule, and cerebral cortex.
Leigh's disease (Fig SK35-9)	On T_2-weighted images there are symmetric areas of increased signal intensity in the basal ganglia, thalamus, brainstem, and cerebellum (seen as low attenuation on CT).	Fatal familial disorder (autosomal recessive) that may be due to an abnormality in pyruvate metabolism and produces bilaterally symmetric foci of necrosis and degeneration leading to multiple neurologic defects.
Wilson's disease (Fig SK35-10)	On T_2-weighted images, areas of increased signal intensity most commonly in the putamen and caudate, but also in the thalamus, dentate nuclei, midbrain, and subcortical white matter. Generalized cortical and central atrophy usually occurs.	Also termed hepatolenticular degeneration, this autosomal recessive disorder of copper metabolism produces the classic syndrome of dysphagia, slowness and rigidity of movements, dysarthria, and tremor that usually occurs during the second or third decade of life. Pathologically, there is softening and atrophy or frank cavitation in the lentiform nuclei.
Hallervorden-Spatz disease (Fig SK35-11)	Decreased signal in the lentiform nuclei and perilentiform white matter (due to excess iron deposition) on T_2-weighted images. There may be areas of increased signal in the periventricular white matter (disordered myelination) and disproportionate atrophy of the brainstem and cerebellum.	Progressive inherited (autosomal recessive) disorder of movement that arises in late childhood or early adolescence and is characterized by abnormal iron deposition in the globus pallidus, reticular zone of the substantia nigra, and red nucleus.

Condition	Imaging Findings	Comments
Adrenoleukodystrophy (Fig SK35-12)	Large, usually symmetric and confluent areas of increased signal intensity on T_2-weighted images that tend to involve the white matter of the occipital, posterior parietal, and temporal lobes.	Metabolic encephalopathy typically affecting boys between ages 4 and 8 years in which there is myelin degeneration involving various parts of the cerebrum, brainstem, and optic nerves, as well as the spinal cord. The neurologic findings of behavioral problems, intellectual impairment, and long tract signs can appear before or after adrenal gland insufficiency.
Mucopolysaccharidoses (see Fig SK34-9)	In severe disease, multiple scattered small areas of increased signal on T_2-weighted images in the periventricular white matter. Central atrophy with dilated ventricles usually occurs.	

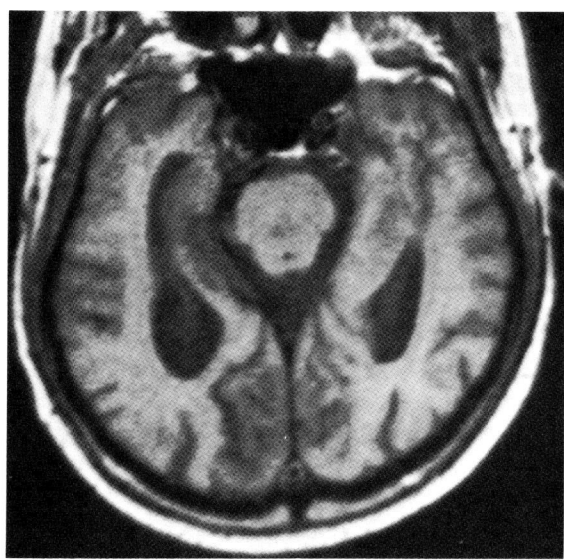

FIG SK35-5. **Alzheimer's disease.** Axial T_1-weighted scan shows bilateral temporal horn dilatation, more marked on the right, and a prominent area of decreased signal intensity in the right hippocampal region.[36]

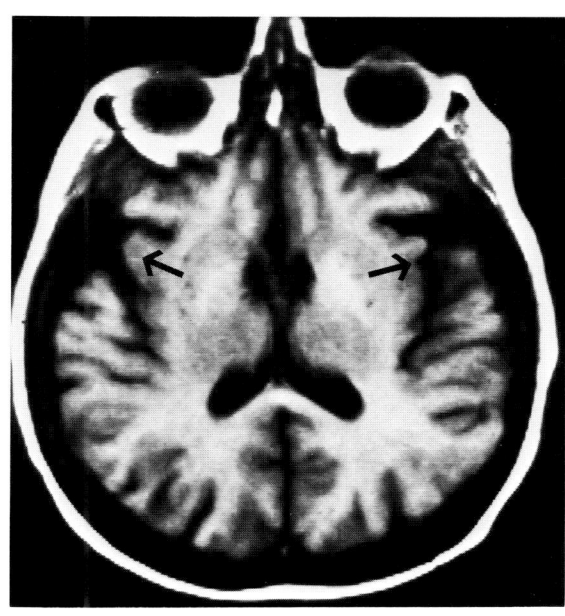

FIG SK35-6. **Pick's disease.**[23]

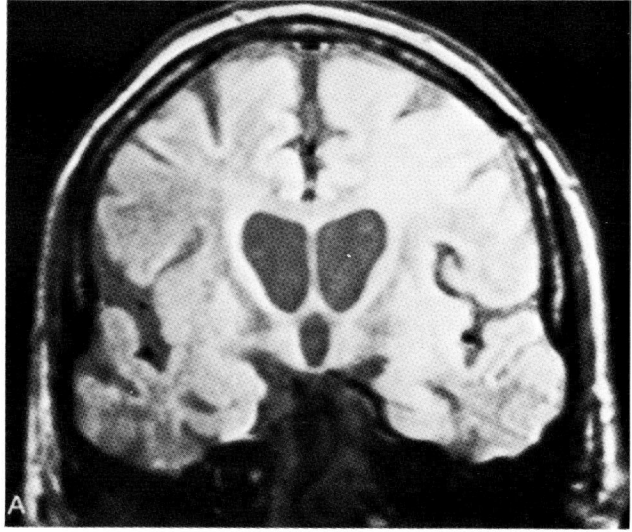

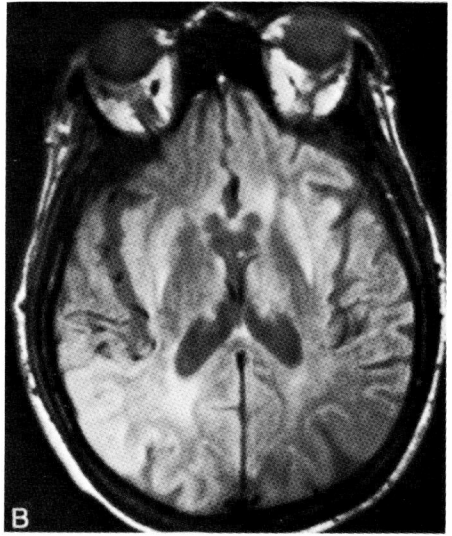

FIG SK35-7. **Huntington's chorea.** (A) Coronal proton-density scan demonstrates atrophy of the caudate nuclei, associated with dilatation of the frontal horns of the lateral ventricles. (B) On an axial scan, the putamen is also small and atrophic bilaterally.[38]

Condition	Imaging Findings	Comments
Nonketotic hyperglycemia	Severe atrophy of the cerebrum and cerebellum. Decreased or absent myelination in supratentorial white matter tracts with sparing of the brainstem and cerebellum.	Inherited disorder of amino acid metabolism in which large quantities of glycine accumulates in body fluids, plasma, urine, and cerebrospinal fluid. Affected persons present in infancy with seizures, abnormal muscle tone, and severe developmental delay.
Phenylketonuria	Widening of sulci and ventricles that may progress to frank atrophy of the cerebrum and cerebellum with confluent widespread white matter lesions on T_2-weighted images.	Accumulation of phenylalanine in the brain, which leads to severe developmental delay and mental retardation.

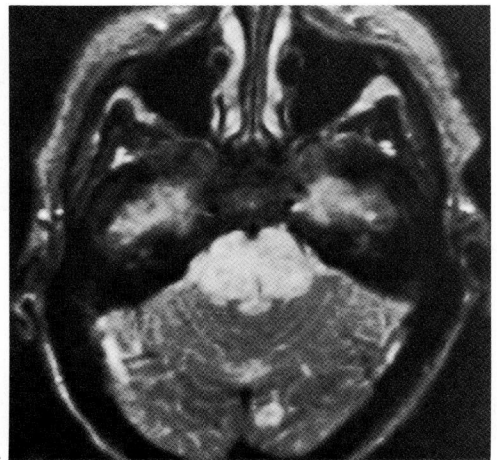 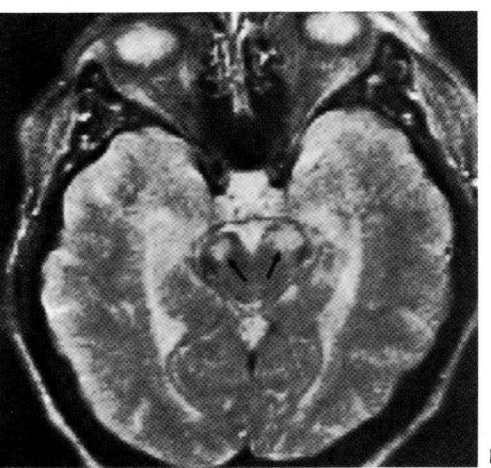

Fig SK35-8. Central pontine myelinolysis. Axial T_2-weighted images show (A) extensive increased signal intensity at the level of the midpons (with sparing of a thin band of tissue in the pontine tegmentum) and (B) symmetric hyperintense lesions in the cerebral peduncles (arrows).[38]

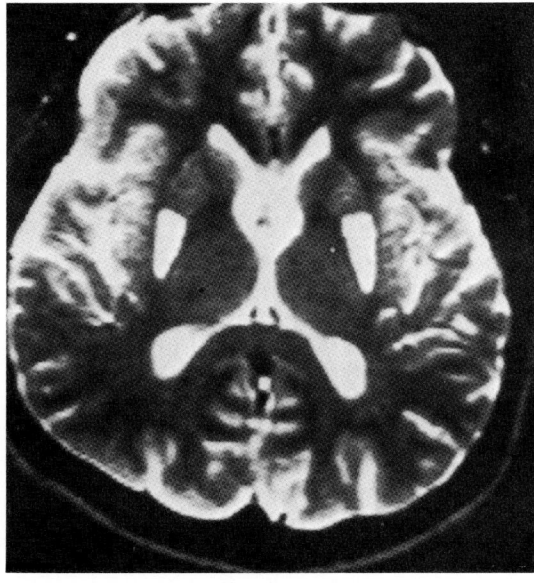 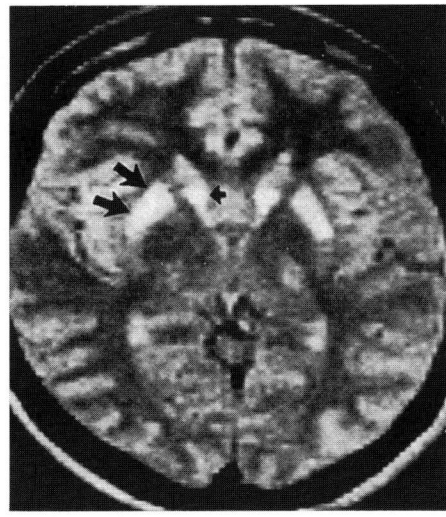

Fig SK35-9. Leigh's disease. Axial T_2-weighted scan shows characteristic prominent hyperintense signal in the putamen.[36]

Fig SK35-10. Wilson's disease. Axial T_2-weighted image shows increased signal intensity in the lenticular nuclei (large arrows) and the posterior aspects of the heads of the caudate nuclei (small arrow).[39]

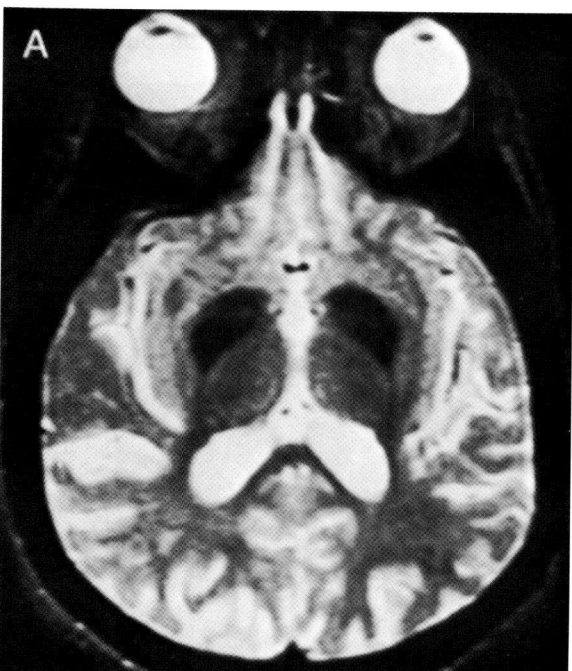
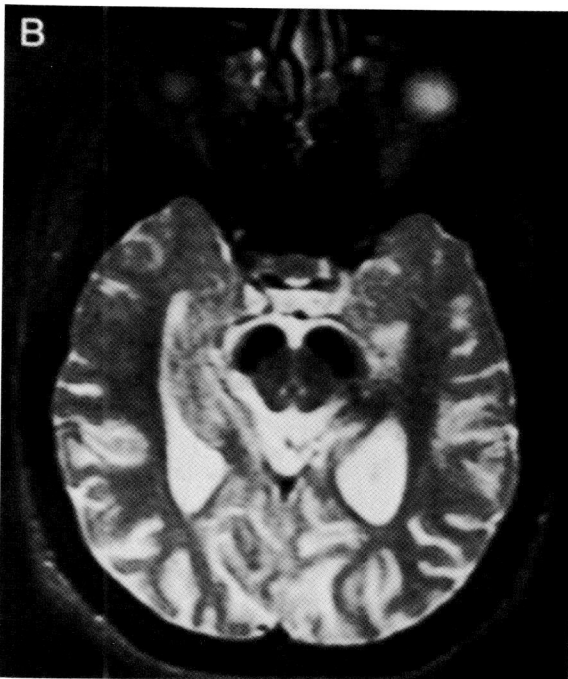

Fɪɢ SK35-11. **Hallervorden-Spatz disease.** Axial T$_2$-weighted images in a 16-year-old show striking hypointense signal in the globus pallidus (A) and substantia nigra (B) bilaterally.[36]

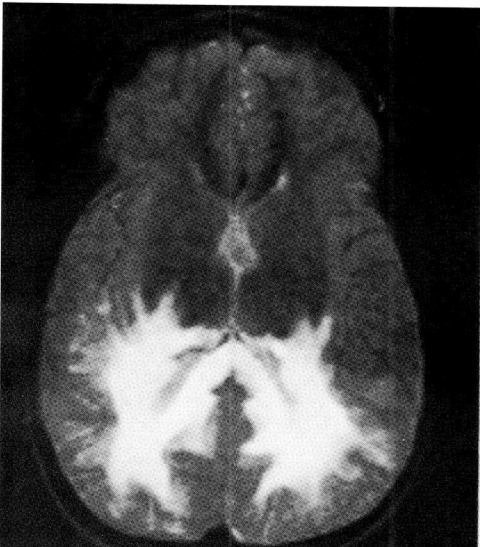

Fɪɢ SK35-12. **Adrenoleukodystrophy.** Axial T$_2$-weighted scan shows bilaterally symmetric hyperintense signal in the white matter of the occipital and parietal lobes. The posterior temporal lobe is also involved and the abnormality extends into the splenium of the corpus callosum.[38]

INTRAVENTRICULAR MASSES

Condition	Imaging Findings	Comments
Choroid plexus papilloma (Fig SK36-1)	Well-defined intraventricular mass, often with lobulated margins, that is hyperdense on CT and only mildly hyperintense on T_2-weighted MR images. Intense homogeneous contrast enhancement.	Uncommon tumor that primarily occurs in children younger than 5 years of age. It most frequently occurs in the lateral ventricles in children and in the fourth ventricle in adults. Calcifications are common. Overproduction of CSF or obstruction of CSF pathways causes hydrocephalus. Parenchymal invasion suggests malignant degeneration to choroid plexus carcinoma.
Colloid cyst (Fig SK36-2)	Smooth, spherical or ovoid mass in the anterior part of the third ventricle that usually has homogeneously high density on CT. Minimal if any contrast enhancement.	Papillomatous lesion containing mucinous fluid with variable amounts of proteinaceous debris, fluid components, and desquamated cells. Classic symptoms are positional headaches related to intermittent obstruction of the foramen of Monro. Most present during adult life, are relatively small (less than 2 cm), and cause dilatation of the lateral ventricles.
Meningioma (Fig SK36-3)	Smoothly marginated mass that is hyperdense on CT and shows marked homogeneous contrast enhancement. On MRI, variable signal intensity and intense contrast enhancement.	Only 1% of meningiomas are intraventricular. They are found most commonly in the atrium, more often on the left than on the right. As with other meningiomas, they most frequently occur in middle-aged or older women.
Ependymoma (Fig SK36-4)	Well-defined mass that typically arises in the floor of the fourth ventricle. It is hyperdense and shows homogeneous enhancement on CT. On MRI, the tumor has a heterogeneous internal texture as a result of the frequent occurrence of calcification, cysts, and necrotic areas in the lesion.	Rare lesion of the first and second decades that affects boys twice as often as girls. Ependymomas are slow-growing but malignant tumors that may expand and infiltrate into the ventricle or adjacent brain substance. They frequently extend through the foramina of Luschka and Magendie into the basal cisterns and cause ventricular and subarachnoid seeding.
Giant cell astrocytoma (Fig SK36-5)	Often lobulated or calcified intraventricular mass that may arise from a subependymal nodule. Uniform contrast enhancement.	This malignant transformation of a hamartoma occurs in about 10% of patients with tuberous sclerosis. It is usually situated in the region of the foramen of Monro. The presence of other subependymal or parenchymal hamartomas strongly suggests this diagnosis.

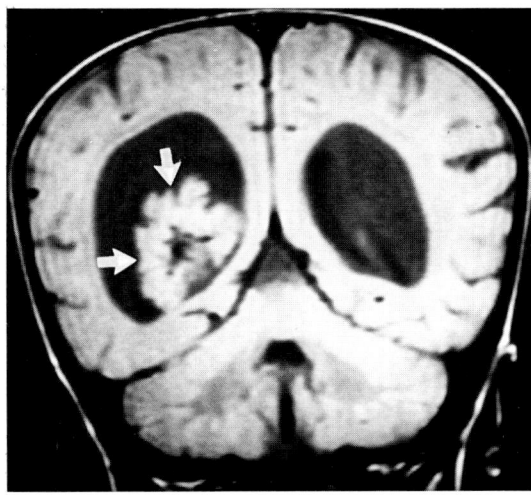

FIG SK36-1. **Choroid plexus papilloma.** T$_1$-weighted coronal image shows a lobulated isointense mass (arrows) in a markedly dilated right lateral ventricle.

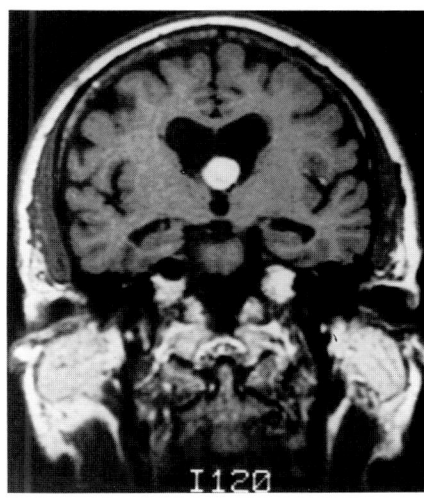

FIG SK36-2. **Colloid cyst.** T$_1$-weighted coronal MR scan shows a hyperintense mass in the third ventricle just posterior to the foramen of Monro. There is ventricular dilatation in this elderly man with a history of recurrent headache.[34]

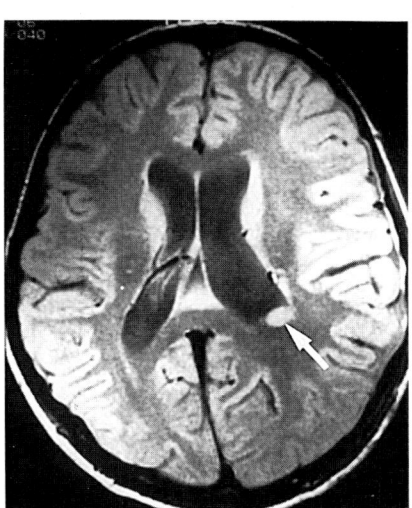

FIG SK36-3. **Intraventricular meningioma.** Well-circumscribed mass (arrow) in the posterior aspect of the left lateral ventricle in a patient with neurofibromatosis.

FIG SK36-4. **Ependymoma.** Large intraventricular mass (arrowheads) located in the third ventricle and anterior horns of both lateral ventricles; there is associated hydrocephalus. Areas of greatest hyperintensity in the tumor represent subacute hemorrhage.[40]

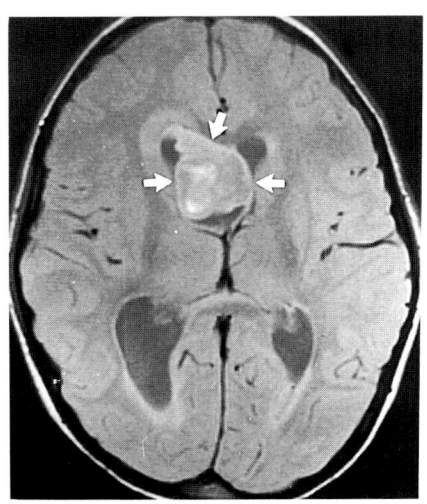

A

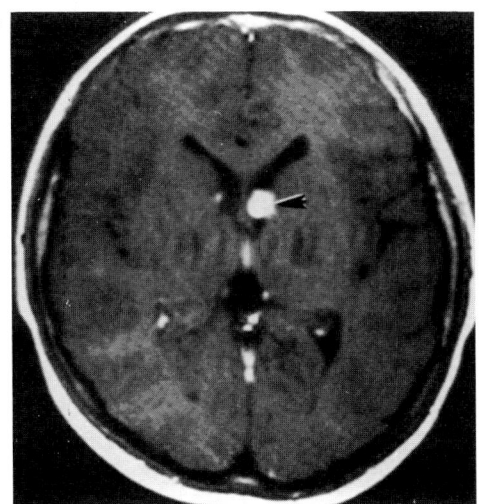

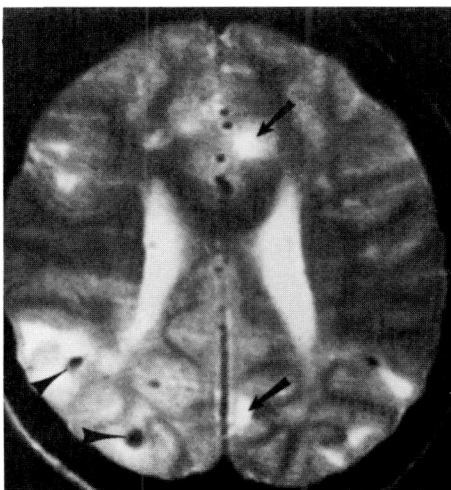

B

FIG SK36-5. **Giant cell astrocytoma.** (A) Contrast-enhanced T$_1$-weighted MR image shows a markedly hyperintense intraventricular mass (arrowhead) in this young boy with clinical stigmata of tuberous sclerosis. (B) T$_2$-weighted image at another level shows characteristic high-signal cortical hamartomas (arrows) as well as dense calcifications (arrowheads).[41]

Condition	Imaging Findings	Comments
Dermoid/epidermoid (Figs SK36-6 and SK36-7)	Intraventricular mass.	MR can identify material within the cyst that has a signal intensity of fat or cerebrospinal fluid, respectively.
Primitive neuroectodermal tumor (Fig SK36-8)	Well-circumscribed mass with intense and homogeneous enhancement.	Cyst formation may occur, especially in infratentorial tumors, and account for the large size of the neoplasm.
Teratoma (Fig SK36-9)	Various epidermal components (fat and calcification) can be identified easily on CT or MRI.	Typically occurs in children less than 1 year old. An elevated serum α-fetoprotein level suggests that the lesion is malignant.
Lymphoma	Variable signal intensity, though most lymphomas are isointense or slightly hyperintense on T_2-weighted images. On CT, the tumor has mildly increased attenuation and shows intense contrast enhancement.	More commonly presents as mass(es) adjacent to the lateral ventricles (often crossing the corpus callosum to the opposite side) or as diffuse infiltration of the parenchyma.
Oligodendroglioma (Fig SK36-10)	Intraventricular mass that may contain calcification.	Adult neoplasm that usually arises in the frontotemporal region.

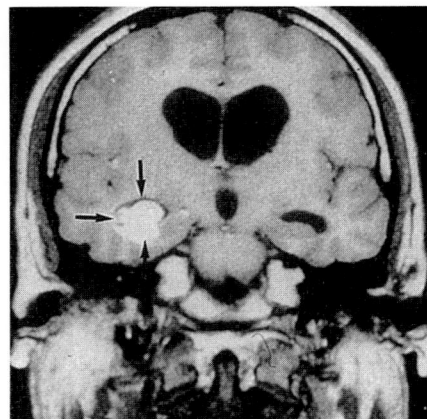

FIG SK36-6. Dermoid cyst. Coronal T_1-weighted MR image shows a hyperintense mass (arrows) filling the dilated right temporal horn. The lateral and third ventricles are enlarged.[42]

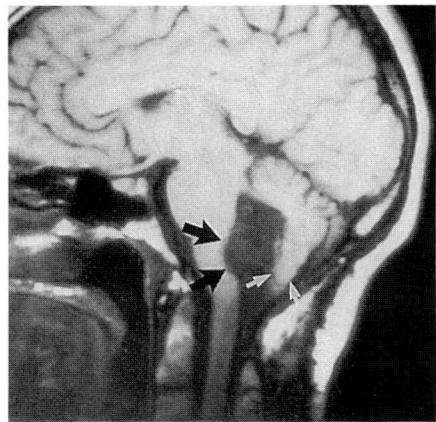

FIG SK36-7. Epidermoid tumor. Sagittal T-weighted MR image shows a large mass filling the fourth ventricle. The mass has a slightly higher signal intensity than CSF. It depresses the brainstem (black arrows) and elevates the tonsil and inferior vermis (white arrows).[42]

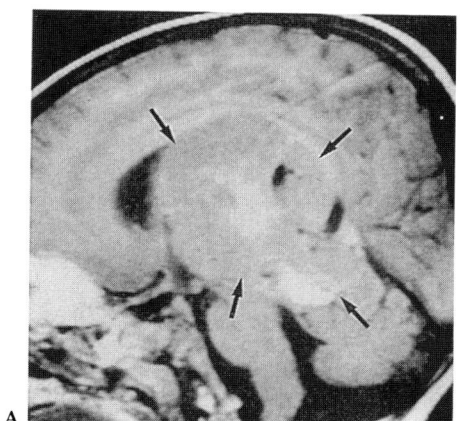
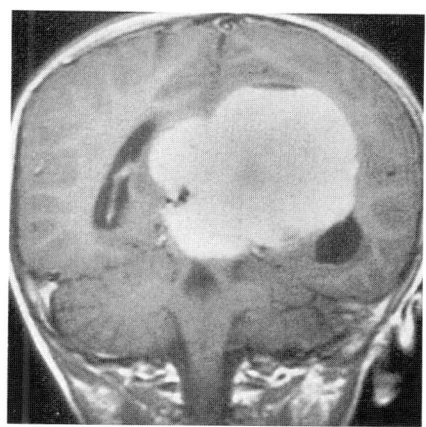

FIG SK36-8. Primitive neuroectodermal tumor. (A) Sagittal T$_1$-weighted MR image shows a large, inhomogeneously isointense mass (arrows) filling the entire body of the left lateral ventricle and compressing the third ventricle, midbrain, and upper vermis of the cerebellum. (B) Coronal T$_1$-weighted scan demonstrates intense enhancement of the lesion.[42]

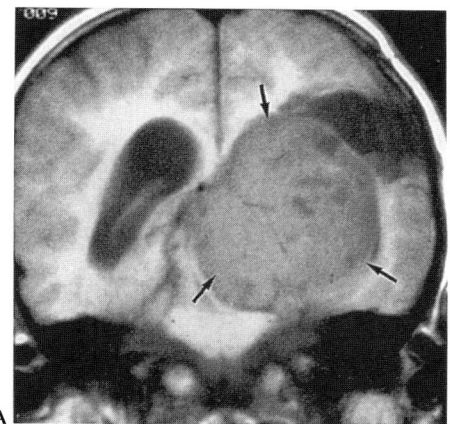
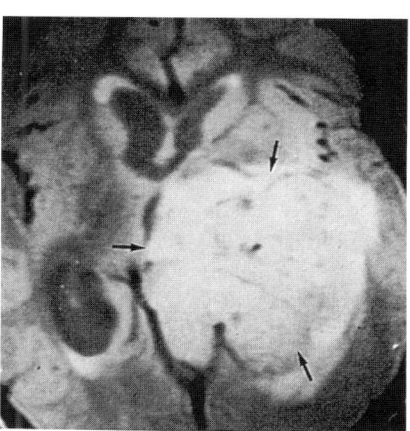

FIG SK36-9. Malignant teratoma. (A) Coronal T$_1$-weighted MR image shows a large, irregular, lobulated mass (arrows) of inhomogeneous hypointensity in the body and occipital horn of the left lateral ventricle. (B) On the axial proton-density-weighted image, the mass is hyperintense (arrows).[42]

Condition	Imaging Findings	Comments
Neurocytoma (neuroblastoma) (Fig SK36-11)	Intraventricular mass that is mainly isointense relative to cortical gray matter on both T_1- and T_2-weighted images. Often contains areas of heterogeneous intensity reflecting tumor calcification (best seen on CT), cystic spaces, and vascular flow voids within the tumor.	Benign primary neoplasm of young adults that tends to occur in the lateral and 3rd ventricles and has a characteristic attachment to the septum pellucidum. On light microscopy it appears identical to oligodendroglioma.
Metastasis (Fig SK36-12)	Intraventricular mass.	Most commonly from melanoma and carcinomas of the lung and breast.

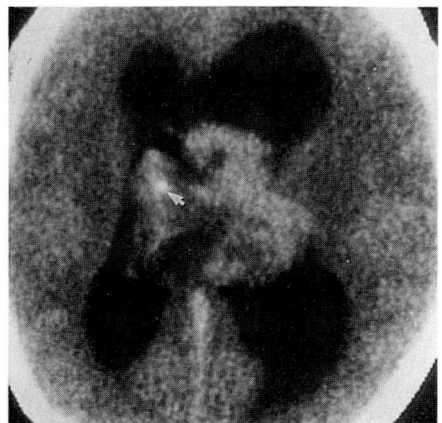
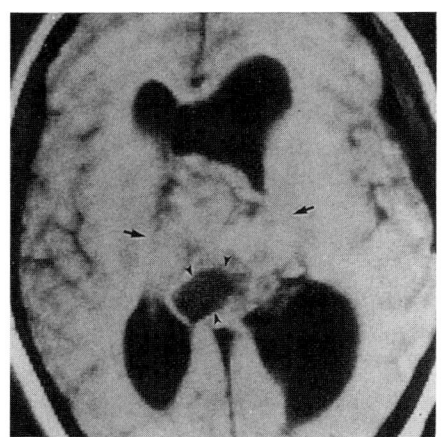

FIG SK36-10. **Oligodendroglioma.** Axial T_1-weighted MR image shows a large lobulated isointense mass (arrows) with cystic components (arrowheads) involving the septum pellucidum and bodies of the lateral ventricles.[42]

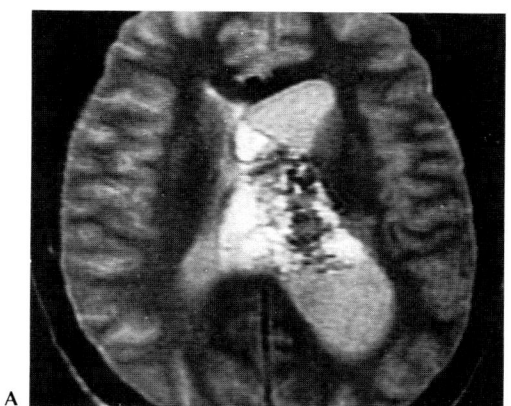
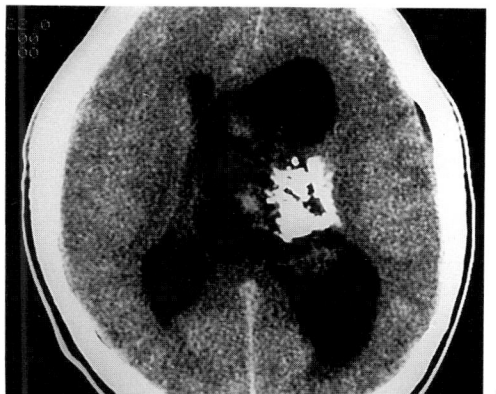

FIG SK36-11. Neurocytoma. (A) Axial T_2-weighted MR image shows the heterogeneous appearance of the lesion, reflecting the presence of cystic spaces and calcifications. (B) CT scan shows coarse, conglomerate calcification and large cystic areas within the intraventricular tumor.[43]

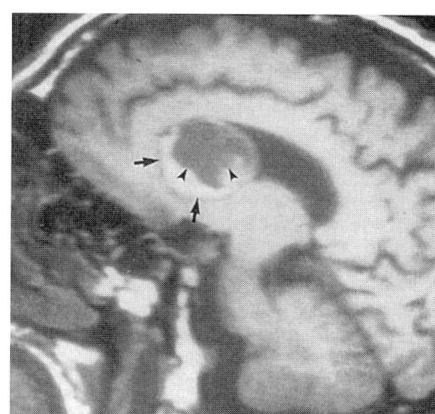

FIG SK36-12. Hemorrhagic metastatic melanoma. Sagittal T_1-weighted MR image shows a round mass filling the left frontal horn near the foramen of Monro. The mass has a hyperintense rim (arrows), most likely representing methemoglobin, and a hypointense center (arrowheads).[42]

ENHANCING VENTRICULAR MARGINS
ON COMPUTED TOMOGRAPHY

Condition	Comments
Meningeal carcinomatosis **(Fig SK37-1)**	Most commonly secondary to oat cell carcinoma of the lung, melanoma, or breast carcinoma. Unlike meningitis, leukemia, or lymphoma, meningeal metastases usually occur in patients with a disseminated malignancy and are seldom associated with fever, leukocytosis, or meningismus.
Leukemia	Meningeal infiltration occurs in up to 10% of patients with acute leukemia. Although systemic chemotherapy, which penetrates the blood-brain barrier ineffectively, fails to prevent cerebral leukemia, the combination of intrathecal methotrexate and whole-brain irradiation effectively eradicates leukemic cells in the central nervous system (except for subarachnoid deposits isolated by adhesions).
Lymphoma **(Fig SK37-2)**	Most common form of intracranial lymphoma, which typically occurs in patients with diffuse histiocytic or undifferentiated lymphoma and poorly differentiated Hodgkin's disease.
Subependymal spread of **primary brain tumor** **(Fig SK37-3)**	Periventricular ''cast'' of tumor may reflect the ependymal seeding or subependymal spread of gliomas or other intracranial neoplasms (eg, medulloblastoma, germinoma).
Inflammatory ventriculitis **(Figs SK37-4 and SK37-5)**	May be secondary to bacterial, fungal, viral, or parasitic infections or to noninfectious inflammatory disease (eg, sarcoidosis).

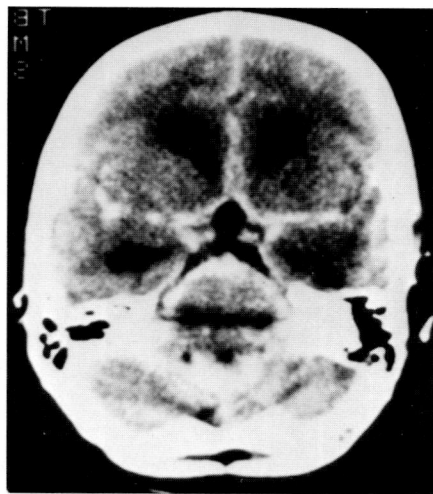

FIG SK37-1. Meningeal carcinomatosis. Generalized enhancement of the meninges with obstructive hydrocephalus.

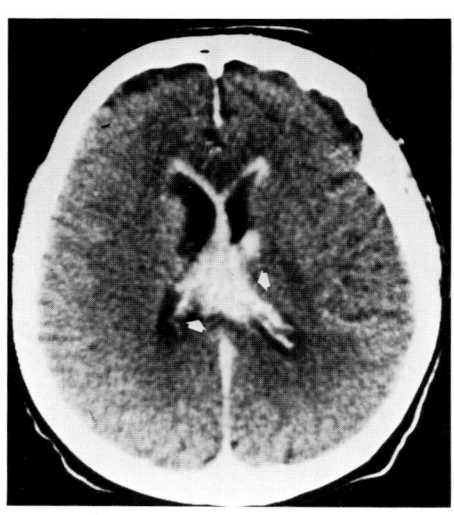

FIG SK37-2. Histiocytic lymphoma. Homogeneously enhancing lesions (arrows) deep in the brain associated with enhancement of ventricular margins.

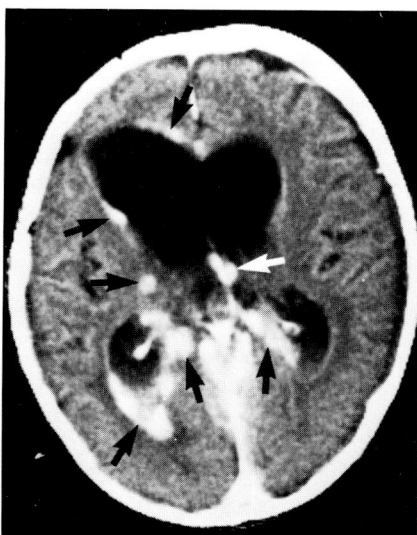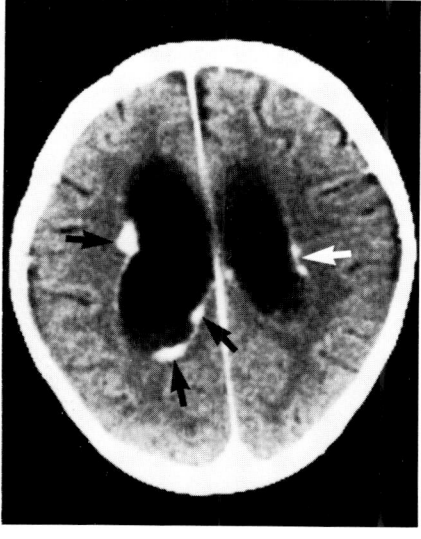

FIG SK37-3. Subependymal metastases. Multiple enhancing ependymal nodules (arrows) in a patient with posterior fossa ependymoblastoma and hydrocephalus.[13]

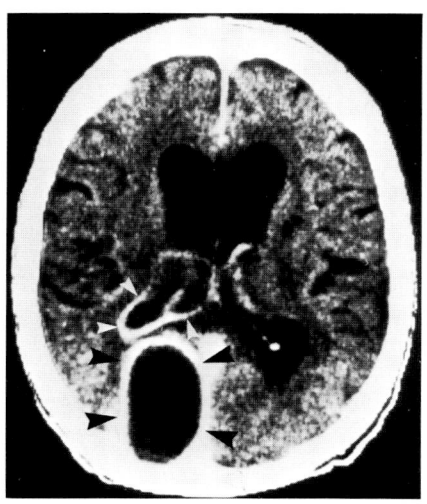

FIG SK37-4. Brain abscess with ventriculitis. CT scan following the intravenous injection of contrast material in a drug addict with lethargy and confusion demonstrates enhancement of the ventricular system (white arrowheads) due to extensive spread of infection. Note the ring-enhancing abscess (black arrowheads) in the right occipital lobe.

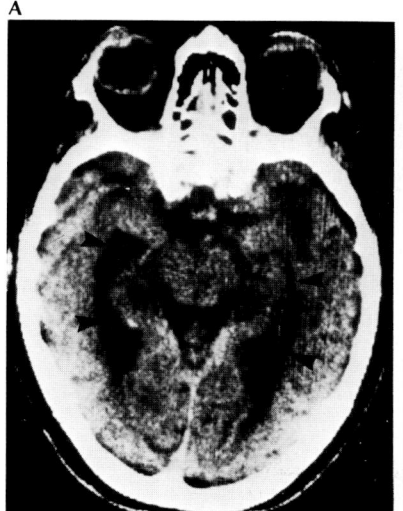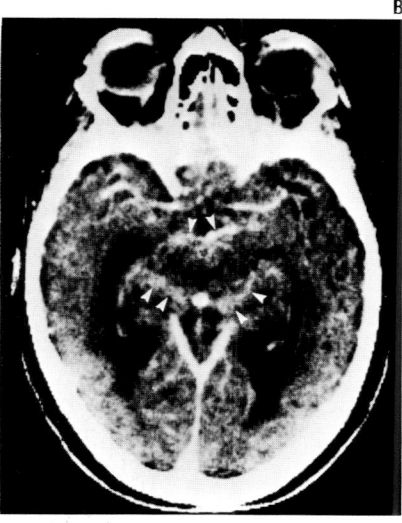

FIG SK37-5. Pneumococcal meningitis. (A) Noncontrast scan shows dilatation of the temporal horns of the lateral ventricles (arrowheads). (B) After the intravenous injection of contrast material, there is enhancement of the meninges in the basal cisterns (arrowheads), reflecting the underlying inflammation due to meningitis. The hydrocephalus in meningitis is due to blockage of the normal flow of cerebrospinal fluid by inflammatory exudate at the level of the aqueduct and the basal cisterns.

MENINGEAL ENHANCEMENT ON MAGNETIC RESONANCE IMAGING

Condition	Comments
Infectious meningitis **(Figs SK38-1 and SK38-2)**	May be secondary to bacterial, fungal, viral, or parasitic infections. MRI is of special value in detecting meningeal inflammation in patients with AIDS.
Meningeal carcinomatosis **(Fig SK38-3)**	Most commonly secondary to oat cell carcinoma of the lung, melanoma, or breast carcinoma. Neoplastic involvement of the leptomeningeal membranes, however, may occur as a complication of any neoplasm arising in the central nervous system or as a metastatic process originating from a distant primary tumor.
Lymphoma **(Fig SK38-4)**	The dramatic increase in the incidence of central nervous system lymphoma in recent years has been attributed to AIDS.
Neurosarcoidosis **(Fig SK38-5)**	Clinically apparent involvement of the central nervous system occurs in 2% to 5% of patients.
Dural venous sinus **thrombosis**	Associated with oral contraceptive use, craniotomy, infection, and, in children, dehydration. In a significant percentage of cases, no etiology can be determined.

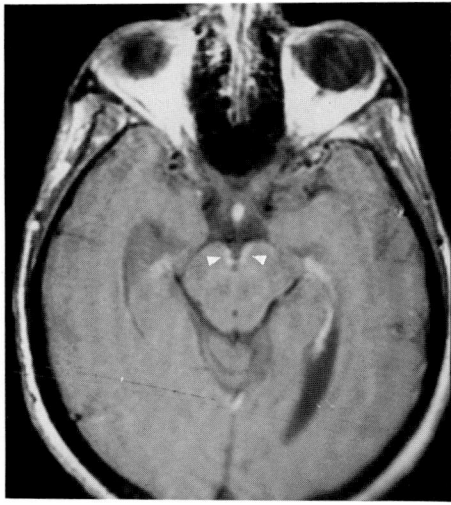

FIG SK38-1. Cryptococcal meningitis in AIDS. Meningeal enhancement along the cerebral peduncles (arrowheads).

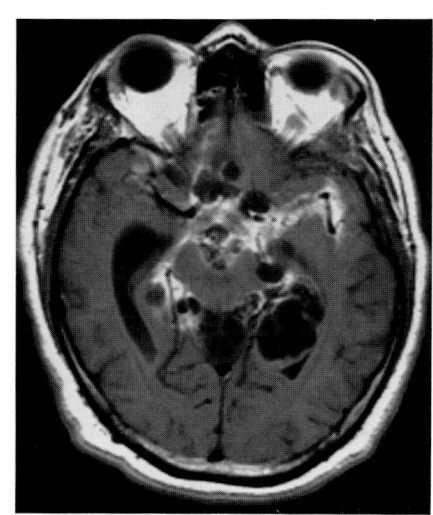

FIG SK38-2. Cysticercosis. Subarachnoid enhancement in the basal cisterns and left sylvian fissure.[44]

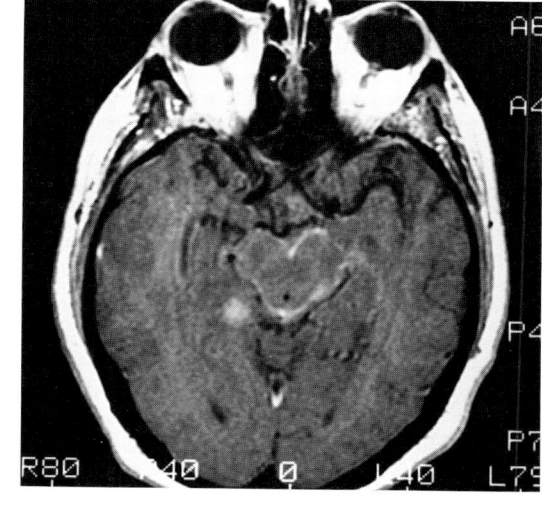

FIG SK38-3. Meningeal carcinomatosis. Enhancement around the midbrain and cerebral peduncles represents pial spread of tumor.[44]

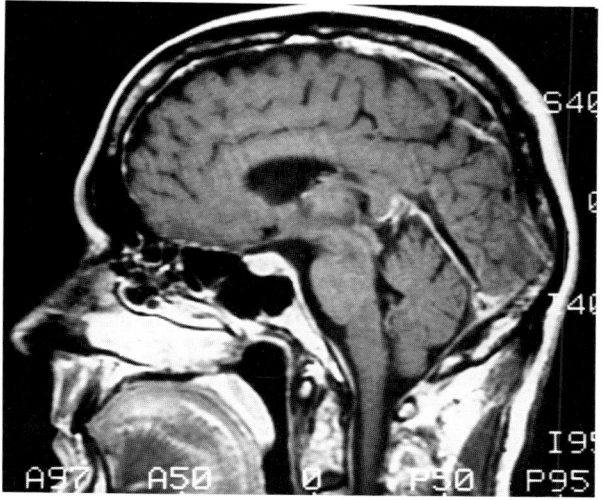

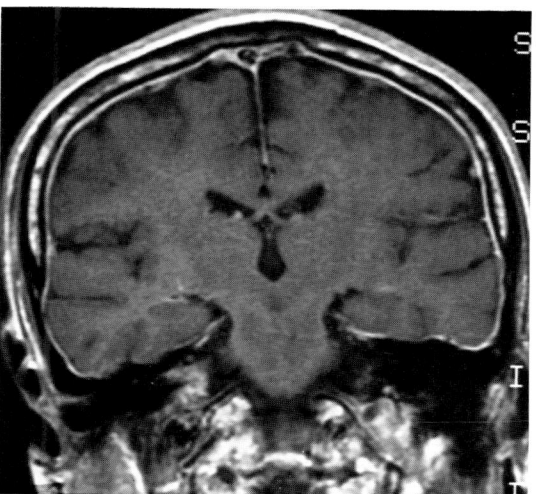

FIG SK38-4. Lymphoma. (A) Sagittal and (B) coronal scans show enhancement of the falx cerebri as well as about the convexity and at the base of the temporal lobes.[44]

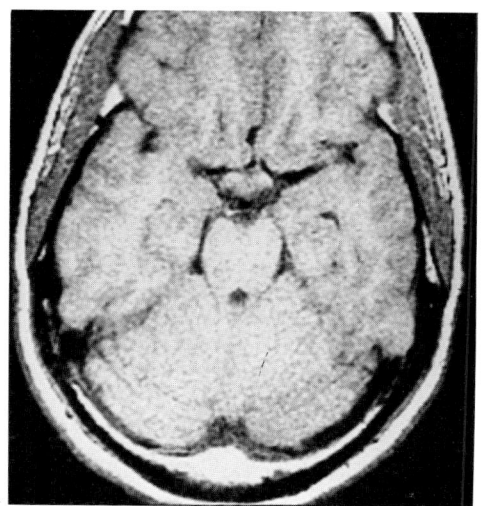

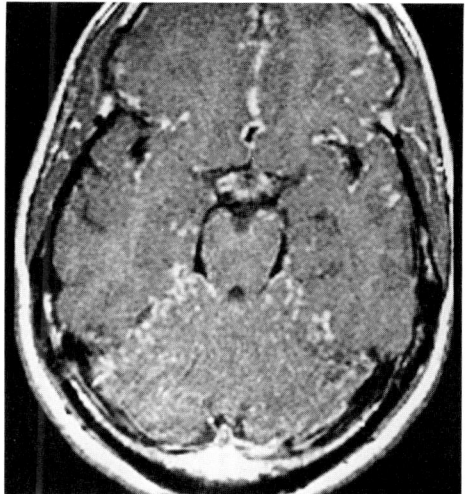

FIG SK38-5. Neurosarcoidosis. (A) Unenhanced image reveals no parenchymal or meningeal abnormalities. (B) An enhanced scan shows diffuse leptomeningeal involvement.[44]

PERIVENTRICULAR CALCIFICATION IN A CHILD
ON COMPUTED TOMOGRAPHY

Condition	Comments
Tuberous sclerosis **(Fig SK39-1)**	Small, round, calcified nodules along the lateral wall of the frontal horn and anterior third ventricle are a hallmark of this inherited neurocutaneous syndrome, which is manifested by the clinical triad of convulsive seizures, mental deficiency, and adenoma sebaceum.
Intrauterine infection **(Fig SK39-2)**	Diffuse calcifications and ventricular enlargement associated with substantial cerebral atrophy and microcephaly typically develop in patients with congenital infections due to cytomegalovirus or toxoplasmosis.

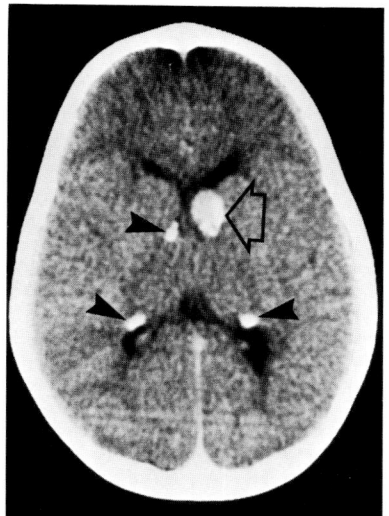

FIG 39-1. Tuberous sclerosis. Multiple calcified hamartomas (solid black arrowheads) lying along the ependymal surface of the ventricles. The open arrow points to a giant cell astrocytoma at the foramen of Monro.

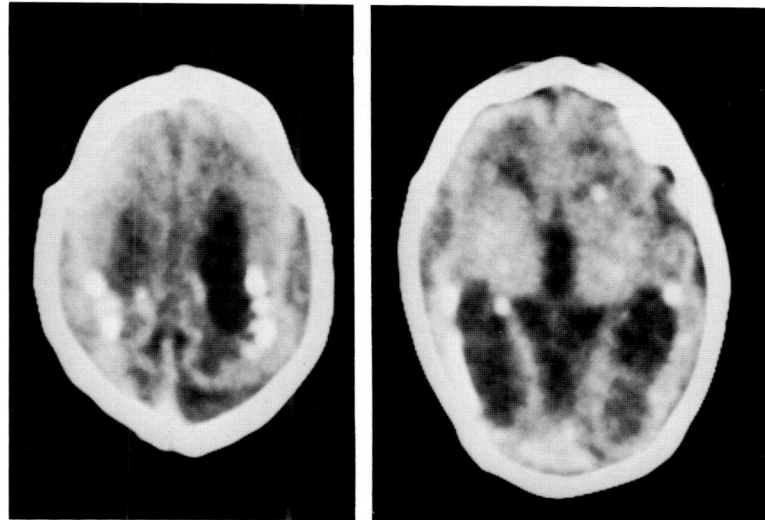

FIG 39-2. Cytomegalovirus infection. Two scans of an infant show multiple periventricular calcifications and dilatation of the ventricular system.

COMMON CONGENITAL MALFORMATIONS OF THE BRAIN ON COMPUTED TOMOGRAPHY AND MAGNETIC RESONANCE IMAGING

Condition	Imaging Findings	Comments
Disorders of neural tube closure (encephalocele/meningocele) (Fig SK40-1)	Herniation of brain, meninges, or both through a variably sized skull defect that is smooth and well defined and tends to have slightly sclerotic margins.	Most frequently involves the occipital bone (70%). Other sites (about 9% each) are the parietal, frontal, and nasal regions.
Disorders of neuronal migration		Congenital malformations of the cerebral wall and cortex that result from deranged migration of neuroblasts and abnormal formation of gyri and sulci. They are believed to arise during weeks 6 to 15 of gestation when successive waves of neuroblasts normally migrate from the subependymal germinal matrix to the surface of the brain to form the standard six-layered cortex.
Lissencephaly (Fig SK40-2)	Abnormal cerebral surface that may be completely smooth and agyric (rare), almost agyric with a few areas of pachygyria (too broad, flattened gyri), or nearly equally agyric and pachygyric.	The cerebrum has an hourglass or figure-of-8 contour because the brain fails to develop opercula. The insulae are exposed, and the middle cerebral arteries course superficially along shallow sylvian grooves. No sylvian triangle is present. The cortical gray matter is thickened (despite a reduced number of cell layers). The white matter is deficient and there is a thin subcortical layer, hypoplasia of the centrum semiovale, and reduced to absent digitations of white matter into the cortex.
Pachygyria (Fig SK40-3)	Abnormally thickened cortical gray matter with coarse, broadened gyri separated by shallow sulci. All or only a part of the brain may be involved.	Pachygyria with no associated agyria is a distinct migrational disorder in which patients live longer than those with lissencephaly, sometimes surviving into later childhood. Nevertheless, they have developmental delay, severe retardation, and seizures. The interface between gray and white matter is abnormally smooth and has incomplete or absent white matter digitations.
Polymicrogyria	Too many gyri of small size separated by wandering sulci.	Because the sulci may not reach the surface of the brain, areas of polymicrogyria may resemble pachygyria on imaging studies and on gross inspection.
Heterotopia (Fig SK40-4)	Single or multiple masses of gray matter of various size and shape in the subependymal or subcortical white matter. These masses maintain the same signal intensity as cortical gray matter on all MR pulse sequences.	Heterotopic rests of gray matter result from arrest of neuronal migration along their paths to the cortex. Heterotopia can be an isolated entity, part of more diffuse migrational disorders, or associated with other malformations.
Schizencephaly (Fig SK40-5)	A pattern varying from unilateral or bilateral slitlike clefts to large, bilateral, fan-shaped defects that extend from the lateral ventricles to the pial surface of the brain.	Full-thickness, transcerebral columns of gray matter that extend in continuity from the subependymal layer of the ventricle to the cortex. Gray matter lines the thin slits (or fan-shaped defects), which are filled with CSF.

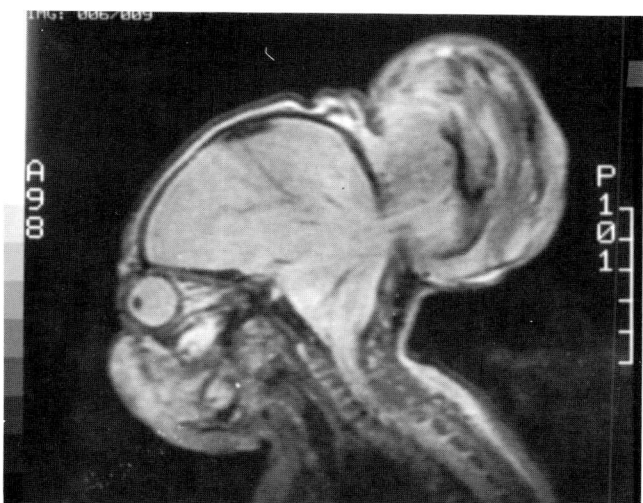

FIG SK40-1. Occipital encephalocele. Parasagittal MR image shows brain parenchyma that has herniated through a posterior calvarial defect. Although the protrusion contains a large vessel, represented by a linear signal void, it is difficult to identify possible ventricular structures because of distortion.[45]

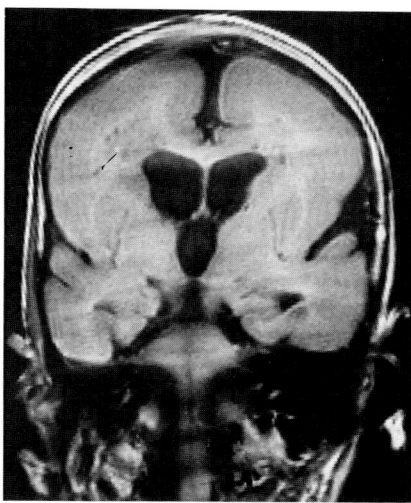

FIG SK40-2. Agyria.[46]

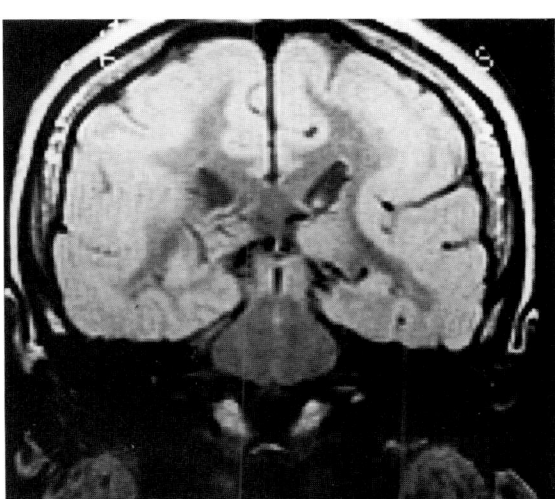

FIG SK40-3. Pachygyria. Coronal MR scan shows broad gyri, an abnormally thick cortex, and poor arborization of white matter.[46]

Condition	Imaging Findings	Comments
Other disorders of organogenesis		
Holoprosencephaly **(Fig SK40-6)**	Spectrum of complex patterns that, in the most severe form, includes a single ventricle and an array of facial deformities.	Complex developmental abnormality of the brain arising from failure of cleavage of the forebrain.
Septo-optic dysplasia **(Fig SK40-7)**	Absence of the septum pellucidum in 50% to 75% of patients. Other findings include flattening of the roof of the frontal horns, pointing of the floors of the lateral ventricles in coronal section, dilatation of the suprasellar cistern and anterior third ventricle, small optic nerves, and small optic chiasm.	Heterogeneous syndrome of optic nerve hypoplasia associated with pituitary/hypothalamic insufficiency (and other endocrine abnormalities) and often with an abnormal corpus callosum, fornix, and infundibulum.
Complete agenesis of the corpus callosum **(Fig SK40-8)**	Increased separation of the lateral ventricles, enlargement of the occipital horns and atria, and upward displacement of the third ventricle.	Although occasionally seen as an isolated lesion, agenesis of the corpus callosum frequently is associated with various other central nervous system malformations and syndromes. Partial agenesis of the corpus callosum may occur.
Lipoma of the corpus callosum **(see Fig SK40-8)**	Focal, midline, nearly symmetric mass of fat in the interhemispheric fissure, usually near the genu of the corpus callosum.	Although asymptomatic in about 10% of cases, most lipomas of the corpus callosum are associated with seizures, mental disturbance, paralysis, or headache. About half the patients have callosal agenesis.
Dandy-Walker malformation **(Fig SK40-9)**	Cystic mass in the posterior fossa associated with a defect in or agenesis of the vermis and separation of the cerebellar hemispheres.	Spectrum of disorders characterized by abnormal development of the cerebellum and fourth ventricle. Commonly associated with hydrocephalus.
Cerebellar aplasia/ hypoplasia **(Fig SK40-10)**	Partial absence of the vermis (usually the inferior lobules) and/or small size or partial absence of one or both cerebellar hemispheres.	Associated findings include absence or decreased size of the cerebellar peduncles (especially the brachium pontis), small size of the brainstem (especially the pons), and enlargement of the surrounding CSF spaces (fourth ventricle, vallecula, cisterna magna, and cerebellopontine angle cisterns).
Chiari malformations		
Chiari I **(Fig SK40-11)**	Caudal displacement of the cerebellar tonsils through the foramen magnum into the cervical spinal canal.	May be associated with hydromyelia (60% to 70%), hydrocephalus (20% to 25%), and basilar impression (25%). No association with myelomeningocele.
Chiari II **(Fig SK40-12)**	Common findings include protrusion of the brainstem downward through the foramen magnum into the upper cervical spinal canal, with the upper spinal cord being driven inferiorly and compacted along its long axis; kinking at the cervicomedullary junction; marked elongation of the fourth ventricle, which descends into the spinal canal along the posterior surface of the medulla; beaked tectum; and hydromyelia.	Complex anomaly affecting the calvarium, spinal column, dura, and hindbrain that is nearly always associated with myelomeningocele. Because of the low position of the medulla and upper spinal cord, the upper cervical nerve roots course upward to their exit foramina, and the lower cranial nerves arise from the medulla in the cervical spinal canal and ascend through the foramen magnum before turning downward to exit their normal foramina.
Chiari III **(Fig SK40-13)**	Herniation of brain contents through a bony defect involving the inferior occiput, foramen magnum, and posterior elements of the upper cervical vertebrae.	Cervico-occipital encephalocele containing nearly all the cerebellum. Variable amounts of brainstem, upper cervical cord, and meninges may be found in the posterior hernia sac.

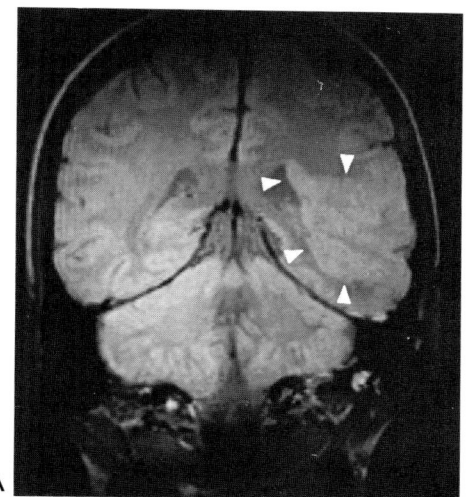
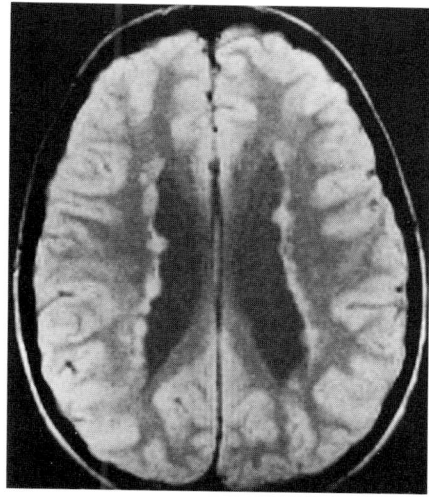

FIG SK40-4. **Heterotopia.** (A) Coronal scan shows hemiatrophy and a gray matter mass bridging from ventricular to cortical surfaces (arrowheads). The intensity of the abnormal bridge of tissue was the same as that of gray matter on all pulse sequences.[46] (B) Gray matter collections lining the subependymal regions of both lateral ventricles.[47]

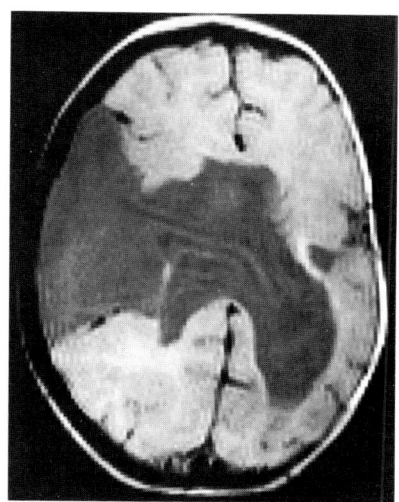
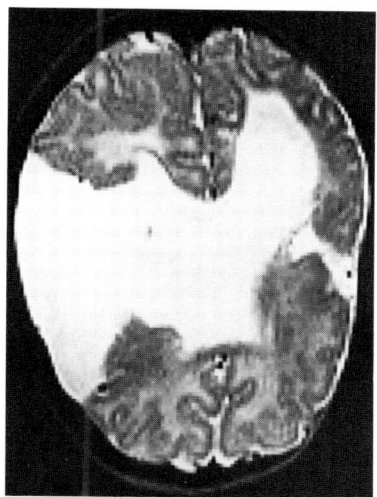

FIG SK40-5. **Schizencephaly.** (A) Proton-density and (B) T_2-weighted MR scans show bilateral full-thickness clefts (more marked on the right) that are lined by gray matter. Note the absence of the septum pellucidum.[46]

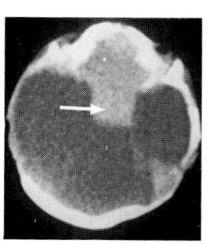
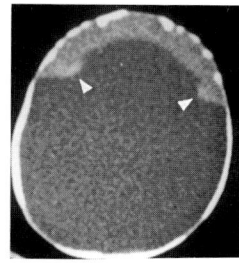

FIG SK40-6. **Holoprosencephaly.** Nonsequential transverse CT scans show a monoventricle with anteriorly fused thalami (arrow). There is absence of the interhemispheric fissure, third ventricle, and corpus callosum. A crescent-shaped anterior cerebral mantle represents the undivided prosencephalon, the posterior margin of which cannot be identified on the CT scan. The monoventricle is distorted by a large compression dorsal cyst, the anterior border of which is approximated by the hippocampal fornix (arrowheads).[45]

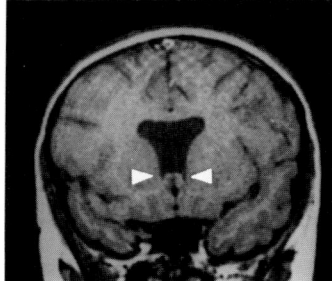

FIG SK40-7. Septo-optic dysplasia. Coronal T$_1$-weighted image shows absence of the septum pellucidum and squared-off frontal horns that have inferior points (arrowheads).[45]

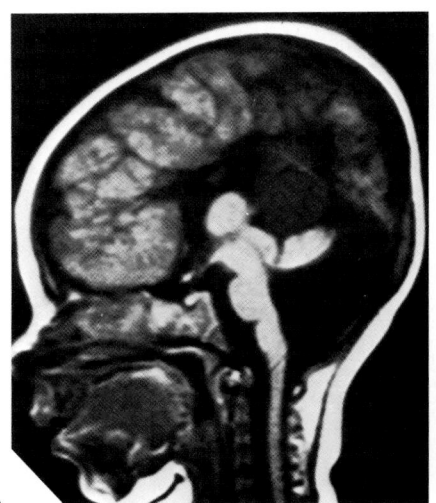
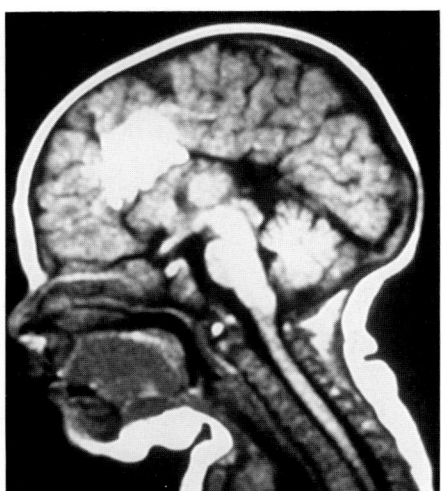

FIG SK40-8. Agenesis of the corpus callosum. (A) Associated findings include a posterior interhemispheric cyst and a Dandy-Walker cyst of the posterior fossa. (B) In this patient, there is a lipoma involving the anterior aspect of the interhemispheric region.[47]

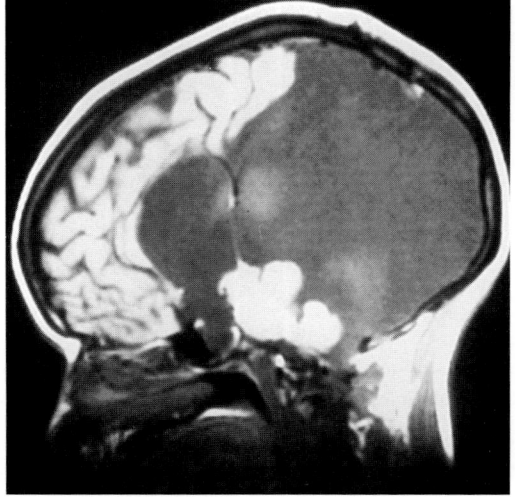
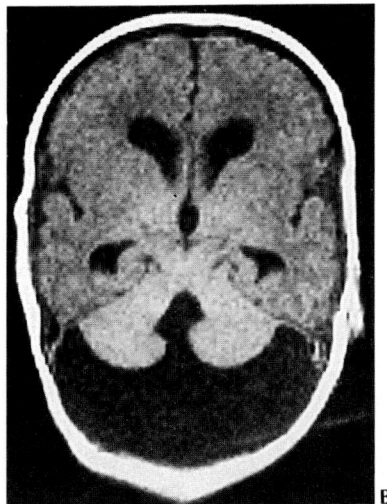

FIG SK40-9. Dandy-Walker malformation. (A) Sagittal and (B) axial[47] MR scans in two different patients show large posterior fossa cystic masses associated with agenesis of the vermis and separation of the cerebellar hemispheres.

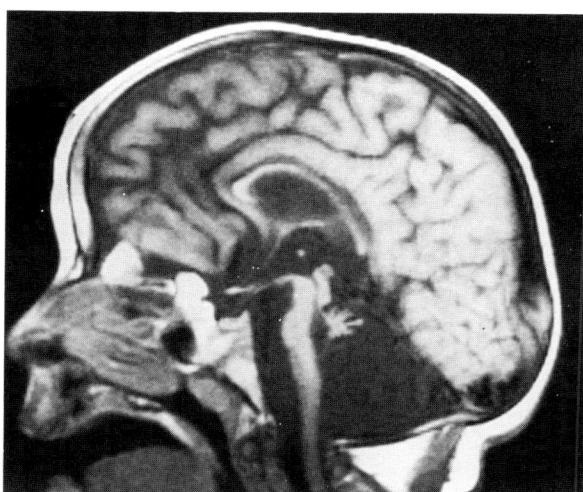

FIG SK40-10. Cerebellar hypoplasia. Sagittal MR scan shows almost total absence of the cerebellum except for a small portion of the superior vermis.[47]

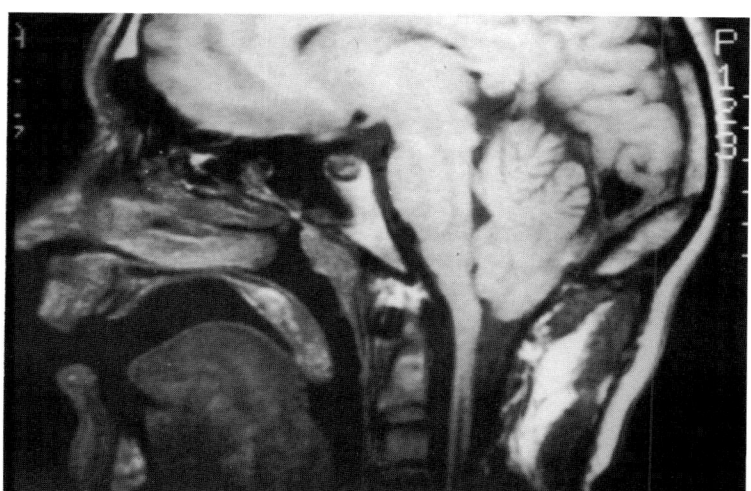

FIG SK40-11. Chiari I malformation. Caudal displacement of the cerebellar tonsils 15 mm below the foramen magnum. Note the associated hydromyelia.

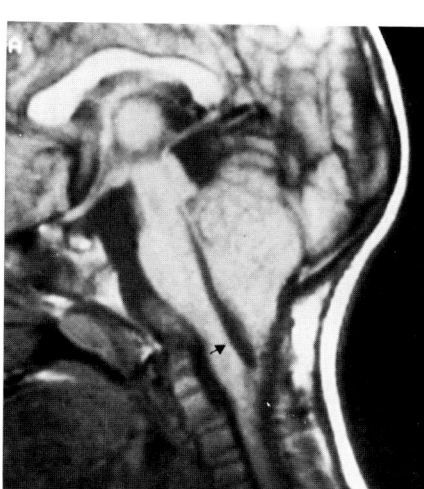

FIG SK40-12. Chiari II malformation. Markedly elongated and inferiorly displaced fourth ventricle (arrow).[47]

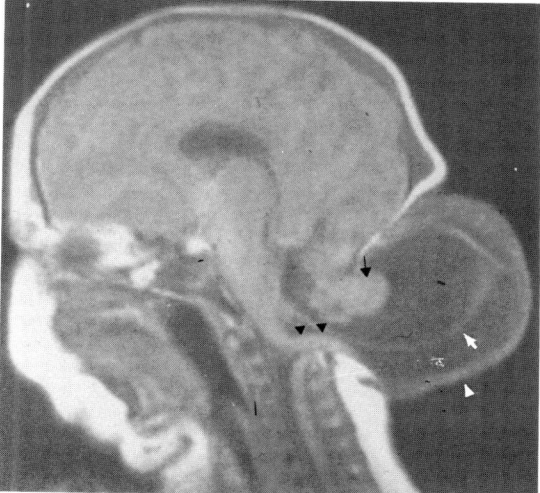

FIG SK40-13. Chiari III malformation with cervico-occipital encephalocele. Sagittal MR scan shows the bony defect involving the inferior occiput, foramen magnum, and posterior elements of C1 and C2 with herniation of the cerebellum (black arrow), dilated posterior aspect of the fourth ventricle (white arrow), brainstem, upper cervical cord (black arrowheads), and meninges (white arrowhead) into the posterior sac.[47]

Condition	Imaging Findings	Comments
Phakomatoses (neurocutaneous syndromes)		Hereditary developmental anomalies characterized by disordered histiogenesis with abnormal cell proliferation in the nervous system and skin.
Neurofibromatosis (Fig SK40-14)	Cranial nerve schwannomas (especially acoustic neuromas) that are often bilateral; meningiomas, frequently bilateral; optochiasmal gliomas (may be bilateral and affect the entire length of the visual apparatus); and cerebral hamartomas.	Autosomal dominant disorder characterized by dysplasia of neural ectodermal and mesodermal tissue. Other cerebral manifestations include orbital dysplasia, in which unilateral absence of a large part of the greater wing of the sphenoid and hypoplasia and elevation of the lesser wing result in a markedly widened superior orbital fissure; brainstem and supratentorial gliomas; arachnoid cysts; and vascular dysplasia with multiple infarctions.
Tuberous sclerosis (Bourneville's disease) (Fig SK40-15)	Cortical, subcortical, white matter, and subependymal tubers; small, round, calcified nodules along the lateral wall of the frontal horn and anterior third ventricle.	Inherited disorder in which the brain is typically involved with hyperplastic nodules of malformed glial-neuroglial tissue. Classic clinical triad of convulsive seizures, mental deficiency, and adenoma sebaceum. Giant cell astrocytoma develops in about 10% of patients; renal angiomyolipomas occur in about half. Large tumors or tubers may obstruct the aqueduct or ventricular foramina and produce hydrocephalus.
Sturge-Weber syndrome (encephalotrigeminal angiomatosis) (see Fig SK8-7)	Undulating parallel plaques of calcification in the brain cortex that appear to follow the cerebral convolutions and most often develop in the parieto-occipital area.	Congenital vascular anomaly in which a localized meningeal venous angioma occurs in conjunction with an ipsilateral facial angioma (port-wine nevus). Clinical findings include mental retardation, seizure disorders, and hemiatrophy and hemiparesis. Hemiatrophy leads to elevation of the base of the skull and enlargement and increased aeration of the ipsilateral mastoid air cells.

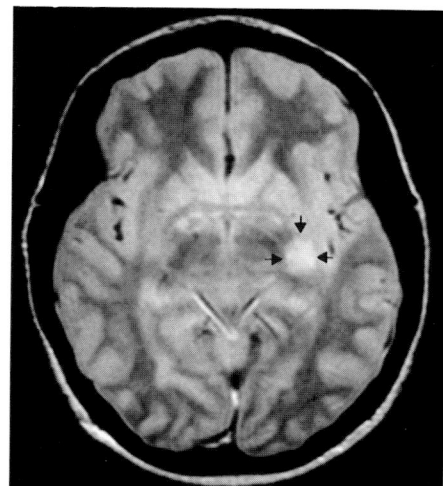

FIG SK40-14. Neurofibromatosis with hamartoma (arrows).

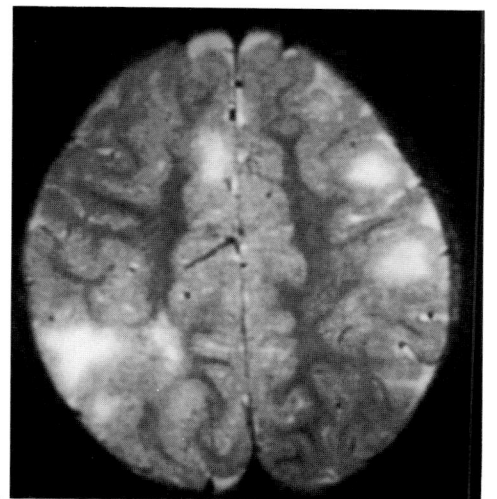

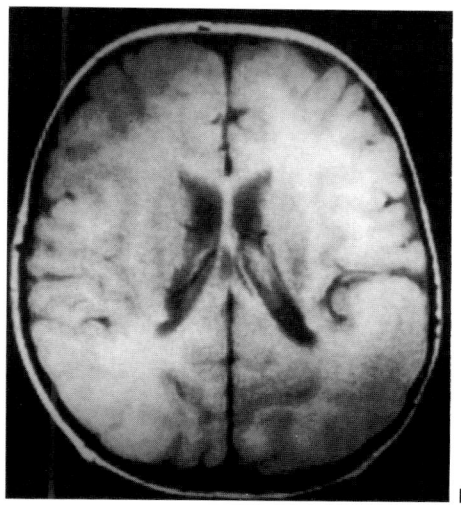

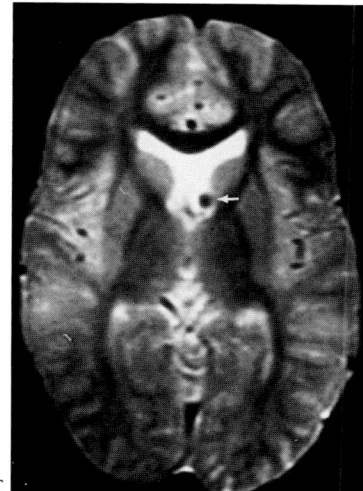

FIG SK40-15. Tuberous sclerosis. (A) High-signal tubers involving both gray and white matter. (B) Multiple, irregular impressions on the lateral ventricles caused by subependymal tubers. (C) Calcified tuber in the wall of the frontal horn producing a signal void (arrow).

MIDLINE CONGENITAL ANOMALIES ON ULTRASONOGRAPHY

Condition	Imaging Findings	Comments
Vein of Galen malformation (Fig SK41-1)	Large, fluid-filled structure that lies between the lateral ventricles and can be followed posteriorly into the straight sinus and the torcular Herophili.	Arteriovenous malformation resulting from failure of the normal embryonic arteriovenous shunts to be replaced by capillaries. Doppler studies can confirm the markedly increased flow in the lesion and permit differentiation of this dilated vessel from a cyst.
Chiari II malformation (Fig SK41-2)	Caudal displacement of the cerebellum and a narrowed and elongated fourth ventricle. Enlarged massa intermedia and often dilation of the third and lateral ventricles.	Complex anomaly affecting the calvarium, spinal column, dura, and hindbrain that is nearly always associated with myelomeningocele. Hydromyelia commonly occurs.
Dandy-Walker syndrome (Fig SK41-3)	Posterior fossa cyst (representing the ballooned fourth ventricle) and partial or complete absence of the vermis with separation of the cerebellar hemispheres.	Occasionally, an arachnoid cyst or an elongated cisterna magna may mimic the Dandy-Walker syndrome, but in these former conditions the vermis and cerebellum are normal. Hydrocephalus may be apparent at birth or develop later.

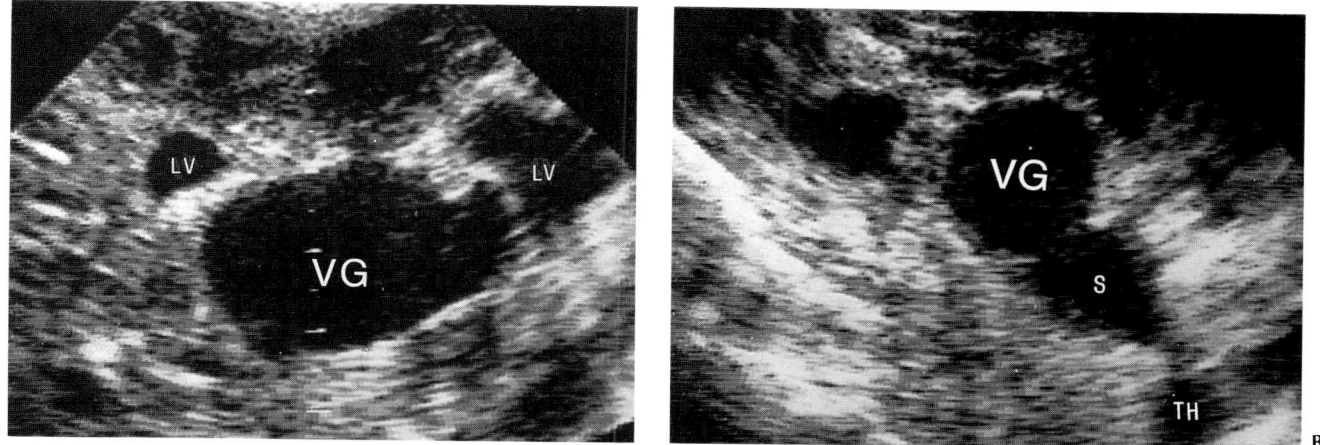

Fig SK41-1. Vein of Galen malformation. (A) Coronal sonogram shows the large vein of Galen (VG) lying between the dilated lateral ventricles (LV). Note the parenchymal atrophy, seen as hypoechoic areas above the vein of Galen. (B) On the sagittal image, the dilated vein of Galen can be followed posteriorly into the straight sinus (S) and the torcular Herophili (TH).[48]

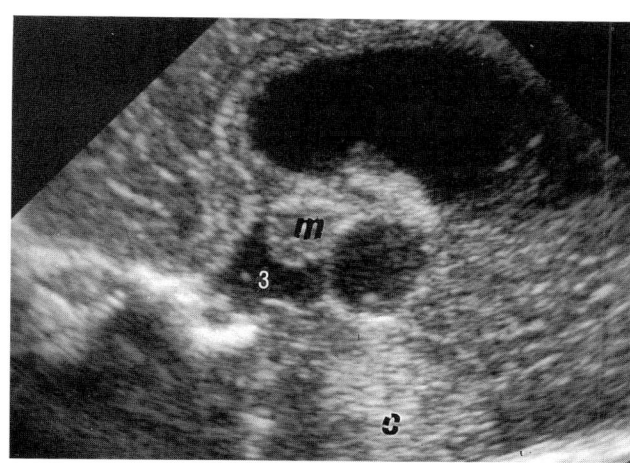

Fig SK41-2. Chiari II malformation. Sagittal sonogram shows the cerebellum (C) and fourth ventricle situated low in the posterior fossa and obliteration of the cisterna magna. An enlarged massa intermedia (M) partially fills the third ventricle (3).[48]

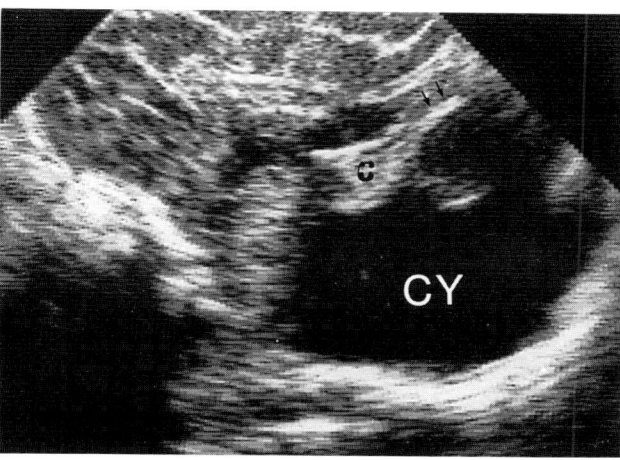

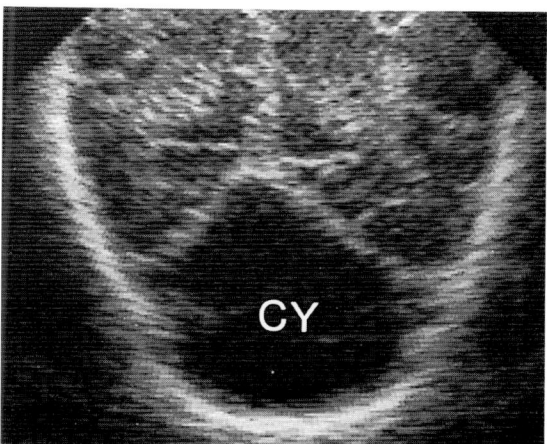

Fig SK41-3. Dandy-Walker syndrome. (A) Sagittal sonogram demonstrates such characteristic features as a posterior fossa cyst (CY) representing the ballooned fourth ventricle and partial or complete absence of the vermis. The often huge cyst displaces the cerebellum (C) and tentorium (arrows) superiorly. (B) Posterior coronal image shows the large cyst (CY) filling the posterior fossa.[48]

Condition	Imaging Findings	Comments
Dandy-Walker variant **(Fig SK41-4)**	Large posterior fossa cyst connected to a partially formed fourth ventricle by a narrow vallecula. The inferior vermis is absent, and the cerebellum is often hypoplastic.	When the separation between the cerebellar hemispheres is very narrow (slitlike), a CT, MR, or ultrasound scan through the posterior fossa is required to establish the communication of the cyst with the fourth ventricle.
Agenesis of the corpus callosum **(Fig SK41-5)**	Increased separation of the lateral ventricles. Enlargement of the occipital horns and atria. Upward displacement of the third ventricle.	Although occasionally seen as an isolated lesion, agenesis of the corpus callosum is frequently associated with various other central nervous system malformations and syndromes.
Lipoma of the corpus callosum **(Fig SK41-6)**	Focal echogenic mass of fat in the interhemispheric fissure, usually near the genu.	About half the patients with lipomas have absence of the corpus callosum, with the echogenic mass lying just above an elevated third ventricle.
Holoprosencephaly **(Fig SK41-7)**	Spectrum of complex patterns that, in the most severe form (alobar), includes a single ventricle and an array of facial deformities.	Complex developmental abnormality of the brain resulting from failure of cleavage of the forebrain into cerebral hemispheres and lateral ventricles.

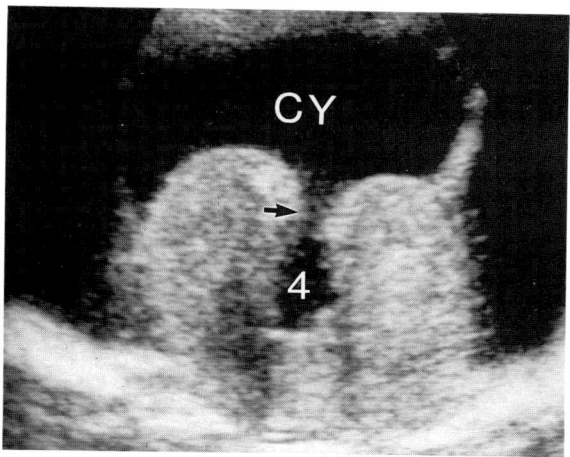

FIG SK41-4. Dandy-Walker variant. Sonogram through the posterior fontanelle demonstrates a large cyst (CY) and fourth ventricle (4), connected by a narrow vallecula (arrowhead).[48]

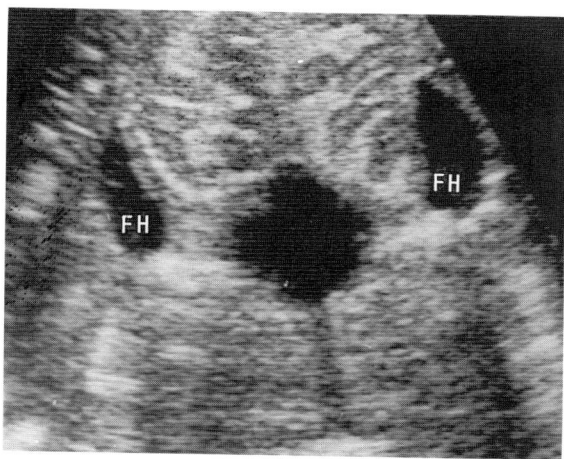

FIG SK41-5. Agenesis of corpus callosum. Coronal sonogram shows separation of the frontal horns (FH), which have concave medial borders.[48]

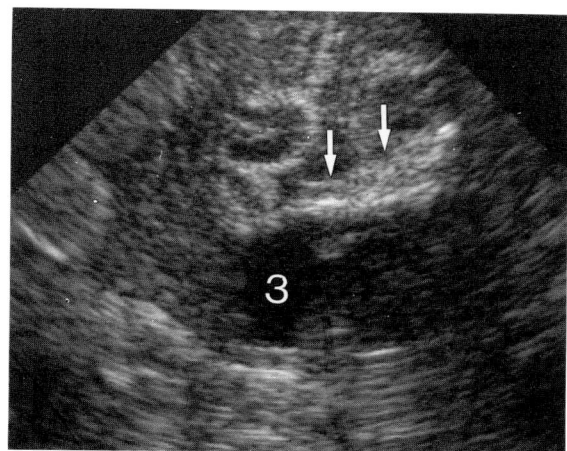

FIG SK41-6. Intracerebral lipoma with absent corpus callosum. Coronal sonogram shows an echogenic area (arrows) superior and to the left of the elevated third ventricle (3).[48]

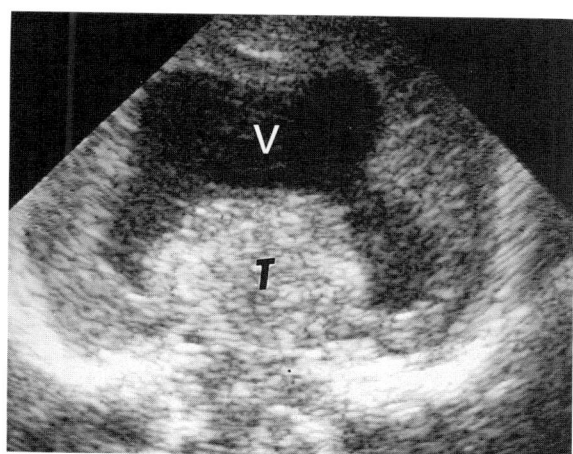

FIG SK41-7. Alobar holoprosencephaly. Posterior coronal sonogram demonstrates the single ventricle (V) and the fused thalami (T).[48]

CENTRAL NERVOUS SYSTEM CHANGES IN ACQUIRED IMMUNODEFICIENCY SYNDROME

Condition	Imaging Findings	Comments
Focal lesions **Toxoplasmosis** **(Figs SK42-1 and SK42-2)**	Single or multiple ring-enhancing lesions. Most commonly located at the corticomedullary junction and in the basal ganglia and white matter. Variable amount of peripheral edema.	This protozoan is the most common opportunistic infection in AIDS patients. Early in their development, the lesions may show more homogeneous enhancement with little mass effect or edema.
Cryptococcosis **(Figs SK42-3 and SK42-4)**	Initially, imaging studies may be negative or show only mild ventricular dilatation. Chronic relapsing infection can result in a parenchymal abscess and meningeal enhancement.	Most common fungal infection of the central nervous system in AIDS. Pathologically, a granulomatous meningitis is the most common manifestation.
Other infections **(Fig SK42-5)**	Single or multiple enhancing lesions.	Herpes simplex encephalitis, tuberculosis, candidiasis, aspergillosis, and bacterial infections.
Lymphoma **(Fig SK42-6)**	Single or multiple masses that often show central necrosis and ring enhancement. Favored sites include the deep white matter of the frontal and parietal lobes, basal ganglia, and hypothalamus.	Lymphoma in AIDS patients has a higher incidence of multiplicity and aggressive behavior. The lesions are frequently found close to the corpus callosum and tend to cross the midline into the opposite hemisphere, a feature that mimics glioblastoma. Unlike glioblastoma and metastases, lymphomas often are associated with only a relatively mild amount of peritumoral edema and mass effect.
Kaposi's sarcoma	Nonspecific enhancing lesion(s).	Rare direct involvement of the brain cannot be distinguished from other masses. Almost all AIDS patients with Kaposi's sarcoma have visible skin lesions.

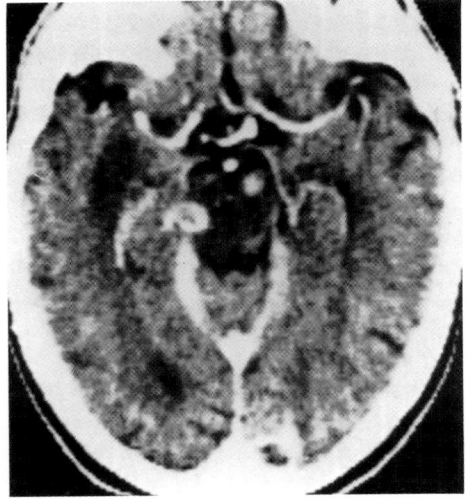

FIG SK42-1. **Toxoplasmosis.** Contrast-enhanced CT scan shows multiple small areas of ring and solid enhancement in the region of the cerebral peduncles and pons. A small round area of enhancement is seen in the left occipital lobe.[49]

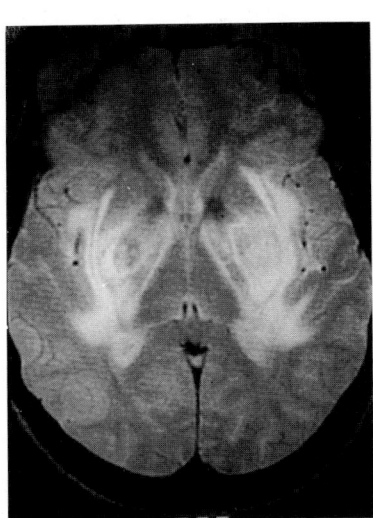

FIG SK42-2. **Toxoplasmosis.** Axial T$_2$-weighted MR scan shows bilateral low-signal masses in the basal ganglia surrounded by extensive edema.

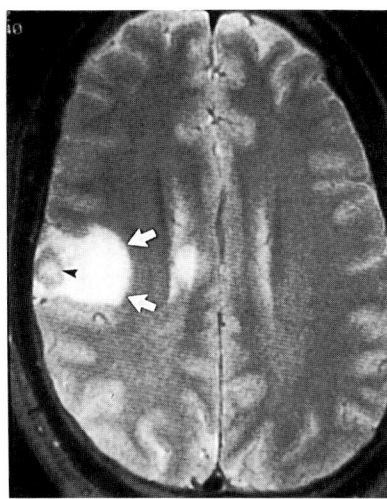

FIG **SK42-3. Cryptococcosis.** Axial T$_2$-weighted MR scan shows a relatively isointense peripheral mass (black arrowheads) with prominent surrounding edema (white arrows).

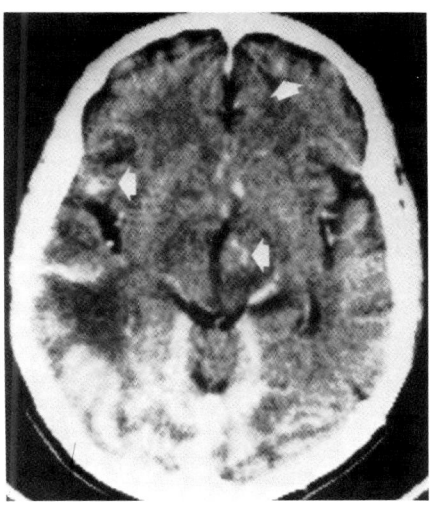

FIG **SK42-4. Cryptococcal meningitis.** Contrast-enhanced CT scan shows dense enhancement of the free edge of the tentorium and prominent enhancement of meninges in the right temporal and both occipital regions. Scattered focal intracerebral areas of enhancement (arrows) were thought to be caused by cryptococcal granulomas.[49]

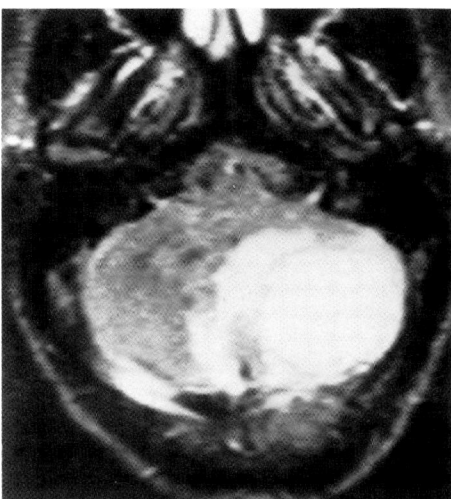

FIG **SK42-5. Streptococcal abscess.** T$_2$-weighted MR scan shows a well-defined, slightly lobulated mass in the left cerebellum. The margin of the abscess has a rim of decreased signal intensity, and there is moderate surrounding edema.[49]

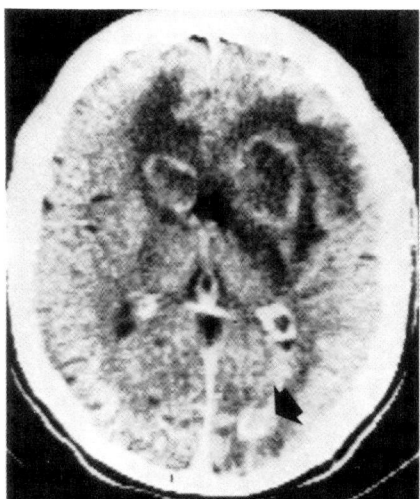

FIG **SK42-6. Lymphoma.** Contrast-enhanced CT scan shows large, bilateral areas of enhancement with surrounding edema in the basal ganglia bilaterally. Another lesion is seen in the left occipital pole (arrow).[49]

Condition	Imaging Findings	Comments
Diffuse atrophy or white matter disease		
Progressive multifocal leukoencephalopathy (PML) (Fig SK42-7)	Round or oval lesions that become larger and more confluent and are often asymmetric. No enhancement or mass effect.	Reactivation of a latent papovavirus in the immunocompromised host that initially tends to involve the subcortical white matter and later spreads to the deeper white matter. The high signal on T_2-weighted MR scans is related to both demyelination and edema.
HIV infection (Fig SK42-8)	Ill-defined, diffuse or confluent patches of abnormal signal intensity without mass effect in the deep white matter of the cerebral hemispheres.	HIV encephalopathy is a progressive subcortical dementia attributed to direct infection of the central nervous system with the virus rather than to an opportunistic infection. Developing in up to 60% of AIDS cases, it typically produces bilateral but not always symmetric lesions that characteristically do not involve the gray matter.
Cytomegalovirus (Fig SK42-9)	Abnormal signal intensity in the ependymal and subependymal regions.	The periventricular changes are better demonstrated on T_1-weighted and proton-density images because on T_2-weighted images the abnormal areas of increased signal intensity may not be clearly differentiated from the normal signal of CSF.

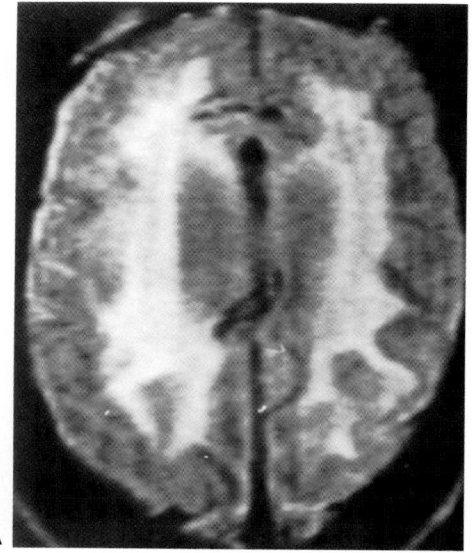
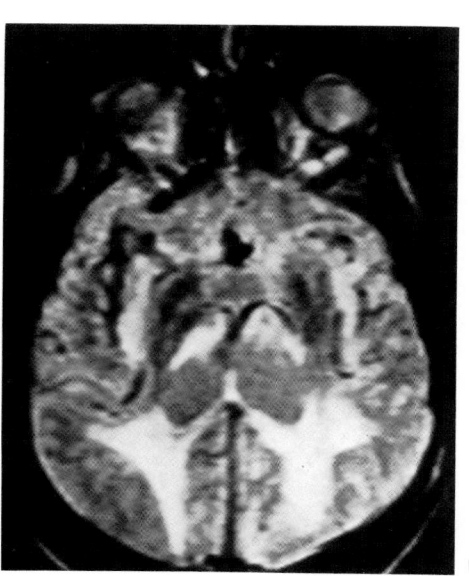

A

B

FIG SK42-7. Progressive multifocal leukoencephalopathy. (A) Initial T_2-weighted MR scan shows irregularly marginated areas of increased signal intensity in the region of the centrum semiovale bilaterally. There is no mass effect, but severe atrophy is seen. (B) Repeat study 3 months later shows progression of the white matter abnormalities, especially in the occipital region.[50]

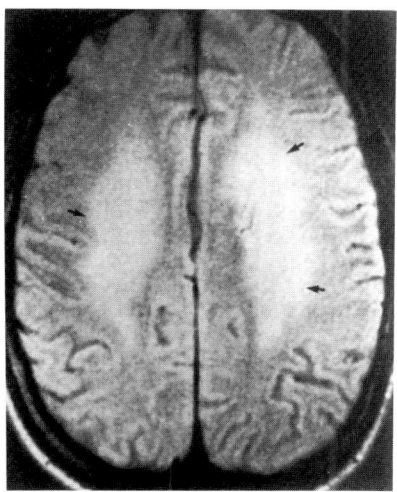

FIG SK42-8. HIV encephalitis. Axial proton-density MR image shows symmetric regions of abnormally increased signal intensity without mass effect in the centrum semiovale bilaterally (arrows).[50]

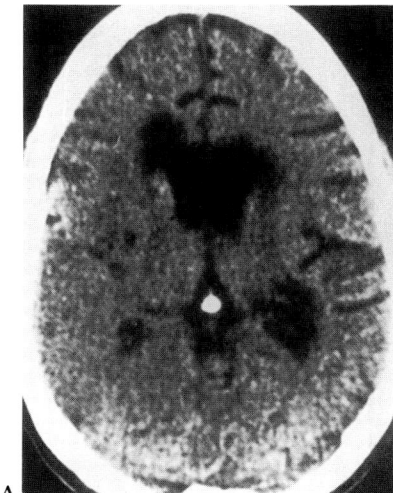

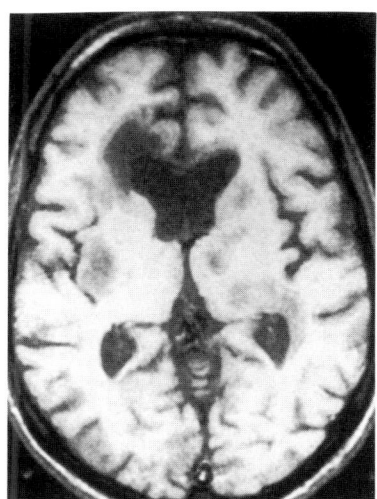

FIG SK42-9. Cytomegalovirus ventriculitis. (A) Nonenhanced CT scan and (B) T_1-weighted MR scan show bilateral periventricular areas of decreased attenuation/signal intensity, which is most marked near the right frontal horn. Note additional bilateral lesions in the basal ganglia.[50]

THICKENING OF THE OPTIC NERVE

Condition	Comments
Optic nerve glioma (Figs SK43-1 and SK43-2)	Most common cause of optic nerve enlargement. Typically causes uniform thickening of the nerve with mild undulation or lobulation. In children (especially preadolescent girls), optic nerve gliomas are usually hamartomas that spontaneously stop enlarging and require no treatment. In older patients, however, these gliomas may have a progressive malignant course despite surgical or radiation therapy. Optic nerve gliomas are a common manifestation of neurofibromatosis (typically low-grade lesions that act more like hyperplasia than neoplasms).
Optic nerve sheath meningioma (Fig SK43-3)	Most commonly occurs in middle-aged women and typically has a greater density, greater enhancement, and less homogeneous appearance than optic nerve gliomas. Other CT features include sphenoid bone hyperostosis and calcification, either eccentric when the tumor is polypoid or on both sides of the optic nerve with a tramline appearance when the tumor circumferentially surrounds the nerve.
Cyst of optic nerve sheath (Fig SK43-4)	Cystic dilatation of the optic nerve sheath produces a mass that is less dense than a meningioma. May develop after irradiation of an optic nerve glioma.

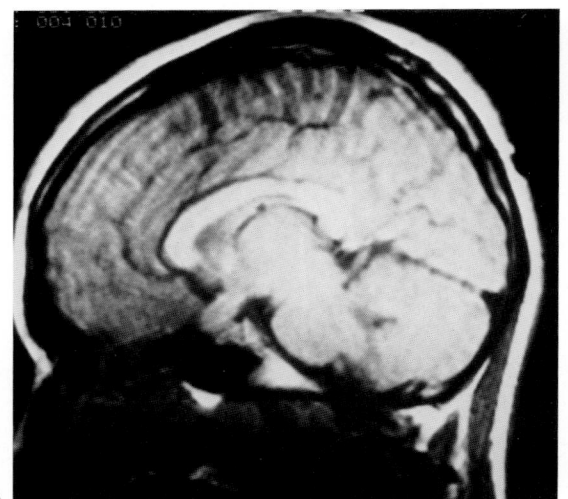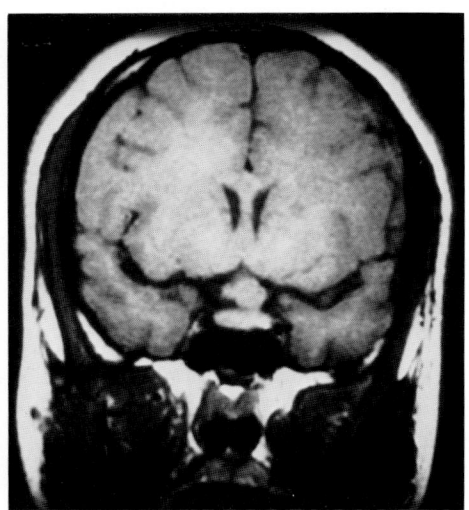

FIG SK43-1. Optic nerve glioma. (A) Sagittal and (B) coronal T₁-weighted MR scans show involvement of the chiasm and left optic nerve.

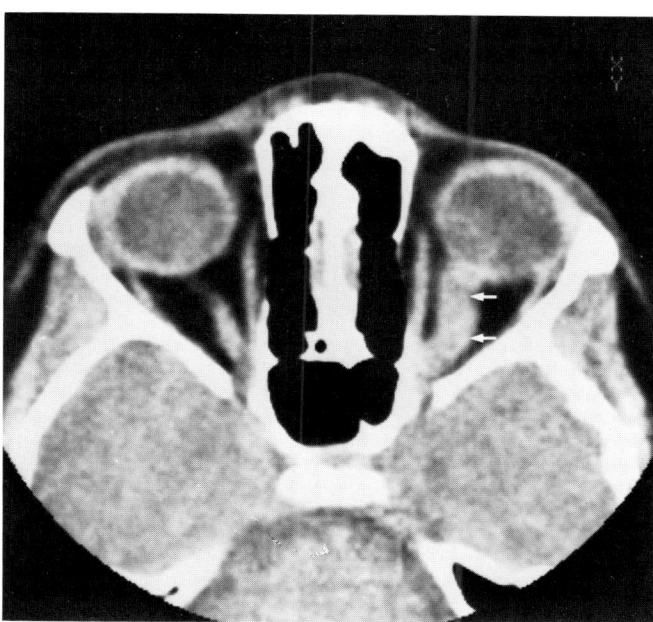

FIG SK43-2. Optic nerve glioma. Diffuse enlargement of the left optic nerve (arrows) in an 8-year-old girl.[13]

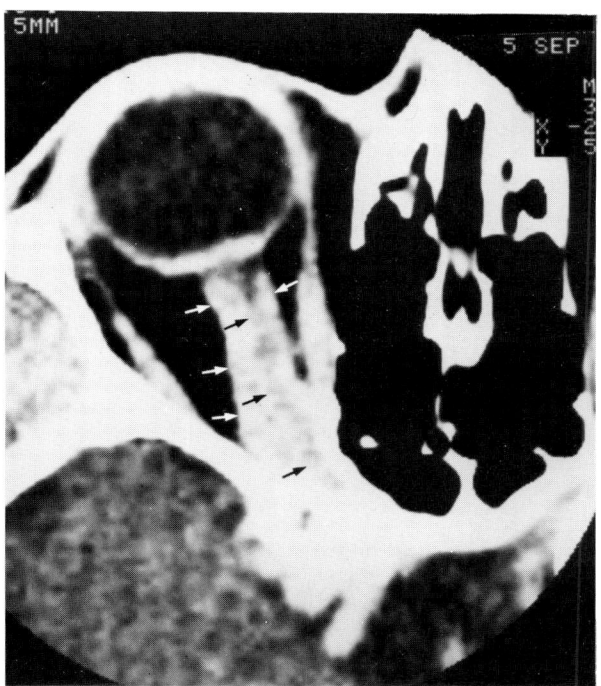

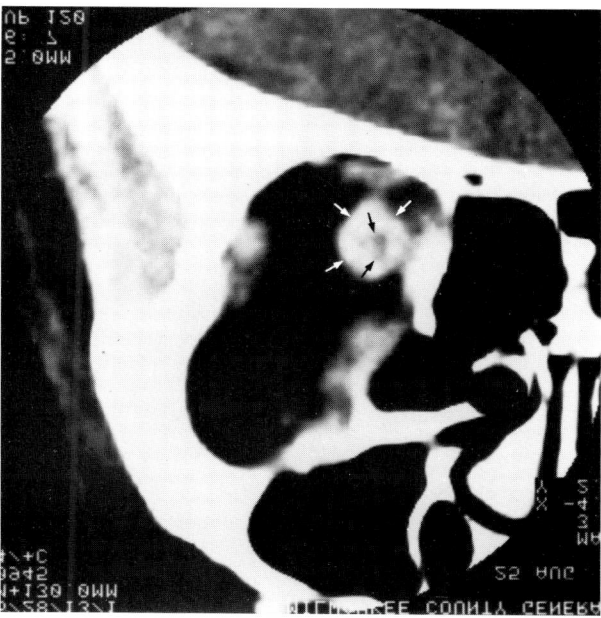

FIG SK43-3. Optic nerve sheath meningioma. (A) Axial scan shows the enhancing tumor (white arrows) along the entire length of the intraorbital optic nerve (black arrows). Note the intracranial portion of the tumor. (B) Coronal scan demonstrates the meningioma (white arrows) surrounding the optic nerve.[13]

Condition	Comments
Optic neuritis	General term referring to thickening of the optic nerve developing from such nonneoplastic processes as multiple sclerosis, infection, ischemia (occlusion of vessels at the anterior portion of the optic nerve associated with temporal arteritis), and degenerative changes resulting from toxic, metabolic, or nutritional factors. After steroid therapy, enlargement of the optic nerve usually resolves.

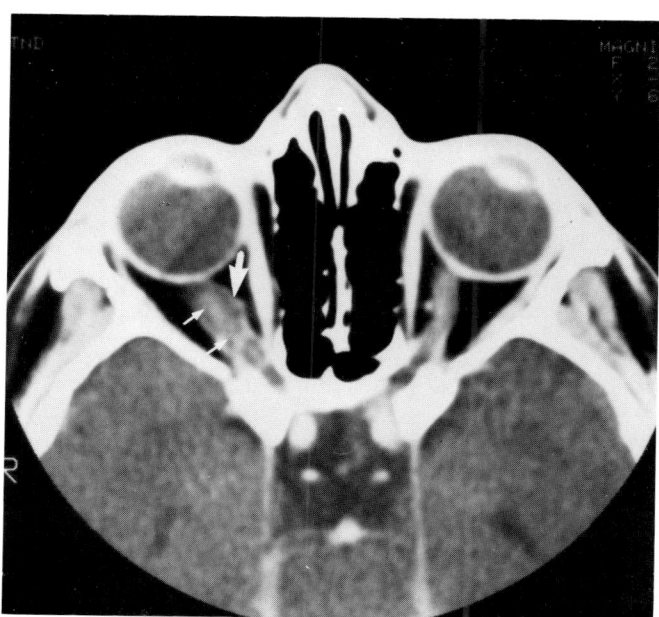

FIG SK43-4. **Cyst of optic nerve sheath.** Large, smoothly marginated retrobulbar mass (arrows) that produced proptosis in this 43-year-old man.[13]

ORBITAL MASSES NOT INVOLVING THE OPTIC NERVE

Condition	Imaging Findings	Comments
Predominantly intraconal masses		
Cavernous hemangioma (Fig SK44-1)	Well-defined intraconal mass that typically occurs lateral to the optic nerve. On CT, the mass is of high density and shows homogeneous contrast enhancement. Calcifications commonly occur, and the lesion may expand bone.	Most common benign orbital neoplasm in adults. They frequently occur in childhood, may cause proptosis, and may be associated with skin or conjunctival lesions. An identical imaging pattern can be seen with the less common lymphangiomas.
Orbital varix (Fig SK44-2)	Fusiform or globular mass that often occurs near the orbital apex. On MRI, high flow usually results in signal void on all imaging sequences, although heterogeneous or even high signal intensity may be seen on T_2-weighted images as a result of turbulent or slow flow, respectively.	Classic history of intermittent exophthalmos associated with crying or coughing. These lesions may be extremely difficult to diagnose because the varix may expand intermittently and not be obvious unless the venous pressure is increased during a Valsalva maneuver.
Orbital pseudotumor (Fig SK44-3)	Most commonly proptosis with no intraorbital abnormality other than a slight increase in fat density. The next most common appearance on CT is diffuse, irregular increased density of the orbital soft tissues with variable contrast enhancement. This nonfocal process tends to involve both intraconal and extraconal regions and obliterates the usual soft-tissue density differences between muscle and fat. Least frequently, there may be a more sharply marginated focal mass that cannot be differentiated from a true neoplasm.	Nonspecific inflammation of orbital tissues that accounts for about 25% of all cases of unilateral exophthalmos. The condition can be remitting or chronic and progressive and may regress spontaneously or respond to steroids. The infiltrative process predominantly involves the tissues immediately behind the globe. On MRI, this chronic inflammatory process usually has low signal on both T_1- and T_2-weighted images, unlike the high signal on T_2-weighted images seen with most other orbital lesions.

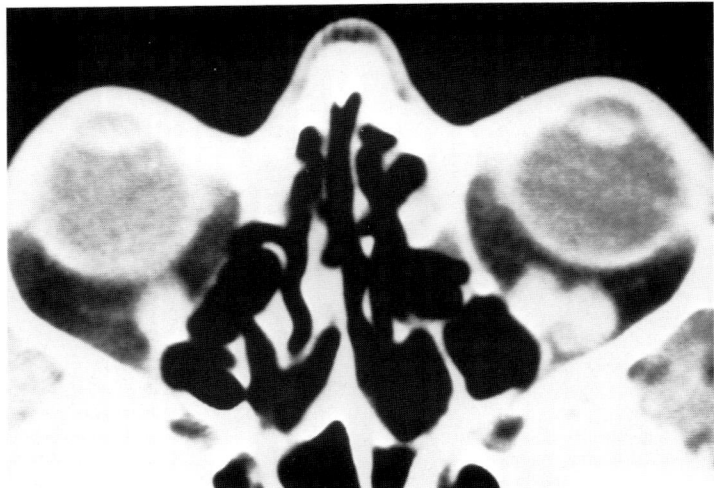

FIG SK44-1. Cavernous hemangioma. Contrast-enhanced CT scan shows a typical homogeneous enhancing intraconal mass.[51]

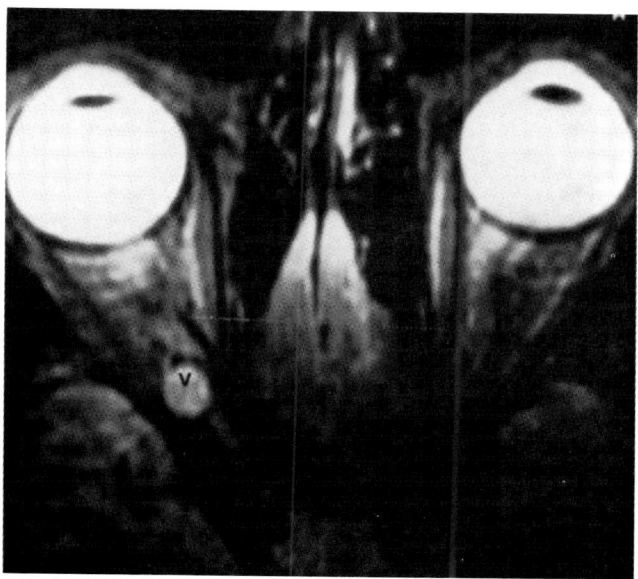

FIG SK44-2. Orbital varix. T_2W MRI scan shows round, hyperintense mass compatible with surgically proved orbital varix (V).[8] •

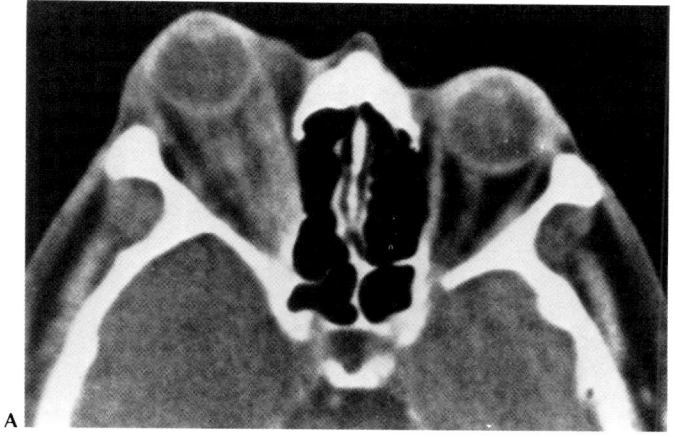

A

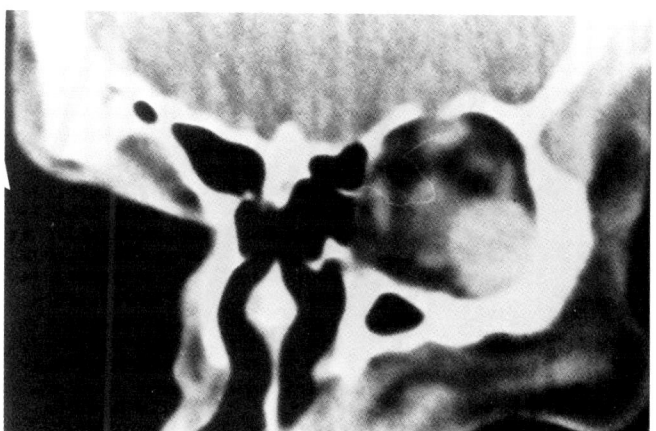

B

FIG SK44-3. Orbital pseudotumor. (A) Axial enhanced CT scan shows a typical poorly defined intraconal mass on the right with marked proptosis.[8] (B) Less common appearance of a focal pseudotumor, predominantly extraconal, in the inferolateral aspect of the right orbit associated with mild proptosis.[8] (C) Proton-density MR scan shows an ill-defined region of relatively low signal intensity behind the globe.

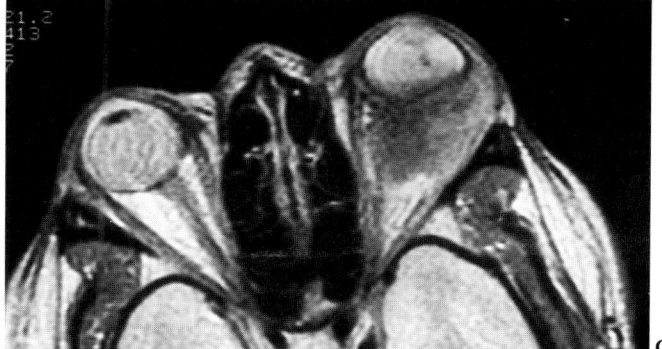

C

Condition	Imaging Findings	Comments
Predominantly extraconal masses **Extension from adjacent structures** Orbital cellulitis/ abscess (Fig SK44-4)	Preseptal cellulitis produces a soft-tissue mass with swelling of the anterior orbital tissues and obliteration of the fat planes. Extension of infection across the fibrous orbital septum into the posterior compartment of the orbit causes edema of the orbital fat and subsequent development of a more discrete mass as the infectious process proceeds.	Acute bacterial infection most often extending from the paranasal sinuses or eyelid. The orbits are predisposed to infections because (1) they are surrounded by the paranasal sinuses that are commonly infected, (2) the thin lamina papyracea offers little resistance to an aggressive process in the ethmoid sinuses, and (3) the veins of the face have no valves and thus serve as another pathway for extension of inflammation into the orbit. In most cases, the cellulitis is confined to the extraconal space; if left untreated, however, it can enter the muscle cone and the intraconal space.
Mucocele (Fig SK44-5)	Paranasal sinus mass that may break through bone and extend into the orbit. On MRI, a mucocele typically has high signal on both T_1- and T_2-weighted images.	Complication of inflammatory disease that probably reflects obstruction of the ostium of the sinus and the accumulation of mucous secretions. Primarily involves the frontal sinuses (65%). About 25% affect the ethmoid sinuses and 10% the maxillary sinuses.
Direct extension of neoplasm (Figs SK44-6 and SK44-7)	Extraorbital mass with extension into the orbit. MRI and CT can define the degree of soft-tissue extension into the orbit; the latter can demonstrate bony destruction.	Neoplasms include carcinomas of the sinuses and nasal cavity, angiofibromas of the pterygopalatine fossa, meningiomas of the floor of the anterior or middle cranial fossa, basal cell carcinomas of the skin, and primary and secondary tumors of the bony orbital wall.

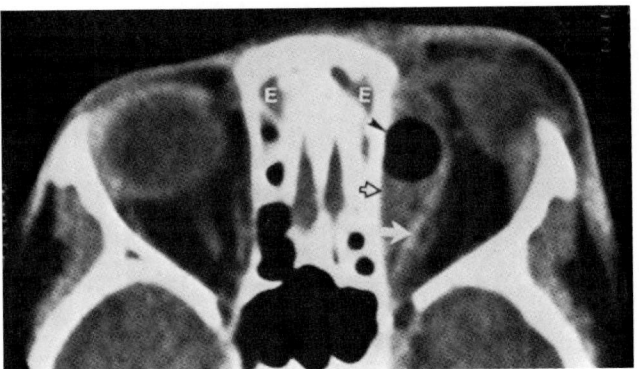

FIG SK44-4. **Orbital subperiosteal abscess.** CT scan shows proptosis of left eye with mucosal thickening of ethmoid air cells (E), with subperiosteal abscess (hollow-arrow). Note air bubble (arrowhead) within abscess and swollen left medial rectus muscle (arrow).[8]

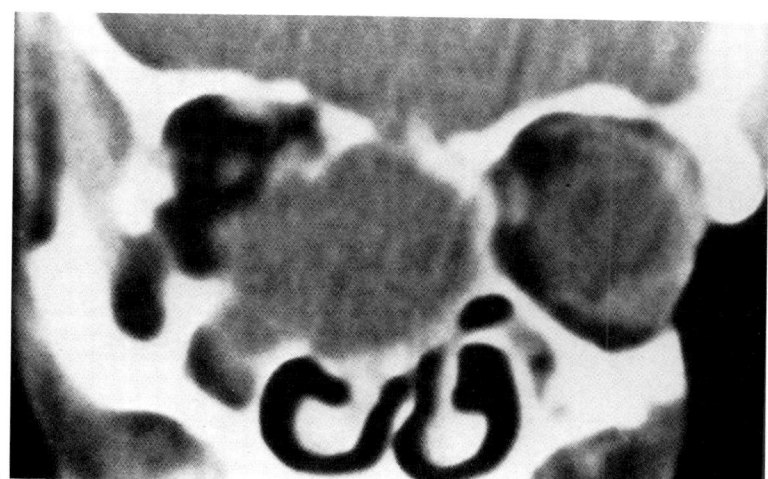

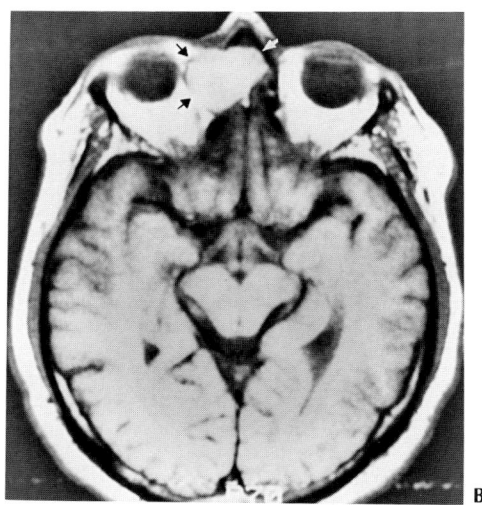

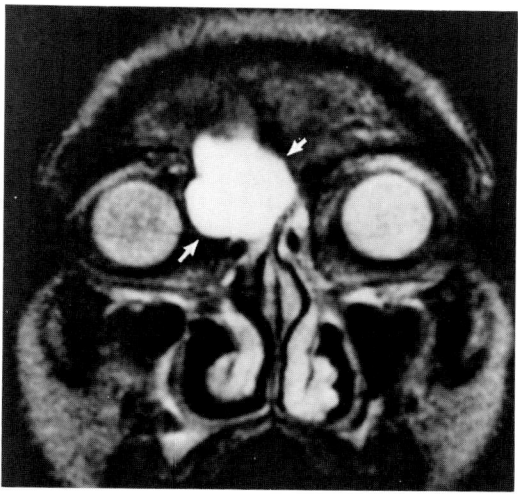

FIG SK44-5. Mucocele. (A) CT scan shows benign expansion of bone by a sharply marginated, lucent, nonenhanced ethmoid mass that has extended into the medial aspect of the right orbit by eroding the lamina papyracea.[8] (B) In another patient, a T_1-weighted MR image shows an expansile, hyperintense abnormality of the anterior ethmoids bilaterally that is greater on the right (arrows).[52] (C) T_2-weighted MR image shows greater signal hyperintensity in the mucocele (arrows) and involvement of the lower right frontal sinus.[52]

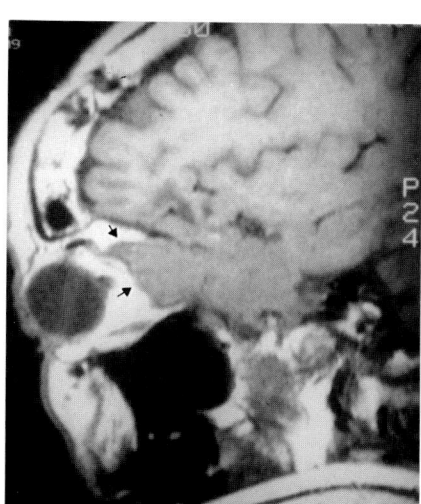

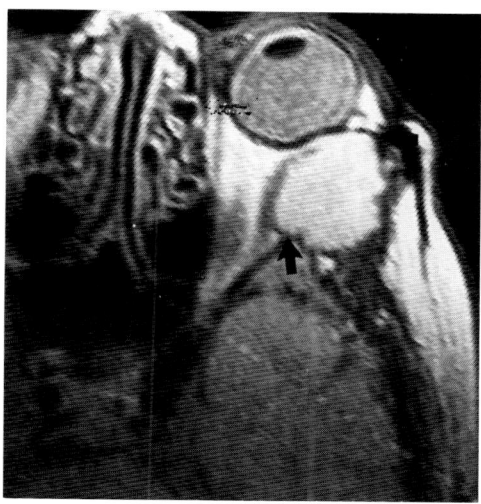

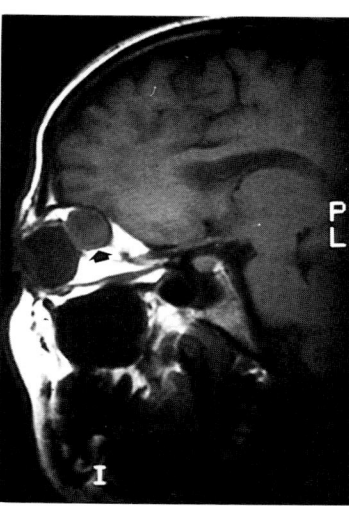

FIG SK44-6. Meningioma. MR image shows a large mass virtually isointense to brain that arose from the planum sphenoidale and extended into the posterior aspect of the orbit (arrows).

FIG SK44-7. Adenoid cystic carcinoma. MR scan shows an ill-defined mass (arrow) invading the lateral rectus muscle and breaking through the lateral wall of the orbit.[51]

FIG SK44-8. Hematogenous metastasis. Well-circumscribed retrobulbar mass (arrow).

Condition	Imaging Findings	Comments
Hematogenous metastases (Fig SK44-8)	Well- or ill-defined masses that are most frequently extraconal, although they may extend into the intraconal region.	Orbital metastases occur in about 10% of patients with generalized malignancy. Primary tumors that most frequently metastasize to the orbit are lung and breast cancers; in children, orbital metastases are seen in 50% of patients with neuroblastoma.
Benign bone lesions	Typically have low signal on all MR sequences.	Osteoma (especially in patients with Gardner's syndrome) and fibrous dysplasia (frequently involves the superolateral aspect of the orbit).
Lacrimal gland tumors (Fig SK44-9)	Soft-tissue mass in the superolateral aspect of the orbit with proptosis and downward displacement of the globe.	About half of primary lacrimal gland masses are of epithelial origin, being equally divided between benign mixed adenomas and carcinomas (most frequently adenoid cystic carcinomas). The remaining 50% include lymphoid lesions, such as dacryoadenitis and pseudotumors. Malignant lacrimal gland lesions generally are more poorly defined and demonstrate invasion of surrounding tissues.
Dacryocystitis	Well-defined, homogeneous mass of fluid intensity in the inferomedial part of the orbit.	Dilatation of the nasolacrimal sac as a result of obstruction or inflammation.
Dermoid cyst (Fig SK44-10)	Well-circumscribed mass that may displace but not infiltrate adjacent structures. Characteristic fat-fluid level is often seen on MRI. May appear as homogeneous high signal on both T_1- and T_2-weighted images.	Congenital lesion arising from epithelial rests that typically presents as painless proptosis and a palpable mass in the upper orbit. The presence of fat excludes most other orbital neoplasms; the dependent fluid excludes lipoma.
Epidermoid cyst	Sharply marginated mass.	Like other extraconal masses, an epidermoid cyst typically has low signal on T_1-weighted images and high signal on T_2-weighted images.
Lymphoma (Fig SK44-11)	Intraconal or extraconal mass that usually has ill-defined margins and may show invasion of surrounding structures.	As with most orbital lesions, lymphomas typically have low signal on T_1-weighted images and high signal on T_2-weighted images.

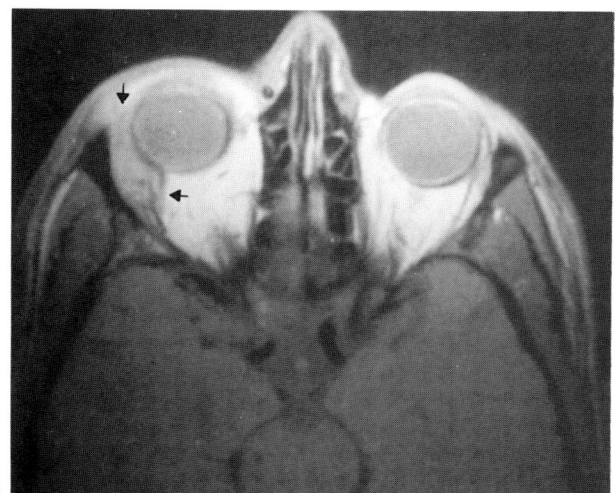
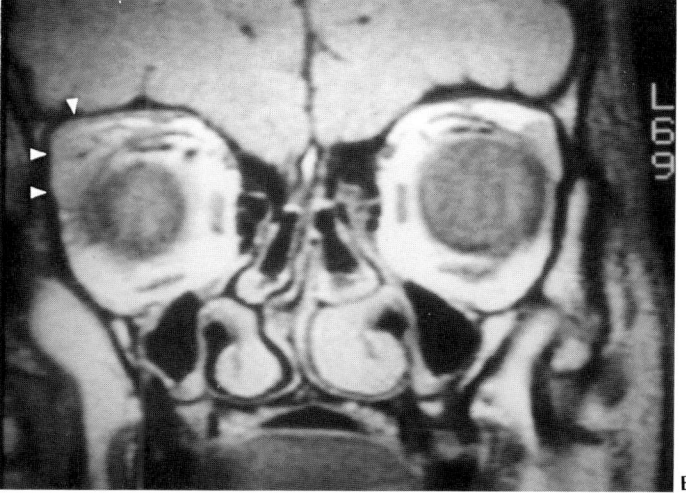

Fig SK44-9. Lacrimal gland tumor. (A) Coronal and (B) axial MR scans show the mass in the superolateral aspect of the right orbit (arrows).

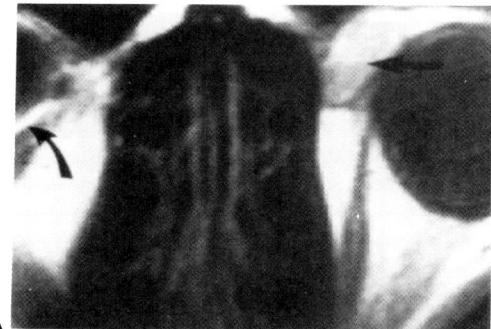
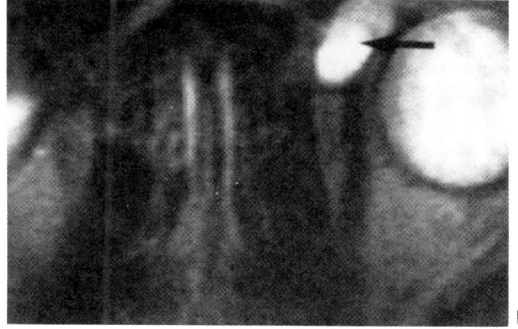

Fig SK44-10. Dermoid cyst. A fat-fluid level (arrows) is seen in this well-defined extraconal lesion on (A) T_1-weighted and (B) T_2-weighted MR images. The artifact in the right orbit (curved arrow) is due to cosmetics.[51]

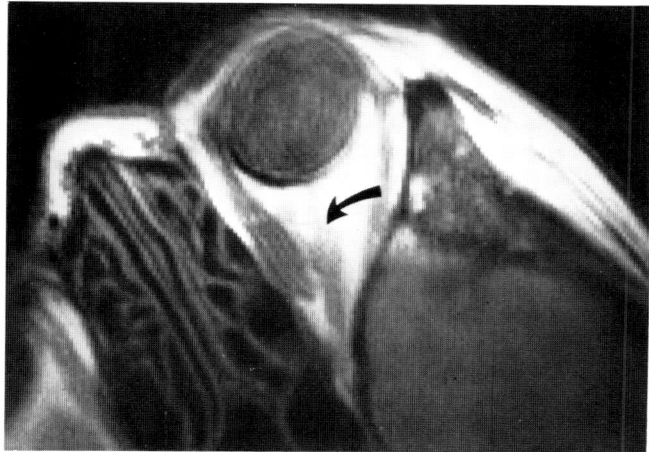
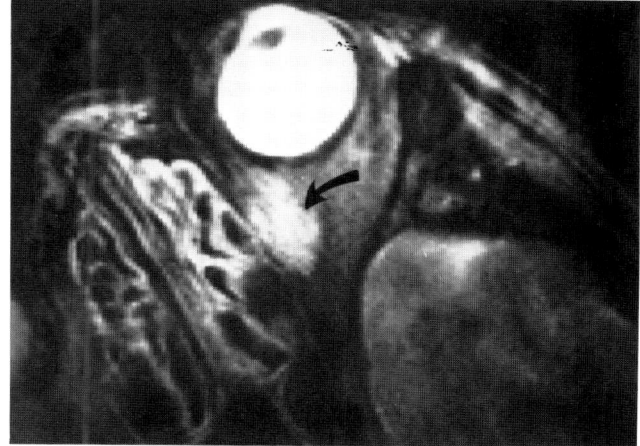

Fig SK44-11. Lymphoma. Ill-defined enlargement of the medial rectus muscle (arrow) that typically has low signal on T_1-weighted images (A) and high signal on T_2-weighted images (B).[51]

THICKENING OF THE RECTUS MUSCLES

Condition	Comments
Thyroid ophthalmopathy (Graves' disease) (Fig SK45-1)	Hypersecretion by fibroblasts of mucopolysaccharides, collagen, and glycoproteins causes binding of water and increased intraorbital pressure, leading to ischemia, edema, and sometimes fibrosis of extraocular muscles. The medial and inferior rectus muscles are usually affected before and to a greater degree than the lateral rectus or superior muscle group. The two eyes may be involved symmetrically or asymmetrically.
Rhabdomyosarcoma (Fig SK45-2)	Uncommon, highly malignant orbital tumor arising from extraocular muscle that typically presents with rapidly progressive exophthalmos in boys under 10 years of age. Appears as a large, noncalcified, enhancing retrobulbar mass, often with adjacent bone destruction. The identification of a displaced, but otherwise normal, optic nerve helps to exclude an optic nerve tumor.
Metastases	Unusual manifestation of infiltration by such neoplasms as lymphoma, leukemia, and neuroblastoma. An orbital neurofibroma may rarely produce a mass thickening the contour of a rectus muscle.
Orbital myositis	Inflammatory process that usually affects multiple muscles in children and a single muscle in adults and presents with rapid onset of proptosis, erythema of the lids, and injection of the conjunctiva. In most cases, steroid therapy causes the enlarged muscles to return to a normal appearance.
Orbital pseudotumor	Inflammatory process that can affect virtually all the intraorbital soft-tissue structures. The variable appearances of this condition include enlargement of one or more extraocular muscles, a discrete or poorly defined intraconal or extraconal mass that may obliterate the muscle-fat planes, enlargement of the lacrimal gland, and scleral thickening. There is generally improvement after steroid therapy.
Infiltrative processes	Orbital cellulitis, Wegener's granulomatosis, lethal midline granuloma, sarcoidosis, foreign body reaction.
Carotid-cavernous fistula	Dilation of the cavernous sinus may cause enlargement of the extraocular muscles due to venous congestion. Typical findings consist of unilateral proptosis and enlargement of the superior ophthalmic vein.

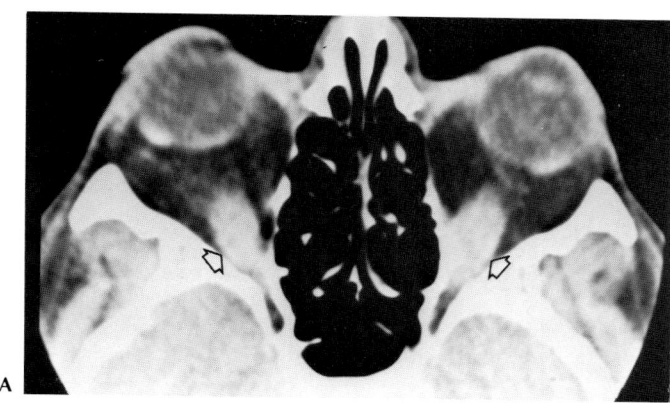

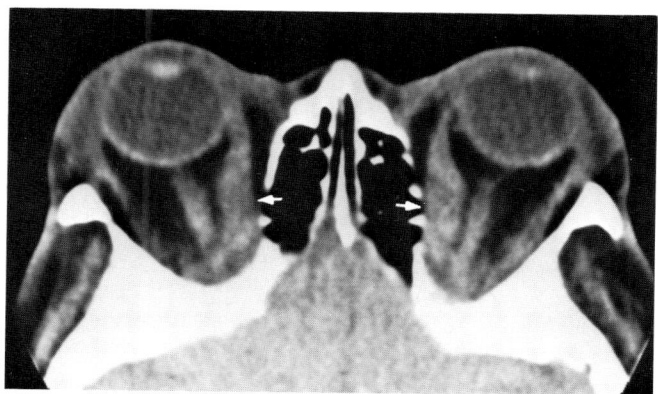

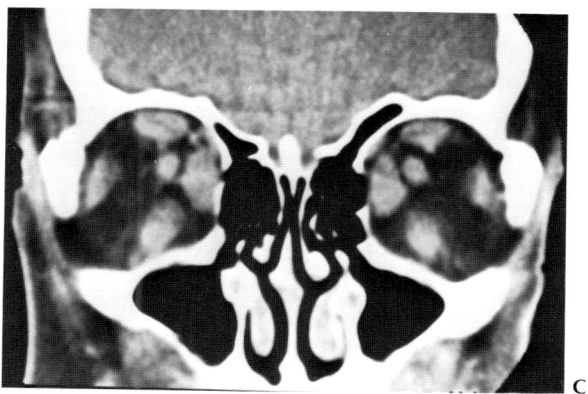

FIG SK45-1. **Thyroid ophthalmopathy.** (A) Axial view shows bilateral thickening of the inferior rectus muscles (arrows). (B) At a higher level, there is thickening of the medial rectus muscles bilaterally (arrows). (C) Coronal view shows thickening of virtually all the rectus muscles on both sides.

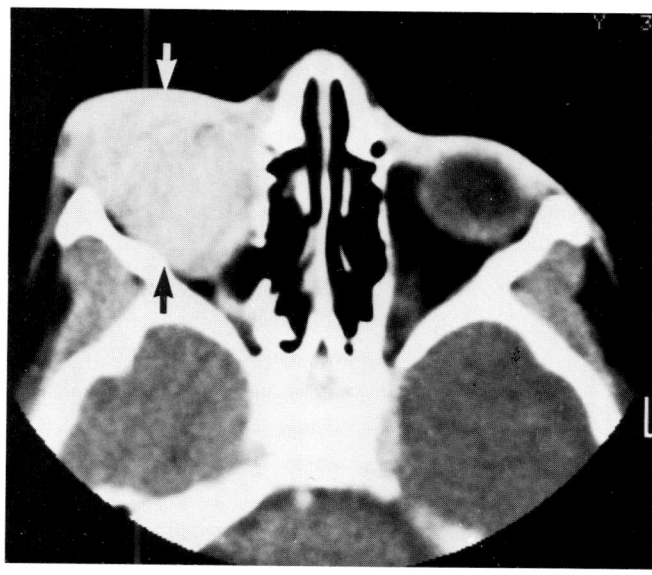

FIG SK45-2. **Rhabdomyosarcoma.** Enhancing tumor (arrows) fills virtually the entire right orbit in a 6-year-old child with rapidly progressing proptosis.[13]

SOURCES

1. Reprinted with permission from ''Hypophosphatasia'' by W James and B Moule, *Clinical Radiology* (1966;17:368–376), Copyright © 1966, Royal College of Radiologists.

2. Reprinted from *Caffey's Pediatric X-Ray Diagnosis*, ed 8, by FN Silverman with permission of Year Book Medical Publishers Inc, © 1985.

3. Reprinted with permission from ''Button Sequestrum Revisited'' by SD Sholkoff and F Mainzer, *Radiology* (1971;100:649–652), Copyright © 1971, Radiological Society of North America Inc.

4. Reprinted with permission from ''The Calvarial 'Doughnut Lesion': A Previously Undescribed Entity'' by T Keats and JF Holt, *American Journal of Roentgenology* (1969;105:314–318), Copyright © 1969, American Roentgen Ray Society.

5. Reprinted with permission from ''The Small Orbit Sign in Supraorbital Fibrous Dysplasia'' by SK Tchang, *Journal of Canadian Association of Radiologists* (1973;24:65–69), Copyright © 1973, Canadian Association of Radiologists.

6. Reprinted from *Introduction to Neuroradiology* by HO Peterson and SA Kieffer with permission of JB Lippincott Company, © 1972.

7. Reprinted with permission from ''Roentgen Findings in Cerebral Paragonimiasis'' by SJ Oh, *Radiology* (1968;90:292–299), Copyright © 1968, Radiological Society of North America Inc.

8. Reprinted from *Head and Neck Imaging* by RT Bergeron, AG Osborn, and PM Som (Eds) with permission of The CV Mosby Company, St Louis, © 1990.

9. Reprinted with permission from ''Paranasal Sinus Obliteration in Wegener's Granulomatosis'' by MR Paling, RL Roberts, and AS Fauci, *Radiology* (1982;144:539–543), Copyright © 1982, Radiological Society of North America Inc.

10. Reprinted with permission from ''Radiation Therapy of Midline Granuloma'' by AS Fauci, RE Johnson, and SM Wolff, *Annals of Internal Medicine* (1976;84:140–147), Copyright © 1976, American College of Physicians.

11. Reprinted with permission from ''Extramedullary Plasmacytoma'' by SI Schabel et al, *Radiology* (1978;128:625–628), Copyright © 1978, Radiological Society of North America Inc.

12. Reprinted with permission from ''Juvenile Nasopharyngeal Fibroma: Roentgenologic Characteristics'' by CB Holman and WE Miller, *American Journal of Roentgenology* (1965;94:292–298), Copyright © 1965, American Roentgen Ray Society.

13. Reprinted from *Cranial Computed Tomography* by AL Williams and VM Haughton with permission of The CV Mosby Company, St Louis, © 1985.

14. Reprinted with permission from ''Lymphoma after Organ Transplantation: Radiological Manifestations in the Central Nervous System, Thorax, and Abdomen'' by DE Tubman, MP Frick, and DW Hanto, *Radiology* (1984;149:625–631), Copyright © 1984, Radiological Society of North America Inc.

15. Reprinted with permission from ''Acquired Immunodeficiency Syndrome: Neuroradiologic Findings'' by WM Kelly and MB Brant-Zawadzki, *Radiology* (1983;149:485–491), Copyright © 1983, Radiological Society of North America Inc.

16. Reprinted with permission from ''Unusual Neuroradiological Features of Intracranial Cysticercosis'' by CS Zee et al, *Radiology* (1980;137:397–407), Copyright © 1980, Radiological Society of North America Inc.

17. Reprinted from *Cranial Computed Tomography* by SH Lee and HCVG Rao (Eds) with permission of McGraw-Hill Book Company, © 1983.

18. Reprinted with permission from ''Virchow-Robin Space: A Path of Spread in Neurosarcoidosis'' by M Mirfakhraee et al, *Radiology* (1986;158:715–720), Copyright © 1986, Radiological Society of North America Inc.

19. Reprinted with permission from ''CT in Hydatid Cyst of the Brain'' by K Abbassioun et al, *Journal of Neurosurgery* (1978;49:408–411), Copyright © 1978, American Association of Neurological Surgeons.

20. Reprinted with permission from ''Adult Supratentorial Tumors'' by SW Atlas, *Seminars in Roentgenology* (1990;25:130–154), Copyright © 1990, Grune & Stratton Inc.

21. Reprinted with permission from ''Intracranial Oligodendrogliomas'' by YY Lee and P Van Tassel, *American Journal of Roentgenology* (1989;152:361–369), Copyright © 1989, American Roentgen Ray Society.

22. Reprinted with permission from ''Colloid Cysts of the Third Ventricle'' by PP Maeder et al, *American Journal of Roentgenology* (1990;155:135–141), Copyright © 1990, American Roentgen Ray Society.

23. Reprinted from *Essentials in Neuroimaging* by B Kirkwood, with permission of Churchill Livingstone, Copyright © 1991.

24. Reprinted with permission from ''The Radiology of Pituitary Adenoma'' by SM Wolpert, *Seminars in Roentgenology* (1984;19:53–69), Copyright © 1984, Grune & Stratton Inc.

25. Reprinted with permission from ''Amenorrhea and Galactorrhea: A Role for MRI'' by LP Mark and WM Haughton, *MRI Decisions* (Jan-Feb 1989:26–32), Copyright © 1989, PW Communications, International. All rights reserved.

26. Reprinted with permission from ''Imaging of Intrasellar, Suprasellar, and Paraseller Tumors'' by RA Zimmerman, *Seminars in Roentgenology* (1990;25:174–197), Copyright © 1990, Grune & Stratton Inc.

27. Reprinted with permission from ''Adult Infratentorial Tumors'' by LT Bilaniuk, *Seminars in Roentgenology* (1990;25:155–173), Copyright © 1990, Grune & Stratton Inc.

28. Reprinted with permission from ''MR Imaging of Primary Tumors of Trigeminal Nerve and Meckel's Cave'' by WTC Yuh et al, *American Journal of Neuroradiology* (1988;9:665–670), Copyright © 1988, Williams & Wilkins Company.

29. Reprinted with permission from ''MRI of the Pituitary Gland: Adenomas'' by SC Patel and WP Sanders, *MRI Decisions* (1990;4:12–20), Copyright © 1990, PW Communications, Int'l. All rights reserved.

30. Reprinted with permission from ''MR Anatomy and Pathology of the Hypothalamus'' by DJ Loes, TJ Barloon, WTC Yuh, et al, *American Journal of Roentgenology* (1991;156:579–585), Copyright © 1991, American Roentgen Ray Society.

31. Reprinted with permission from ''Paragangliomas of the Jugular Bulb and Carotid Body'' by T Vogl et al, *American Journal of Roentgenology* (1989;153:583–587), Copyright © 1989, American Roentgen Ray Society.

32. Reprinted with permission from ''MRI of the Jugular Foramen'' by DL Daniel and LP Mark, *MRI Decisions* (1991;5:2–11), Copyright © 1991, PW Communications, Int'l. All rights reserved.

33. Reprinted with permission from ''CT, MR, and Pathology in HIV Encephalitis and Meningitis'' by MJD Post et al, *American Journal of Roentgenology* (1988;151:373–380), Copyright © 1988, American Roentgen Ray Society.

34. Reprinted with permission from ''Imaging Decisions in the Evaluation of Headache'' by CE Johnson and RD Zimmerman, *MRI Decisions* (1989;3:2–16), Copyright © 1989, PW Communications, International. All rights reserved.

35. Courtesy of Bruce H. Braffman, MD.

36. Reprinted from *MR and CT Imaging of the Head, Neck and Spine, 2nd Edition*, by RE Latchaw (Ed.), with permission of CV Mosby Company, Copyright © 1991.

37. Reprinted with permission from "Multiple System Atrophy (Shy-Drager Syndrome): MR Imaging" by B Pastakia, R Polinsky, G DiChiro, et al, *Radiology* (1986;159:499–502), Copyright © 1986, Radiological Society of North America.

38. Reprinted from *Clinical Magnetic Resonance Imaging* by RR Edelman and JR Hesselink (Eds) with permission of WB Saunders Company, © 1990.

39. Reprinted with permission from "Wilson's Disease of the Brain, MR Imaging" by AM Aisen, W Martel, TO Grabielsen, et al, *Radiology* (1985;157:137–141), Copyright © 1985, Radiological Society of North America.

40. Reprinted with permission from "Intracranial Ependymoma and Subependymoma: MR Manifestations" by GP Spoto et al, *American Journal of Neuroradiology* (1990;11:83–91), Copyright © 1990, American Society of Neuroradiology.

41. Reprinted with permission from "Gd-DTPA-Enhanced Cranial MR Imaging in Children: Initial Clinical Experience and Recommendations for Its Use" by AD Elster and GD Rieser, *American Journal of Neuroradiology* (1989;10:1027–1030), Copyright © 1989, American Society of Neuroradiology.

42. Reprinted with permission from "Intraventricular Mass Lesions of the Brain: CT and MR Findings" by RD Tien, *American Journal of Roentgenology* (1991;157:1283–1290), Copyright © 1991, American Roentgen Ray Society.

43. Reprinted with permission from "Intraventricular neurocytoma: Radiological Features and Review of the Literature" by SK Goergen, MF Gonzales and CA McLean, *Radiology* (1992;182:787–792), Copyright © 1992, Radiological Society of North America.

44. Reprinted with permission from "Intracranial Meningeal Pathology: Use of Enhanced MRI" by MR Ross, DO Davis, AS Mark, *MRI Decisions* (1990;4:24–33), Copyright © 1990, PW Communications, International. All rights reserved.

45. Reprinted with permission from "Congenital Central Nervous System Anomalies" by LB Poe, LL Coleman, F Mahmud, *Radiographics* (1989;9:801–826), Copyright © 1989, Radiological Society of North America Inc.

46. Reprinted with permission from "Magnetic Resonance Imaging of Disturbances in Neuronal Migration: Illustration of an Embryologic Process" by AS Smith et al, *Radiographics* (1989;9:509–522), Copyright © 1989, Radiological Society of North America Inc.

47. Reprinted with permission from "Common Congenital Brain Anomalies" by SE Byrd and TP Naidich, *Radiologic Clinics of North America* (1988;26:755–772), Copyright © 1988, WB Saunders Company.

48. Reprinted with permission from "Sonography of Congenital Midline Brain Malformations" by KC Funk and MJ Siegel, *Radiographics* (1988;8:11–25), Copyright © 1988, Radiological Society of North America, Inc.

49. Reprinted with permission from "CNS Complications of AIDS: CT and MR Findings" by RG Ramsey and GK Geremia, *American Journal of Roentgenology* (1988;151:449–454), Copyright © 1988, American Roentgen Ray Society.

50. Reprinted with permission from "Encephalitis Caused by Human Immunodeficiency Virus: CT and MR Imaging Manifestations with Clinical and Pathologic Correlation" by HS Chrysikopoulos et al, *Radiology* (1990;175:184–191), Copyright © 1990, Radiological Society of North America Inc.

51. Reprinted with permission from "Surface-Coil MR Imaging of Orbital Neoplasms" by JA Sullivan and SE Harms, *American Journal of Neuroradiology* (1986;7:29–34), Copyright © 1986, Williams & Wilkins Company.

52. Reprinted with permission from "Mucoceles of the Paranasal Sinuses: MR Imaging with CT Correlation" by P Van Tassel et al, *American Journal of Roentgenology* (1989;153:407–412), Copyright © 1989, American Roentgen Ray Society.

Spine Patterns

2

GENERALIZED VERTEBRAL OSTEOPOROSIS

Condition	Comments
Osteoporosis of aging (senile or postmenopausal osteoporosis) (Fig SP1-1)	Most common form of generalized osteoporosis. As a person ages, the bones lose density and become more brittle, fracturing more easily and healing more slowly. Many elderly persons are also less active and have poor diets that are deficient in protein. Females are affected more often and more severely than males, since postmenopausal women have deficient gonadal hormone levels and decreased osteoblastic activity.
Drug-induced osteoporosis (Fig SP1-2)	Patients receiving large doses of steroids over several months often develop generalized osteoporosis. Patients treated with 15,000 to 30,000 U of heparin for 6 months or longer also may develop generalized osteoporosis (possibly due to a direct local stimulating effect of heparin on bone resorption).
Deficiency states **Protein deficiency (or abnormal protein metabolism)**	Inability to produce adequate bone matrix in such conditions as malnutrition, nephrosis, diabetes mellitus, Cushing's syndrome, and hyperparathyroidism. Also patients with severe liver disease (hepatocellular degeneration, large or multiple liver cysts or tumors, biliary atresia). Pure dietary protein deficiency is rare in developed countries.
Vitamin C deficiency (scurvy)	Scurvy is now rarely seen in adults, though it can develop in severely malnourished individuals, especially elderly persons. There must be a prolonged period of vitamin C deficiency before symptoms become manifest. Osteoporosis is prominent in the axial skeleton, especially the spine. Biconcave deformities of vertebral bodies, condensation of bone at the superior and inferior vertebral margins, and centralized osteopenia are identical to the changes of osteoporosis in other disorders.
Intestinal malabsorption	Underlying mechanism in such conditions as sprue, scleroderma, pancreatic disease (insufficiency, chronic pancreatitis, mucoviscidosis), Crohn's disease, decreased absorptive surface of the small bowel (resection, bypass procedure), infiltrative disorders of the small bowel (eosinophilic enteritis, lactase deficiency, lymphoma, Whipple's disease), and idiopathic steatorrhea.
Endocrine disorders (Fig SP1-3)	Hypogonadism (especially Turner's syndrome and menopause); adrenocortical abnormality (Cushing's syndrome, Addison's disease); nonendocrine steroid-producing tumor (eg, oat cell carcinoma); diabetes mellitus; pituitary abnormality (acromegaly, hypopituitarism); thyroid abnormality (hyperthyroidism and hypothyroidism).

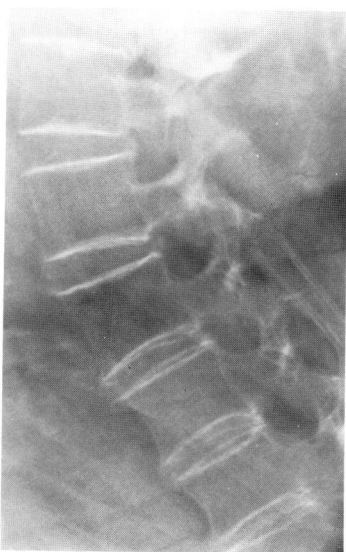

Fig SP1-1. Osteoporosis of aging. Generalized demineralization of the spine in a postmenopausal woman. The cortex appears as a thin line that is relatively dense and prominent (picture-frame pattern).

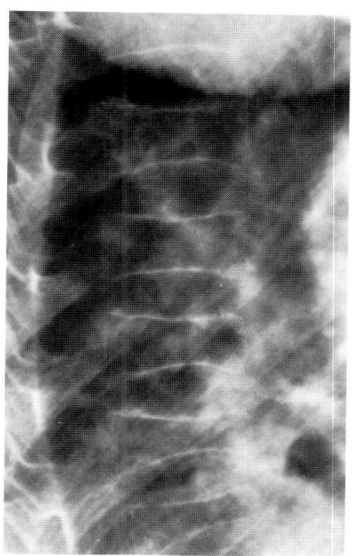

Fig SP1-2. Steroid-induced osteoporosis. Lateral view of the thoracic spine in a patient on high-dose steroid therapy for dermatomyositis demonstrates severe osteoporosis with thinning of cortical margins and biconcave deformities of vertebral bodies.

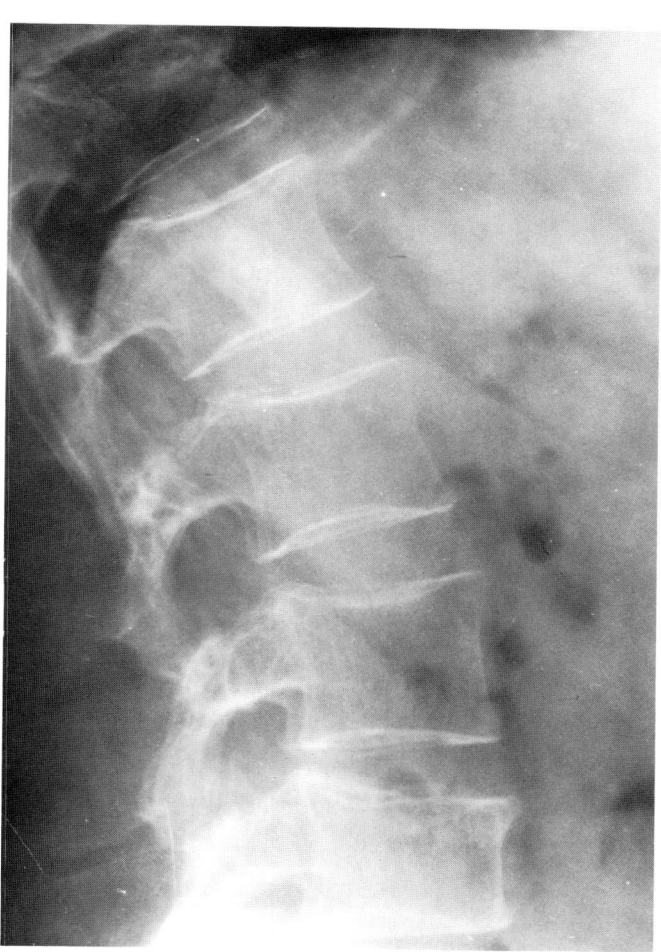

Fig SP1-3. Cushing's syndrome due to adrenal hyperplasia. Marked demineralization and an almost complete loss of trabeculae in the lumbar spine. The vertebral end plates are mildly concave and the intervertebral disk spaces are slightly widened. Note the compression of the superior end plate of L4.[1]

Condition	Comments
Neoplastic disorders **(Fig SP1-4)**	Diffuse cellular proliferation in the bone marrow with no tendency to form discrete tumor masses may produce generalized skeletal deossification simulating postmenopausal osteoporosis in adults with multiple myeloma or diffuse skeletal metastases and in children with acute leukemia. Pressure atrophy produces cortical thinning and trabecular resorption.
Anemia **(Fig SP1-5)**	Extensive marrow hyperplasia within the vertebral bodies produces a decrease in the number of trabeculae, thinning of the subchondral bone plates, accentuation of vertical trabeculation, and biconcave or central squared-off vertebral depressions. This appearance can be seen with thalassemia and sickle cell disease, as well as in severe iron deficiency anemia.
Ankylosing spondylitis	In longstanding disease, osteoporosis of the vertebral bodies becomes apparent and may be severe. Biconcave deformities of the vertebral bodies may develop.
Osteogenesis imperfecta **(Fig SP1-6)**	Inherited generalized disorder of connective tissue with multiple fractures, hypermobility of joints, blue sclerae, poor teeth, deafness, and cardiovascular disorders such as mitral valve prolapse or aortic regurgitation. In the spine, osteoporosis, ligamentous laxity, and posttraumatic deformities may result in severe kyphoscoliosis. Vertebral bodies are flattened and may be biconvex or wedge shaped anteriorly.
Neuromuscular diseases **and dystrophies**	Decreased muscular tone leading to osteoporosis, bone atrophy with cortical thinning, scoliosis, and joint contractures occurs in congenital disorders and such acquired conditions as spinal cord disease and immobilization for chronic disease or major fracture. Lack of the stress stimulus of weight bearing is the underlying cause of the generalized disuse atrophy termed space flight osteoporosis.
Homocystinuria **(Fig SP1-7)**	Inborn error of methionine metabolism that causes a defect in the structure of collagen or elastin and a radiographic appearance similar to that of Marfan's syndrome. Striking osteoporosis of the spine and long bones (extremely rare in Marfan's syndrome).

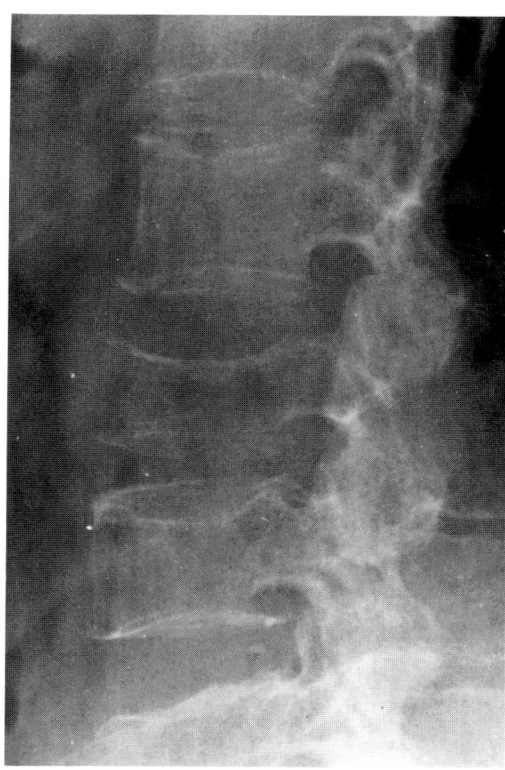

FIG SP1-4. Multiple myeloma. Diffuse myelomatous infiltration causes generalized demineralization of the vertebral bodies and a compression fracture of L2.

A

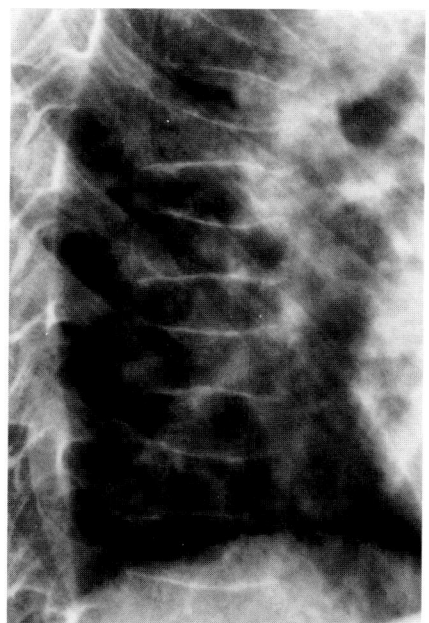

B

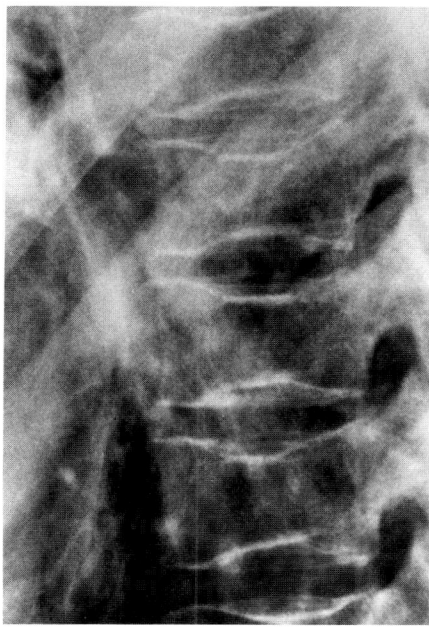

FIG SP1-5. Sickle cell anemia. (A) Biconcave indentations on both the superior and inferior margins of the soft vertebral bodies produce the characteristic fish vertebrae. (B) Localized steplike central depressions of multiple vertebral end plates.

FIG SP1-6. Osteogenesis imperfecta. In addition to generalized osteoporosis, some vertebrae show biconcave deformities whereas others demonstrate anterior wedging.[2]

Condition	Comments
Lipid storage diseases	Gaucher's disease and Niemann-Pick disease. Accumulation of abnormal quantities of complex lipids in the bone marrow produces a generalized loss of bone density and cortical thinning.
Hemochromatosis	Iron-storage disorder often associated with diffuse osteoporosis of the spine and vertebral collapse. About half the patients have a characteristic arthropathy that most frequently involves the small joints of the hand. Hepatosplenomegaly and portal hypertension are common.
Idiopathic juvenile osteoporosis (Fig SP1-8)	Rare condition characterized by the abrupt onset of generalized or focal bone pain in children 8 to 12 years of age. Osteoporosis of the spine, particularly in the thoracic and lumbar regions, may be combined with vertebral collapse. The disease is usually self-limited with spontaneous clinical and radiologic improvement.

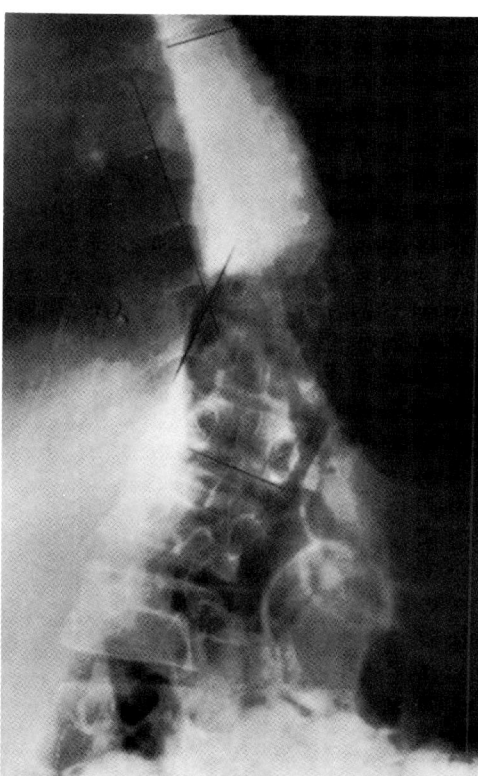

FIG SP1-7. Homocystinuria. Scoliosis and osteoporosis.[2]

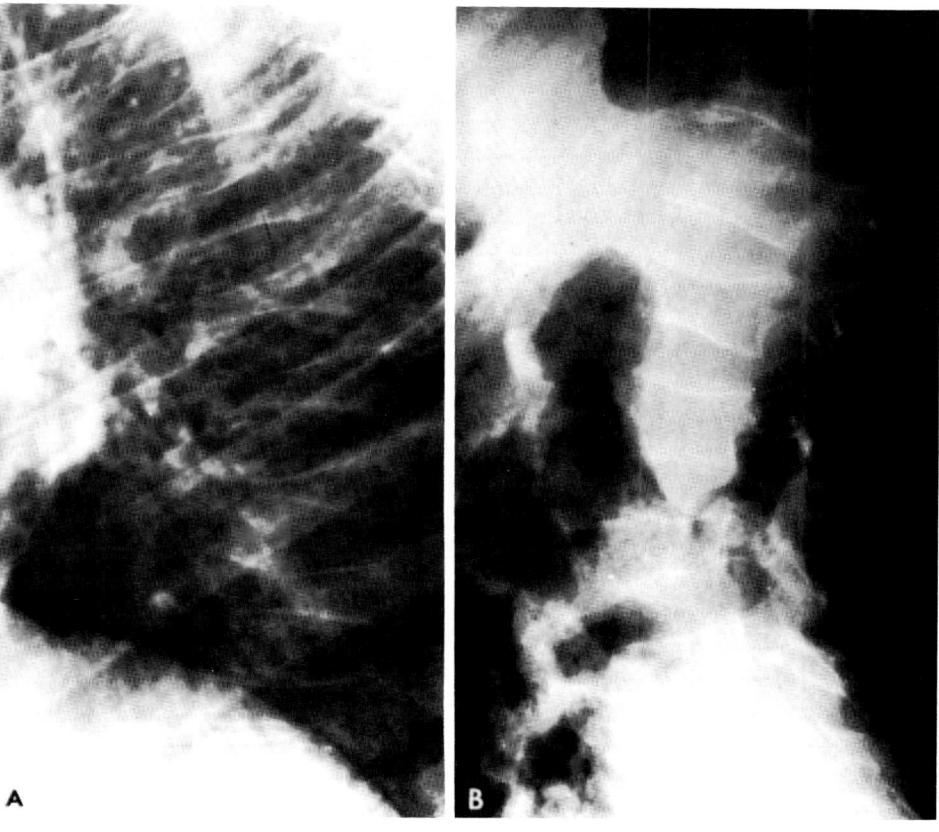

FIG SP1-8. Idiopathic juvenile osteoporosis. Lateral radiographs of (A) thoracic and (B) lumbar regions of the spine show striking osteoporotic lucency associated with severe compression and collapse of multiple vertebral bodies. Note the ballooning of several disk spaces.[2]

LYTIC LESION OF A VERTEBRAL BODY
OR POSTERIOR ELEMENTS

Condition	Imaging Findings	Comments
Osteoblastoma (Figs SP2-1 and SP2-2)	Expansile lucent (or opaque) lesion that grows rapidly, readily breaking through the cortex and producing a sharply defined soft-tissue component that is often circumscribed by a thin calcific shell.	Rare bone neoplasm that involves the vertebral column (most frequently the neural arches and spinous processes) in about half of patients. Most frequently occurs in the second decade of life and produces a dull aching pain, tenderness, and soft-tissue swelling. May contain some internal calcification.
Hemangioma (Fig SP2-3)	Demineralized and occasionally expanded vertebral body with characteristic multiple coarse linear striations running vertically.	Benign, slow-growing tumor composed of vascular channels. Usually asymptomatic and identified in middle-aged patients. The coarse vertical trabecular pattern may extend into the pedicles and laminae. Soft-tissue and intraspinal extension of the tumor or secondary hemorrhage can produce a paraspinal mass.
Aneurysmal bone cyst (Fig SP2-4)	Expansile, trabeculated, lucent lesion that primarily involves the posterior elements. There may be extension into or primary involvement of a vertebral body.	Consists of numerous blood-filled arteriovenous communications, rather than being a true neoplasm. Most frequently occurs in children and young adults and presents as mild pain of several months' duration, swelling, and restriction of movement. May cross a vertebral interspace and involve adjacent vertebrae.

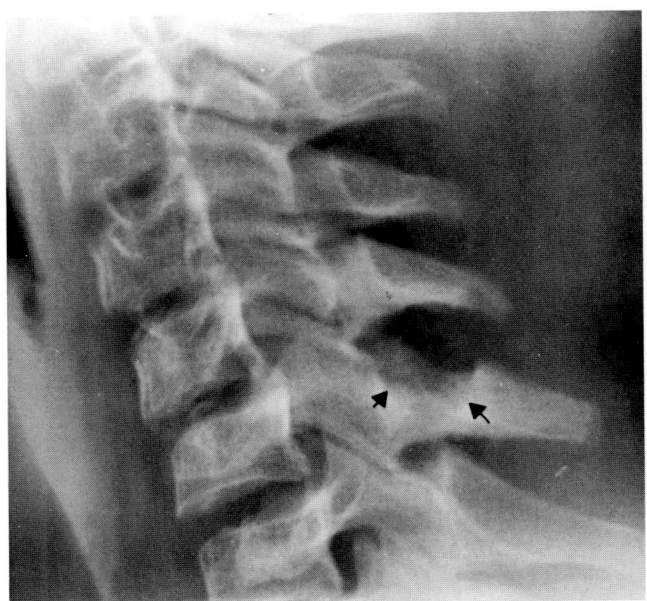

FIG SP2-1. **Osteoblastoma** of the cervical spine. Sharply defined, erosive lesion (arrows) involves the superior margin of a lower cervical spinous process.

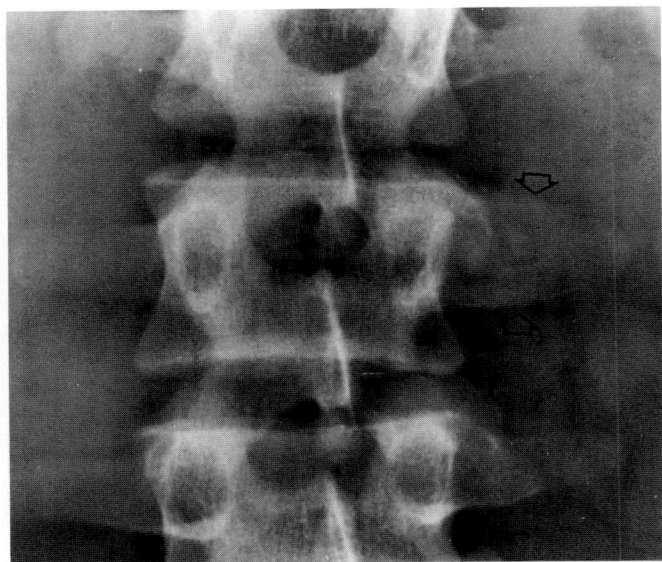

FIG SP2-2. **Osteoblastoma** of the lumbar spine. Well-circumscribed, expansile lesion (arrows) involves the left transverse process of a midlumbar vertebra.

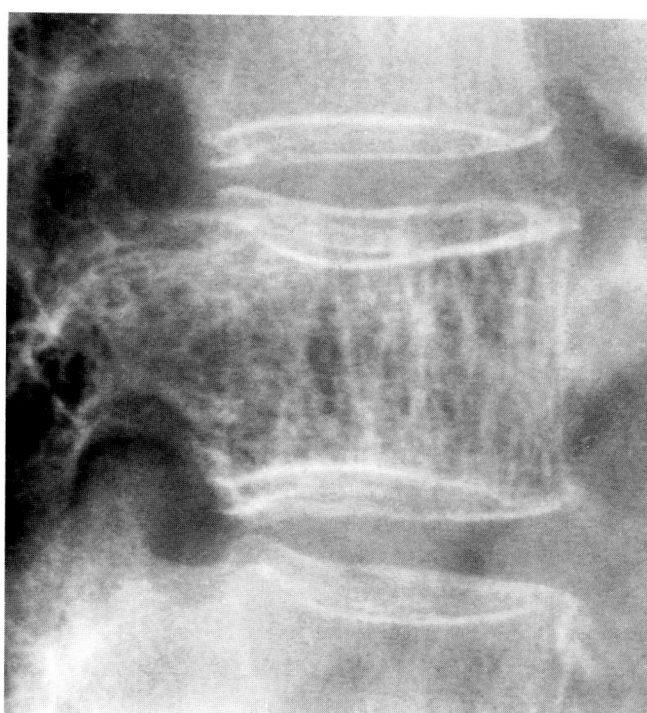

FIG SP2-3. **Hemangioma** of a vertebral body. Multiple coarse, linear striations run vertically in the demineralized vertebral body.

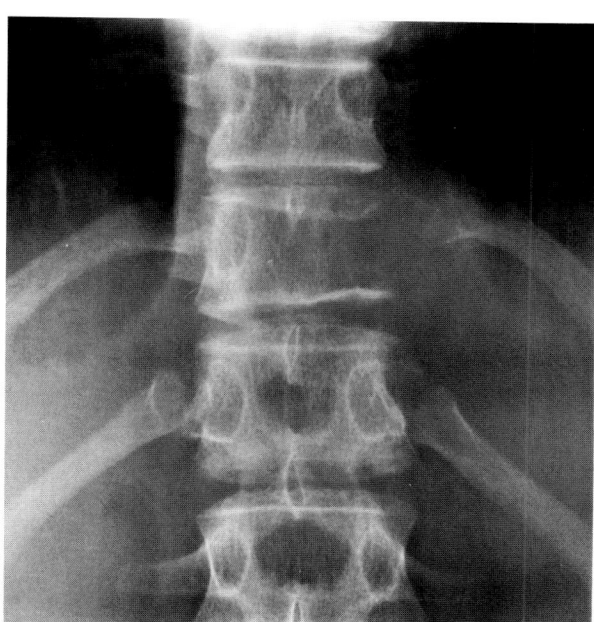

A

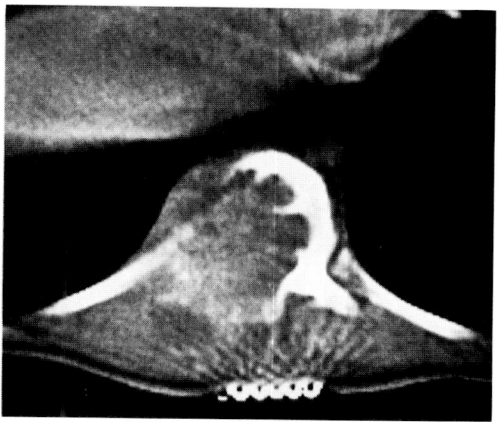

B

FIG SP2-4. **Aneurysmal bone cyst** of a thoracic vertebral body. (A) Destruction of the body and posterior elements. No peripheral shell of bone can be recognized. (B) CT scan shows irregular destruction suggesting a malignant process.[3]

Condition	Imaging Findings	Comments
Giant cell tumor (Fig SP2-5)	Slow-growing lucent lesion that often has ill-defined margins and may progress to vertebral collapse.	Most giant cell tumors of the spine occur in the sacrum, where the tumor has an expansile appearance.
Chordoma (see Figs SK9-4 and SK10-4)	Bulky mass causing ill-defined bone destruction or cortical expansion. Flocculent calcifications may develop in a large soft-tissue mass.	Arises from remnants of the notocord and primarily involves the sacrococcygeal region (50%) and clivus (30%). The remainder of the tumors occur elsewhere in the spine. Locally invasive, but does not metastasize.
Eosinophilic granuloma (see Fig SP6-7)	Bubbly, lytic, expansile lesions of both vertebral bodies and posterior elements can occur without significant collapse.	Most common manifestation is the characteristic collapse of a vertebral body (vertebra plana). A paraspinal mass can simulate a soft-tissue abscess related to vertebral osteomyelitis.
Fibrous dysplasia	Expansile lesion with a ground-glass or purely lytic appearance.	Infrequent manifestation. Vertebral collapse or a posteriorly expanding fibrous-tissue mass can result in cord compression.
Hydatid (echinococcal) cyst (Fig SP2-6)	Single or multiple expansile lytic lesions containing trabeculae. May be associated with cortical erosion and a soft-tissue mass.	Bone involvement occurs in about 1% of patients and most commonly affects the vertebral bodies, pelvis, and sacrum. Infiltration of daughter cysts into the bone produces a multiloculated appearance that resembles a bunch of grapes. Rupture into the spinal canal may produce neurologic abnormalities, including paraplegia.
Metastases (Fig SP2-7)	Single or multiple areas of bone destruction of variable size with irregular and poorly defined margins.	Spinal metastases typically destroy the pedicles (unlike multiple myeloma, in which the pedicles are infrequently destroyed). Because almost half the mineral content of a bone must be lost before it is detectable on plain radiographs, radionuclide bone scanning is far more sensitive for screening.

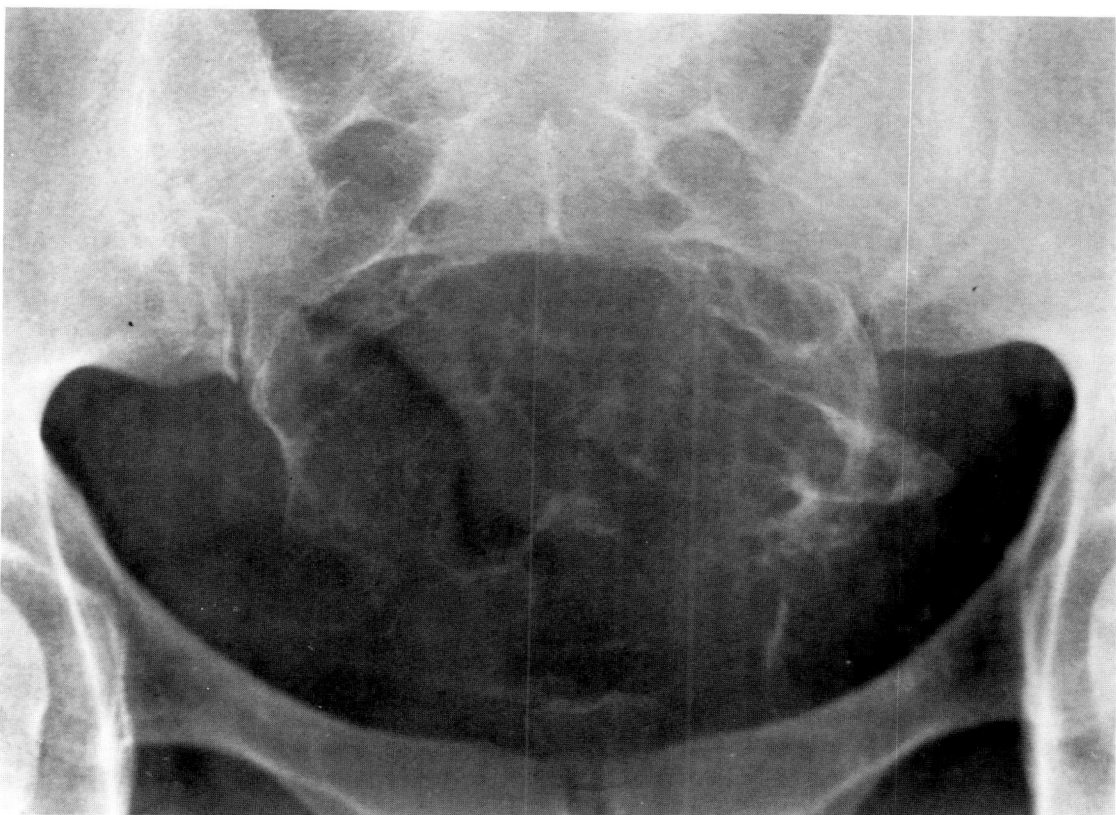

FIG SP2-5. **Giant cell tumor** of the sacrum. Huge expansile lesion.

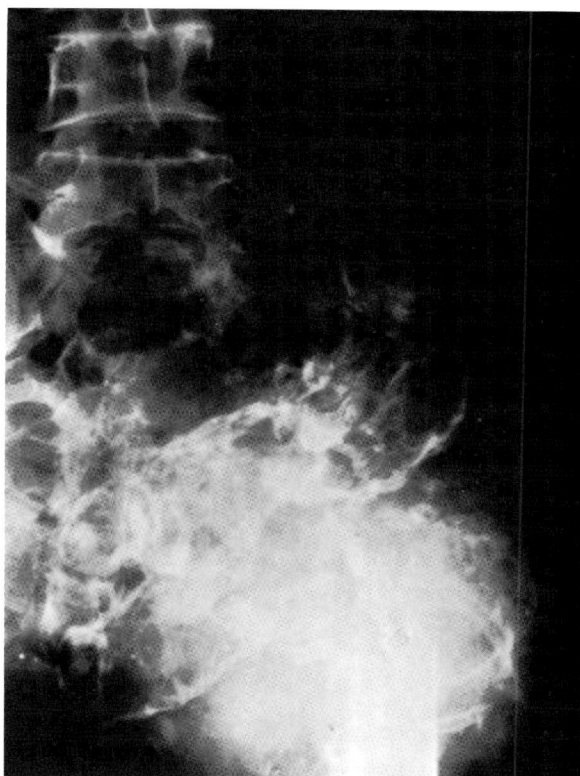

FIG SP2-6. **Echinococcosis.** Expansile, bubbly, lytic lesions of the pelvis, sacrum, and proximal femur associated with deformity, osseous fragmentation, and soft-tissue swelling.[2]

Condition	Imaging Findings	Comments
Plasmacytoma	Multicystic expansile lesion with thickened trabeculae. Primarily involves the vertebral body.	Involved vertebral body may collapse and disappear completely or the lesion may extend across the intervertebral disk to invade the adjacent vertebral body (simulating infection). Multiple myeloma causes generalized decreased bone density and destructive changes involving multiple vertebral bodies and often results in multiple vertebral compression fractures (see Fig SP6-2).
Lymphoma (Fig SP2-8)	Patchy osteolysis, with or without associated osteosclerosis.	Single or multiple lesions may have well- or ill-defined margins. Vertebral compression fractures may occur.
Osteomyelitis (see Figs SP6-3 and SP6-4)	Earliest sign is subtle erosion of the subchondral bony plate with loss of the sharp cortical outline. This may progress to total destruction of the vertebral body associated with a paravertebral soft-tissue abscess. Unlike neoplastic processes, osteomyelitis usually affects the intervertebral disk space and often involves adjacent vertebrae.	Osteomyelitis is caused by a broad spectrum of infectious organisms that reach bone by hematogenous spread, extension from a contiguous site of infection, or direct introduction (trauma or surgery). Because the earliest changes are usually not evident on plain radiographs until at least 10 days after the onset of symptoms, radionuclide bone scanning is the most valuable imaging modality for early diagnosis (increased isotope activity reflects the inflammatory process and increased blood flow).

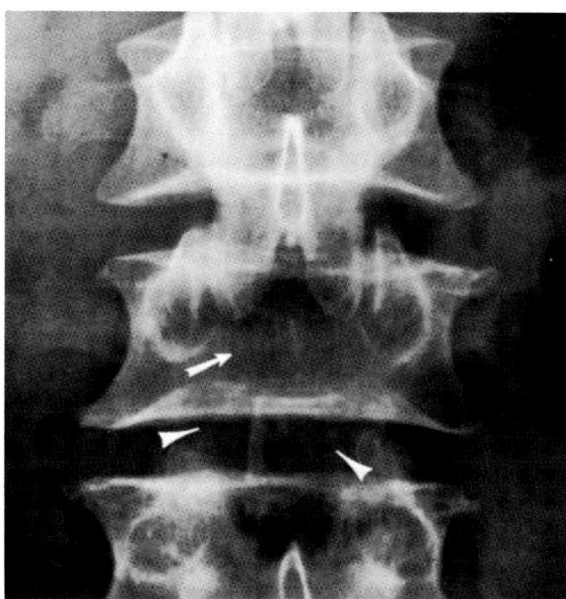

FIG SP2-7. **Metastasis.** Osseous destruction (arrowheads) of a portion of the pedicles, the entire lamina, the inferior articulating processes, and the spinal process produces the appearance of an empty vertebral body (arrow).[2]

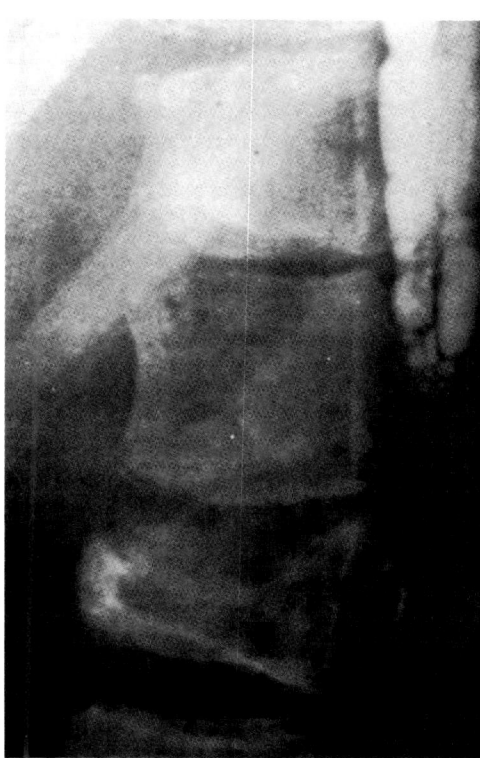

FIG SP2-8. **Lymphoma.** Lateral radiograph of the thoracolumbar junction shows lucency of multiple vertebral bodies with destruction and collapse. There is some patchy sclerosis and evidence of a previous myelogram.[2]

OSTEOSCLEROTIC VERTEBRAL LESIONS

Condition	Imaging Findings	Comments
Bone island (enostosis/endosteoma)	Circular or triangular areas of dense compact bone in the vertebral body (occasionally the posterior elements) that are usually homogeneous with a well-defined margin but infrequently show radiating spicules.	Asymptomatic, completely benign, and detected in about 1% of individuals. May present a diagnostic dilemma when seen in a patient with a known malignancy and possible metastases. Typically shows no activity on radionuclide bone scans (unlike metastases), though some bone islands may demonstrate isotope uptake.
Osteoblastic metastases (Fig SP3-1)	Single or multiple ill-defined areas of increased density that may progress to complete loss of normal bony architecture. Vary from a small, isolated round focus of sclerotic density to a diffuse sclerosis involving most or all of a bone (eg, ivory vertebral body).	Osteoblastic metastases are most commonly secondary to lymphoma and carcinomas of the breast and prostate. Other primary tumors include carcinomas of the gastrointestinal tract, lung, and urinary bladder. Osteoblastic metastases are generally considered to be evidence of slow growth in a neoplasm that has allowed time for reactive bone proliferation.
Paget's disease (Fig SP3-2)	In the reparative stage, there is a mixed lytic and sclerotic pattern with cortical thickening and enlargement of affected bone. In the sclerotic stage, there may be a uniform increased density (eg, ivory vertebra).	The purely sclerotic phase is less common than the combined destructive and reparative stages. An ivory vertebra may simulate osteoblastic metastases or Hodgkin's disease, though in Paget's disease the vertebra is also expanded.
Osteomyelitis (chronic or healed) (Fig SP3-3)	Thickening and sclerosis of bone with an irregular outer margin surrounding a central ill-defined area of lucency.	After a variable period (10 to 12 weeks), regenerative changes appear in the bone with sclerosis or eburnation. The severity of osteosclerotic response is variable. Although extensive sclerosis has been described as typical of pyogenic rather than tuberculous infection, this appearance may also be evident in tuberculosis, particularly in black patients. With early and proper treatment of pyogenic infection, a completely radiodense (ivory) vertebra may be produced.
Osteoid osteoma (Fig SP3-4)	Small, round or oval lucent nidus surrounded by a large, dense sclerotic zone of cortical thickening. The nidus may only be detectable on tomography.	Benign bone tumor that usually develops in young men. Classic clinical symptom is local pain that is worse at night and is dramatically relieved by aspirin. In the spine, osteoid osteomas most commonly arise in the posterior elements and are often associated with scoliosis. Surgical excision of the nidus is essential for cure. (It is not necessary to remove the reactive calcification.)

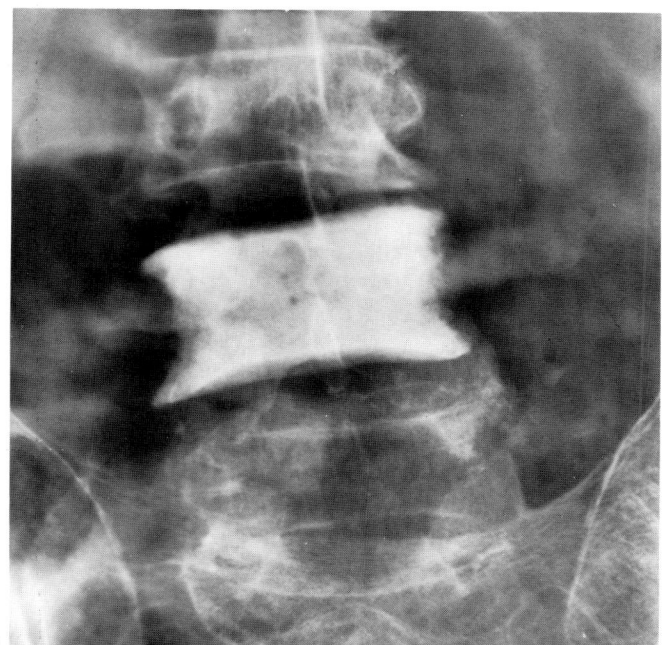

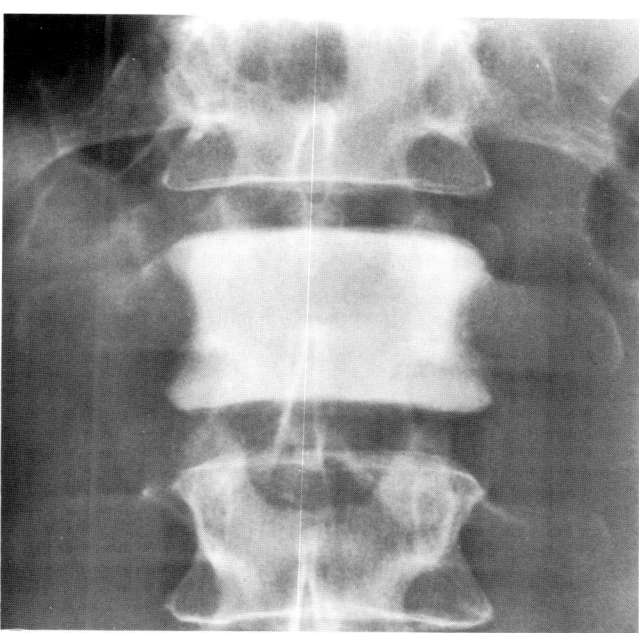

A   B

FIG SP3-1. **Osteoblastic metastases** (ivory vertebrae). (A) Carcinoma of the prostate. (B) Lymphoma.

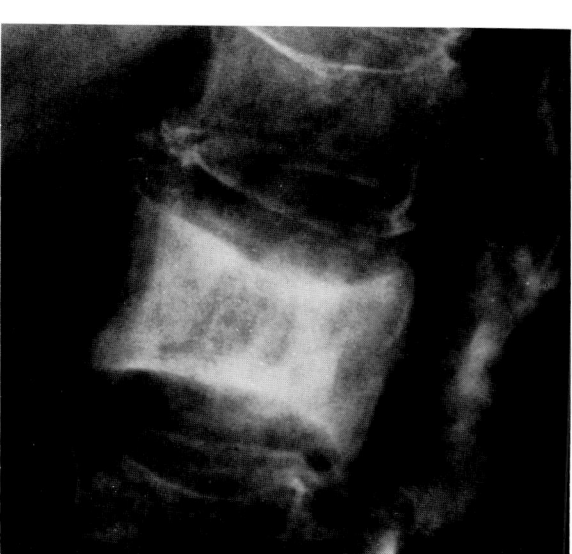

FIG SP3-2. **Paget's disease.** Sclerotic vertebral body with associated enlargement and cortical thickening.[4]

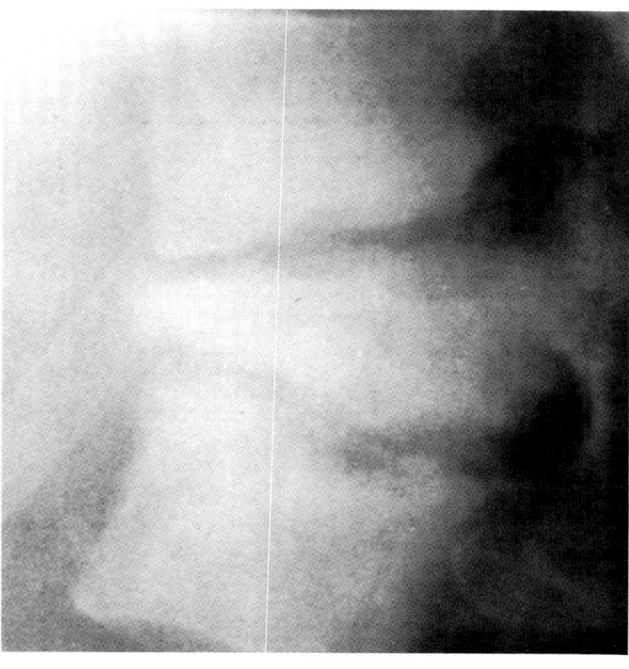

FIG SP3-3. **Chronic osteomyelitis.** There is destruction and collapse of bone with reactive sclerosis and narrowing of two intervertebral disk spaces. Note the poorly defined or fuzzy diskovertebral junctions associated with this pyogenic infection.[2]

Condition	Imaging Findings	Comments
Osteochondroma (exostosis)	Cartilage-covered osseous excrescence that arises from the surface of a bone. Typically, there is a blending of the cortex of an osteochondroma with that of normal bone.	Although the spine is affected infrequently, lesions developing in the vertebral column or ribs can cause spinal cord compression. Vertebral osteochondromas primarily involve the posterior elements, especially the spinous processes, and tend to arise in the lumbar and cervical regions. Rapid growth or the development of localized pain suggests malignant degeneration to chondrosarcoma.
Multiple myeloma	Generalized patchy or uniform bone sclerosis.	Very rare manifestation. Scattered, slow-growing osteoblastic lesions with dense plasmacytic infiltrates and normal laboratory findings may be termed *plasma-cell granuloma.*
Mastocytosis (Fig SP3-5)	Scattered sclerotic foci (simulating metastases) or uniform ivory vertebra.	Caused by diffuse deposits of mast cells in the bone marrow. Episodic release of histamine from mast cells causes typical symptoms of pruritis, flushing, tachycardia, asthma, and headaches, as well as an increased incidence of peptic ulcers. There often is hepatosplenomegaly, lymphadenopathy, and pancytopenia.
Osteopoikilosis (Fig SP3-6)	Multiple sclerotic foci (2 mm to 2 cm) producing a typical speckled appearance.	Rare asymptomatic hereditary condition that infrequently involves the spine but tends to affect the small bones of the hands and feet, the pelvis, and the epiphyses and metaphyses of long bones.
Melorheostosis (Fig SP3-7)	Irregular sclerotic thickening of the cortex, usually confined to one side of a single bone or to multiple bones of one extremity.	Rare disorder. Axial involvement may be accompanied by fibrolipomatous lesions in the spinal canal. In the extremities, sclerosis typically begins at the proximal end of the bone and extends distally, resembling wax flowing down a burning candle.
Congenital stippled epiphyses (chondrodysplasia punctata) (Fig SP3-8)	Multiple punctate calcifications occurring in epiphyses before the normal time for appearance of ossification centers.	Rare condition that most commonly involves the hips, knees, shoulders, and wrists. Affected bones may be shortened, or the process may regress and leave no deformity. Abnormalities of vertebral end plates may cause the vertebral bodies to have an irregular shape and lead to the development of kyphoscoliosis.
Tuberous sclerosis (Fig SP3-9)	Dense sclerotic foci that may be discrete and round, ovoid, or flame-shaped. In the spine, the pedicles and posterior portions of the vertebral bodies are most often involved.	Rare inherited disorder presenting with the clinical triad of convulsive seizures, mental deficiency, and adenoma sebaceum. Associated with renal and intracranial hamartomas and characteristic scattered intracerebral calcifications.
Callus formation	Localized increase in bone density about a healed or healing fracture.	History of trauma is helpful in making this diagnosis.

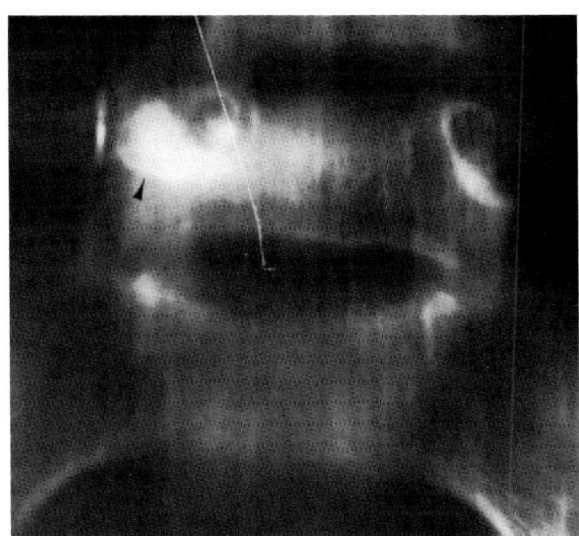

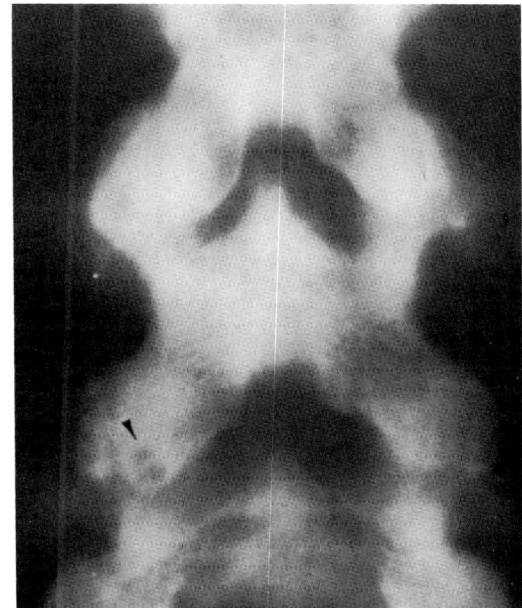

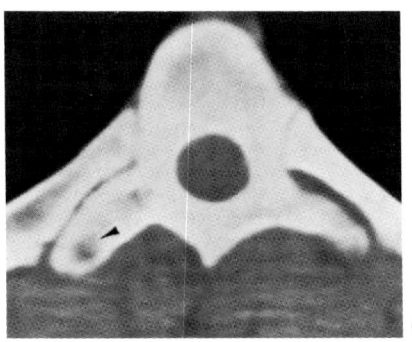

FIG SP3-4. Osteoid osteoma. (A) Sclerotic lesion of a pedicle (arrowhead). (B) Radiolucent nidus (arrowhead) in an inferior articular process. (C) Axial CT scan clearly shows the radiolucent nidus in a transverse process.[2]

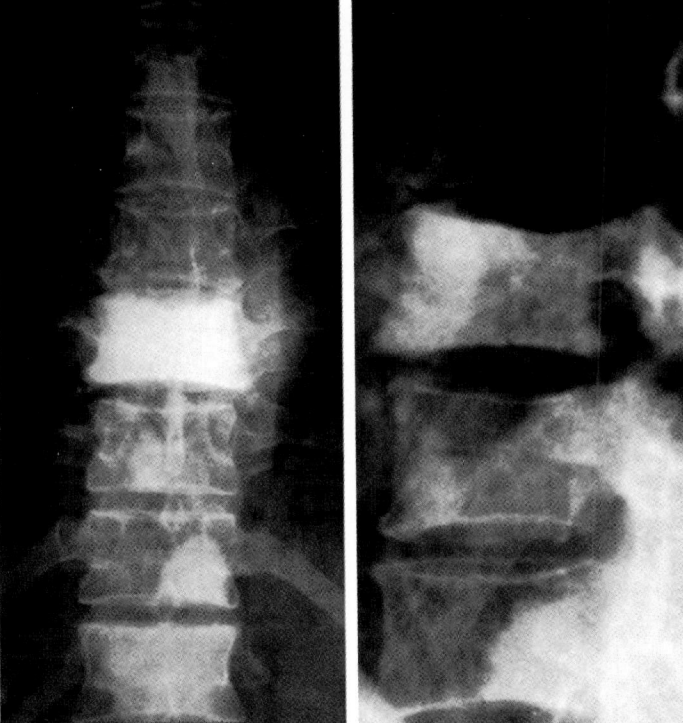

FIG SP3-5. Mastocytosis. (A) Frontal and (B) lateral radiographs of the thoracic region of the spine show focal osteosclerotic lesions associated with paravertebral swelling.[2]

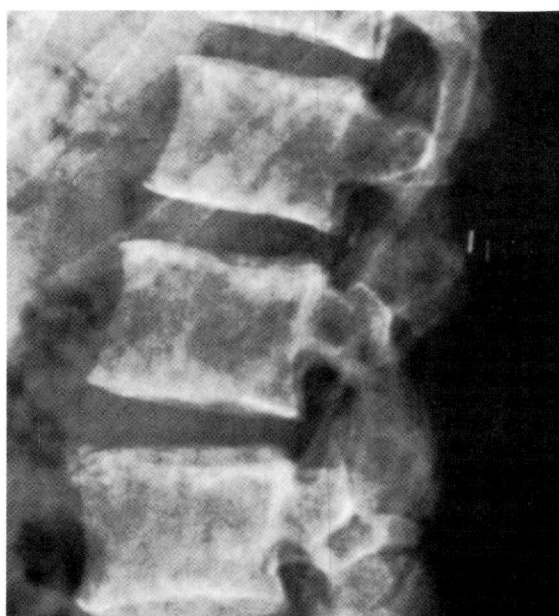

FIG SP3-6. Osteopoikilosis. Multiple sclerotic foci in the margins of the vertebral bodies and posterior elements.[2]

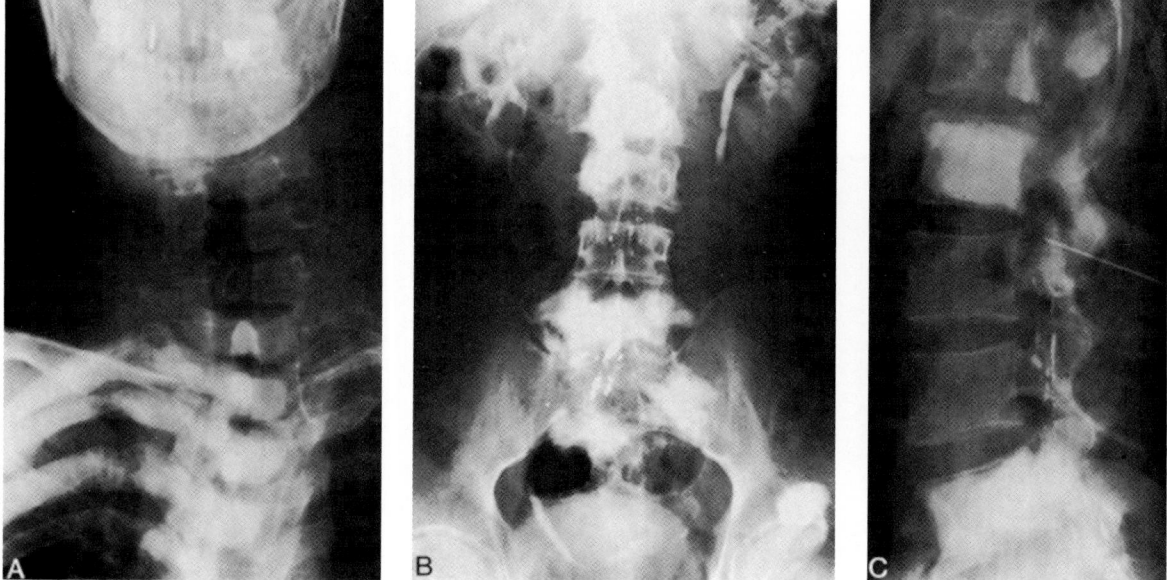

FIG SP3-7. Melorheostosis. Three radiographs of the axial skeleton show hyperostosis and enostoses involving the upper right ribs, the thoracic and lumbar vertebrae, the sacrum, and the ilium. Quadriparesis developed in this 21-year-old man because of a diffuse intramedullary lipoma in the spinal cord.[2]

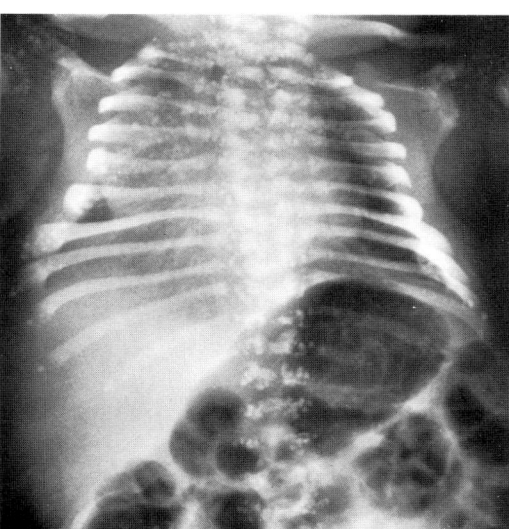

FIG SP3-8. **Congenital stippled epiphyses.** Multiple small punctate calcifications of various sizes involve virtually all the epiphyses in this view of the chest and upper abdomen.

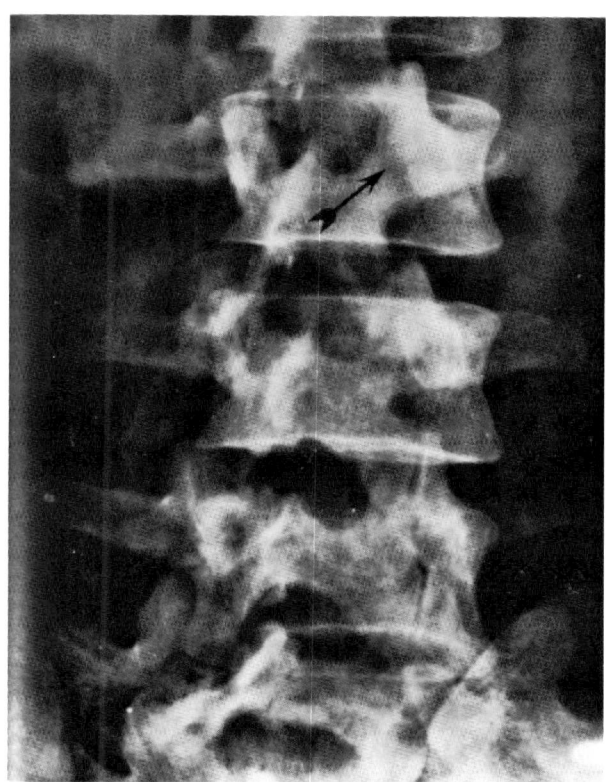

FIG SP3-9. **Tuberous sclerosis.** Left oblique view shows a homogeneously dense left pedicle and superior articular facet (arrow). This was an incidental finding on excretory urography.[2]

GENERALIZED VERTEBRAL OSTEOSCLEROSIS

Condition	Imaging Findings	Comments
Myelofibrosis (myelosclerosis, myeloid metaplasia) (Fig SP4-1)	About half the patients have a widespread, diffuse increase in bone density (ground-glass appearance) that primarily affects the spine, ribs, and pelvis. Increased radiodensity or condensation of bone at the inferior and superior margins of the vertebral body can produce a "sandwich" appearance.	Hematologic disorder in which gradual replacement of marrow by fibrosis produces a varying degree of anemia and a leukemoid blood picture. Most commonly idiopathic, though a large percentage of patients have antecedent polycythemia vera. Extramedullary hematopoiesis causes massive splenomegaly, often hepatomegaly, and sometimes tumor-like masses in the posterior mediastinum. Uniform obliteration of fine trabecular margins of the ribs results in sclerosis simulating jail bars crossing the thorax.
Osteoblastic metastases (Fig SP4-2)	Generalized diffuse osteosclerosis.	Primarily lymphoma and carcinomas of the prostate and breast.
Paget's disease (Fig SP4-3)	Diffuse osteosclerosis may develop in advanced stages of polyostotic disease.	Although the radiographic appearance may simulate that of osteoblastic metastases, characteristic cortical thickening and coarse trabeculation should suggest Paget's disease.
Sickle cell anemia	Diffuse sclerosis with coarsening of the trabecular pattern may be a late manifestation reflecting medullary infarction.	Initially, generalized osteoporosis due to marrow hyperplasia. Common findings include typical "fish vertebrae," a high incidence of acute osteomyelitis in the extremities (often caused by *Salmonella* infection), splenomegaly, and extramedullary hematopoiesis.
Osteopetrosis (Albers-Schönberg disease, marble bones) (Fig SP4-4)	Symmetric, generalized increase in bone density involving the entire skeleton. Typical patterns in the spine are a "bone-within-a-bone" appearance (a miniature bone inset in each vertebral body) and "sandwich" vertebrae (increased density at the end plates). In the extremities, lack of modeling causes widening of the metaphyseal ends of tubular bones.	Rare hereditary bone dysplasia in which failure of the resorptive mechanism of calcified cartilage interferes with its normal replacement by mature bone. Varies in severity and age of clinical presentation from a fulminant, often fatal condition at birth to an essentially asymptomatic form that is an incidental radiographic finding. Although radiographically dense, the involved bones are brittle, and fractures are common even with trivial trauma. Extensive extramedullary hematopoiesis (hepatosplenomegaly and lymphadenopathy).

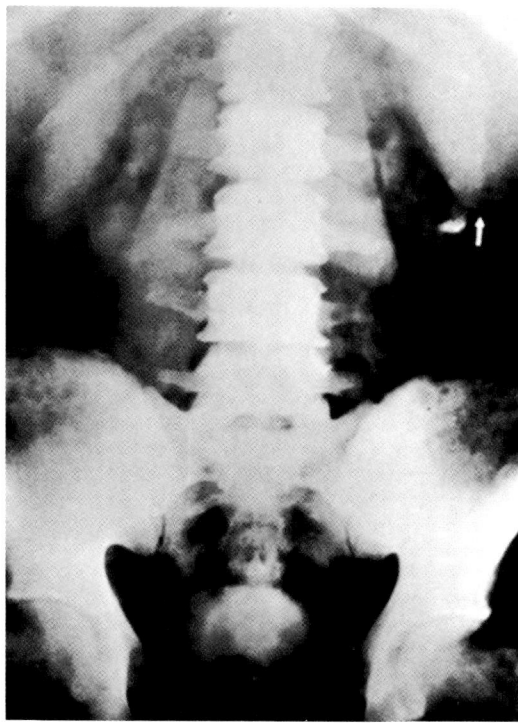

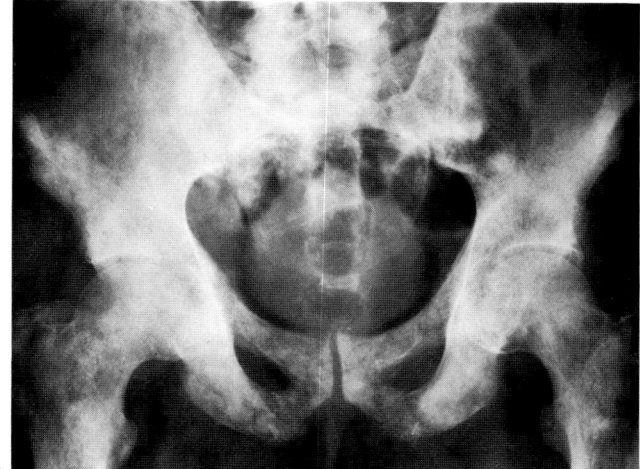

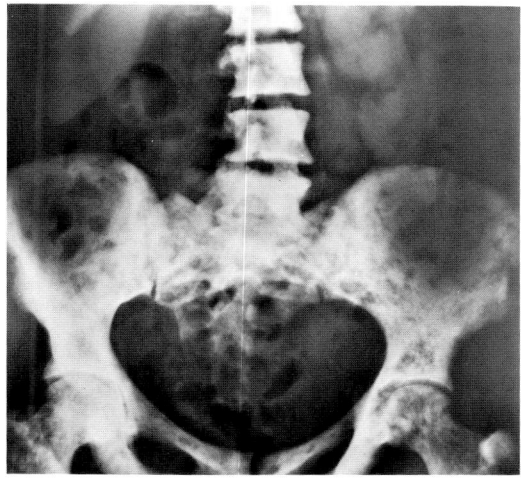

FIG SP4-1. **Myelofibrosis.** Uniform sclerosis of the spine and pelvis seen on a film from an excretory urogram. The renal function is obviously diminished, and the spleen is enlarged (arrow).[2]

FIG SP4-2. **Osteoblastic metastases.** (A) Carcinoma of the prostate. (B) Carcinoma of the breast.

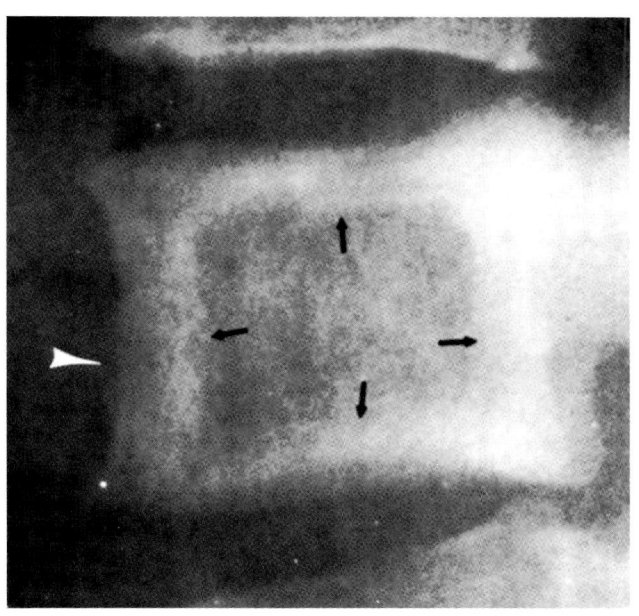

FIG SP4-3. **Paget's disease.** Picture-frame vertebral body with condensation of bone along its peripheral margins (arrows). There is straightening of the anterior surface of the bone (arrowhead) and involvement of the pedicles.[2]

Condition	Imaging Findings	Comments
Pyknodysostosis	Diffuse dense, sclerotic bones. Characteristically there is mandibular hypoplasia with loss of the normal mandibular angle and craniofacial disproportion.	Rare hereditary bone dysplasia. Patients have short stature, but hepatosplenomegaly is infrequent. Numerous wormian bones may simulate cleidocranial dysostosis. Unlike osteopetrosis, in the long bones the medullary cavities are preserved and there is no metaphyseal widening.
Fluorosis **(Fig SP4-5)**	Dense skeletal sclerosis most prominent in the vertebrae and pelvis. Obliteration of individual trabeculae may cause affected bones to appear chalky white. There is often calcification of interosseous membranes and ligaments (paraspinal, iliolumbar, sacrotuberous, and sacrospinous). Vertebral osteophytosis can lead to encroachment of the spinal canal and neural foramina.	Fluorine poisoning may result from drinking water with a high concentration of fluorides, industrial exposure (mining, smelting), or excessive therapeutic intake of fluoride (treatment of myeloma or Paget's disease). Periosteal roughening, hyperostosis, and bony excrescences often develop at sites of muscular and ligamentous attachments at the iliac crests, ischial tuberosities, and long bones.
Mastocytosis **(see Fig SP3-6)**	Diffuse sclerosis; single ivory vertebra; or scattered, well-defined sclerotic foci simulating metastases.	Caused by diffuse deposits of mast cells in the bone marrow. Episodic release of histamine from mast cells causes typical symptoms of pruritus, flushing, tachycardia, asthma, and headaches, as well as an increased incidence of peptic ulcers. There often is hepatosplenomegaly, lymphadenopathy, and pancytopenia.
Renal osteodystrophy **(Fig SP4-6)**	Thick bands of increased density adjacent to the superior and inferior margins of vertebral bodies producing the characteristic "rugger jersey" spine.	Other findings include generalized demineralization of vertebral bodies producing archlike contour defects of the end plates (simulating osteoporosis) and herniation of disk material into the vertebral bodies because of weakening of the diskovertebral junction related to subchondral resorption.
Multiple myeloma	Uniform sclerosis of bone.	Very rare manifestation.

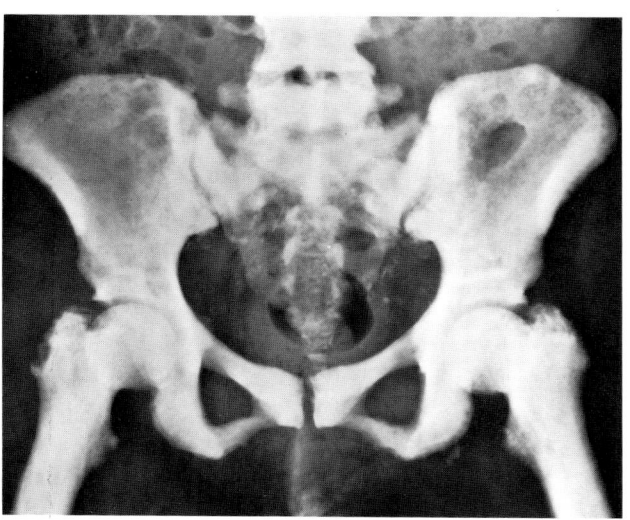

FIG SP4-4. Osteopetrosis. Generalized sclerosis of the lower spine, pelvis, and hips in a 74-year-old woman with the tarda form of this condition.

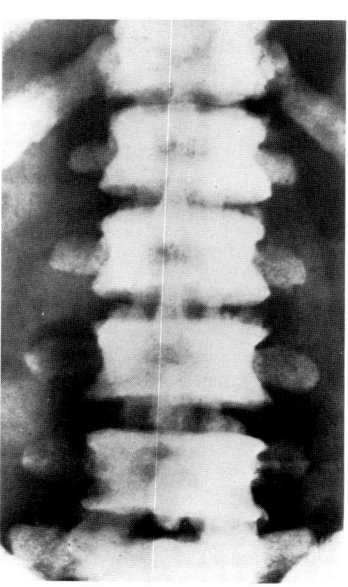

FIG SP4-5. Fluorosis. Diffuse vertebral sclerosis with obliteration of individual trabeculae.[5]

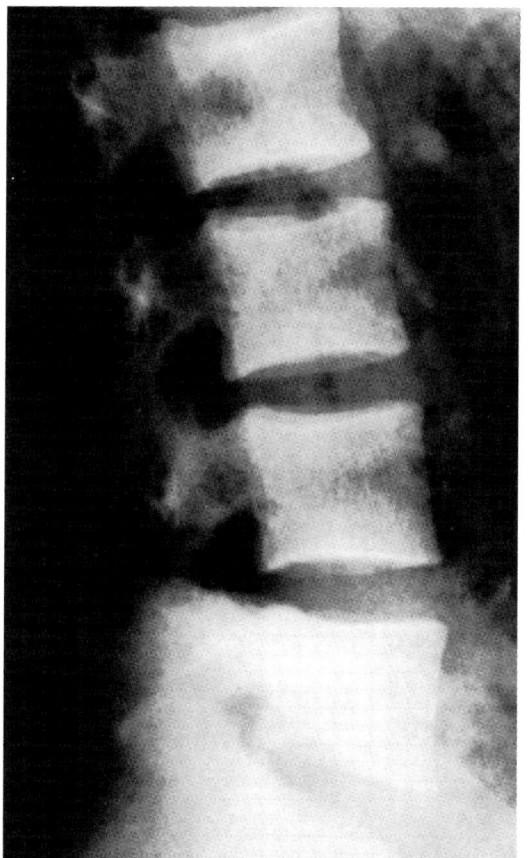

FIG SP4-6. Renal osteodystrophy. Areas of increased sclerosis subjacent to the cartilaginous plates produce the characteristic "rugger jersey" spine in this patient with chronic renal failure.[2]

INCREASE IN SIZE OF ONE OR MORE VERTEBRAE

Condition	Comments
Acromegaly **(Fig SP5-1)**	Appositional bone growth results in a generalized increase in the size of the vertebral bodies. Hypertrophy of cartilage widens the intervertebral disk spaces, while hypertrophy of soft tissue may lead to an increased concavity (scalloping) of the posterior aspects of the vertebral bodies.
Paget's disease **(Fig SP5-2)**	Generalized enlargement of affected vertebral bodies. Increased trabeculation, which is most prominent at the periphery of the bone, produces a rim of thickened cortex and a picture-frame appearance. Dense sclerosis of one or more vertebral bodies (ivory vertebrae) may present a pattern simulating osteoblastic metastases or Hodgkin's disease, though in Paget's disease the vertebrae are also enlarged.
Congenital **(Fig SP5-3)**	Fusion or partial fusion of two or more vertebral bodies (block vertebra) is a frequent occurrence. The underlying bone is otherwise normal. Congenital fusion can usually be differentiated from that resulting from disease because the total height of the combined fused bodies is equal to the normal height of two vertebrae less the intervertebral disk space.
Neuromuscular deficit	Increased height of the vertebral bodies related to the absence of normal vertical stress may develop in patients who cannot bear weight (eg, paralysis, Down's syndrome, rubella syndrome).
Benign bone tumor	Expansion of a vertebral body may result from hemangioma, aneurysmal bone cyst, osteoblastoma, or giant cell tumor.
Fibrous dysplasia	Proliferation of fibrous tissue in the medullary cavity may infrequently involve the spine and cause one or more vertebral bodies to expand. Complications include vertebral collapse and spinal cord compression.

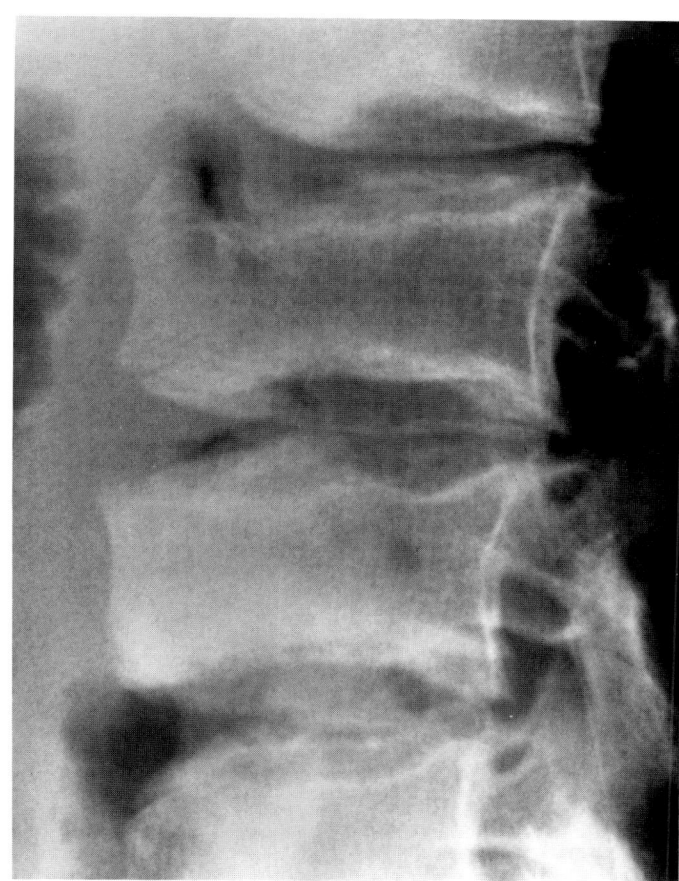

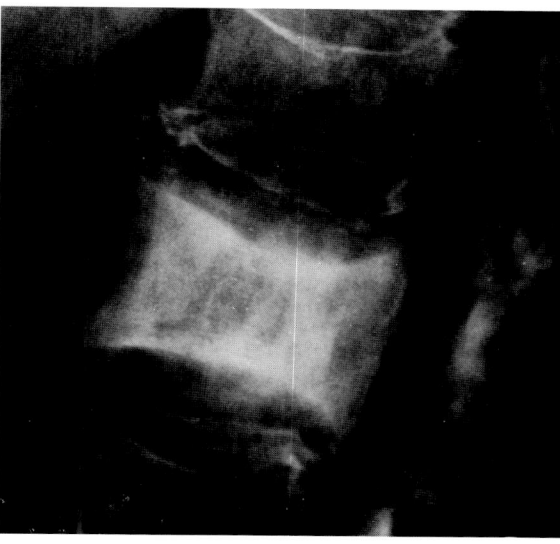

FIG SP5-2. Paget's disease. Enlargement and cortical thickening of a vertebral body, producing an ivory vertebra.[4]

FIG SP5-1. Acromegaly. Enlargement of all vertebral bodies, especially in the anteroposterior direction. Note the mild posterior scalloping.

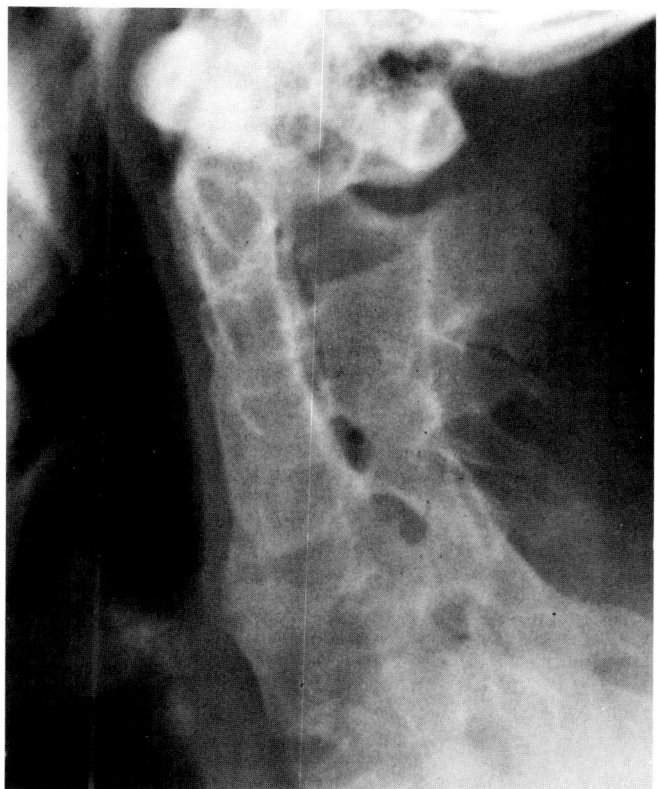

FIG SP5-3. Block vertebrae. Essentially complete fusion of the cervical spine into a solid mass in a patient with Klippel-Feil deformity.

LOSS OF HEIGHT OF ONE OR MORE VERTEBRAL BODIES

Condition	Imaging Findings	Comments
Osteoporosis (Fig SP6-1)	Smooth, archlike indentations of the vertebral end plates that are most marked centrally in the region of the nucleus pulposus. Primarily involves the lumbar and lower thoracic spine (where weight-bearing stress is directed toward the axes of the vertebral bodies).	Regardless of the cause (most commonly senile or postmenopausal osteoporosis, steroid therapy), as the bone density of the vertebral body decreases the cortex appears as a thin line that is relatively dense and prominent, producing a picture-frame pattern. In addition to the typical "fish vertebrae" appearance, osteoporotic vertebral bodies may demonstrate anterior wedging and compression fractures. The characteristic concave contours of the superior and inferior disk surfaces result from expansion of the nucleus pulposus into the weakened vertebral bodies.
Hyperparathyroidism	Generalized demineralization of the vertebral bodies produces archlike contour defects of the superior and inferior vertebral surfaces, simulating osteoporosis.	Subchondral resorption at the diskovertebral junctions produces areas of structural weakening that allow herniation of disk material into the vertebral body (cartilaginous or Schmorl's nodes). In patients with hyperparathyroidism secondary to renal failure, thick bands of increased density adjacent to the superior and inferior margins of vertebral bodies produce the characteristic "rugger jersey" spine.
Osteomalacia	Archlike contour defects of the superior and inferior surfaces of multiple vertebral bodies, simulating osteoporosis.	Insufficient mineralization of the vertebral bodies. In osteomalacia secondary to renal tubular disorders, hyperostosis may be more prominent than deossification. This results in a striking thickening of the cortices and increased trabeculation of spongy bone. Nevertheless, the bony architecture is abnormal and is prone to fracture with relatively minimal trauma.
Multiple myeloma (Fig SP6-2)	Generalized skeletal deossification simulating osteoporosis or destructive changes mimicking metastases. Severe loss of bone substance in the spine often results in multiple vertebral compression fractures.	Decreased bone density and destructive changes are usually limited to the vertebral bodies, sparing the pedicles (lacking red marrow) that are frequently destroyed by metastatic disease. Because multiple myeloma causes little or no stimulation of new bone formation, radionuclide bone scans may be normal even with extensive skeletal infiltration.
Metastases	Destructive process involving not only the vertebral bodies but also the pedicles and neural arches. Pathologic collapse of vertebral bodies frequently occurs in advanced disease.	Destruction of one or more pedicles may be the earliest sign of metastatic disease and aids in differentiating this process from multiple myeloma (pedicles are much less often involved). Because cartilage is resistant to invasion by metastases, preservation of the intervertebral disk space may help to distinguish metastases from an inflammatory process.

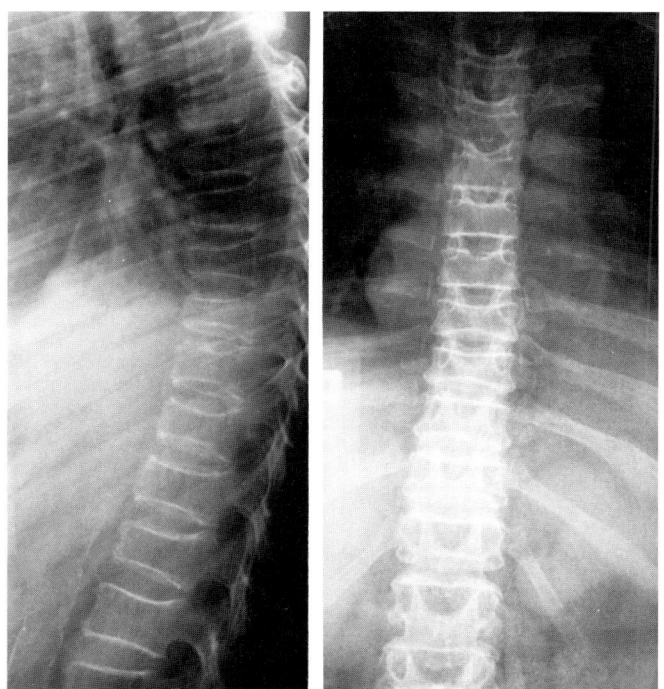

FIG SP6-1. Severe osteoporosis. (A) Lateral and (B) frontal views of the thoracolumbar spine show striking demineralization and compression of multiple vertebral bodies in a 14½-year-old girl treated with steroids for 5 years for chronic glomerulonephritis. The height age of the girl was only 9 years at this time.[6]

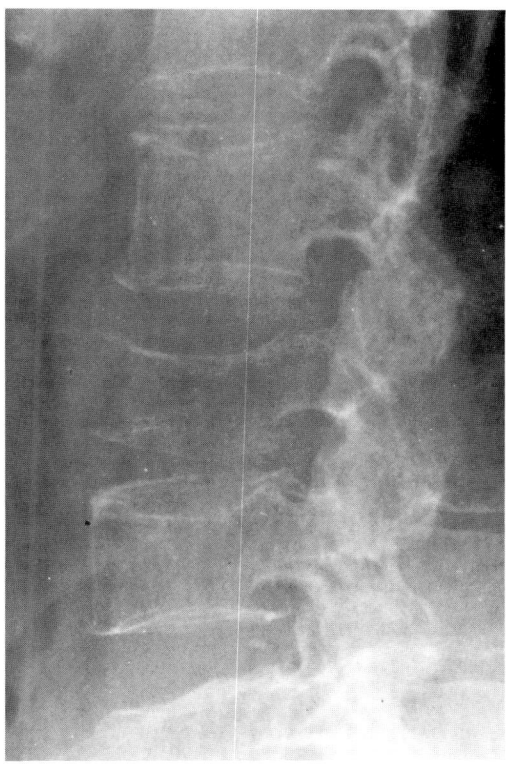

FIG SP6-2. Multiple myeloma. Diffuse myelomatous infiltration causes generalized demineralization of the vertebral bodies and a compression fracture of L2.

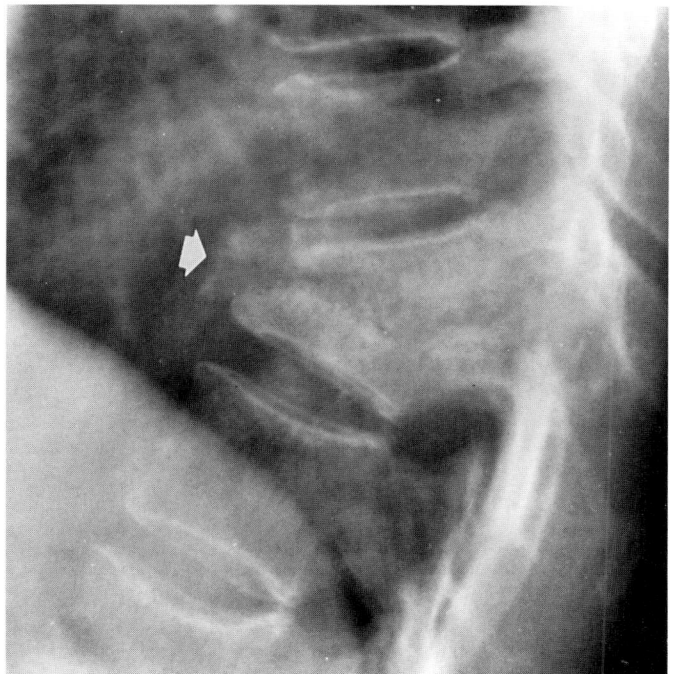

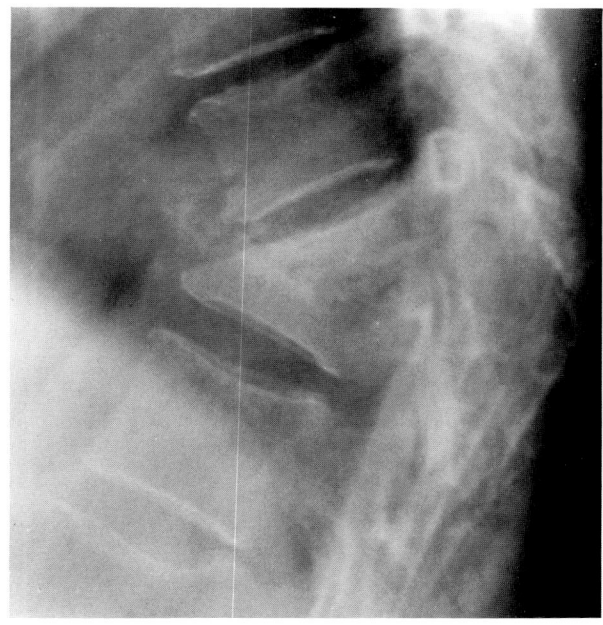

FIG SP6-3. Tuberculous osteomyelitis of the thoracic spine. (A) Initial film demonstrates vertebral collapse and anterior wedging of adjacent midthoracic vertebrae (arrow). The residual intervertebral disk space can barely be seen. (B) Several months later there is virtual fusion of the collapsed vertebral bodies, producing a characteristic sharp kyphotic angulation (gibbous deformity).

Condition	Imaging Findings	Comments
Osteomyelitis **Pyogenic**	Various radiographic patterns including disk space narrowing, loss of the normally sharp adjacent subchondral plates, areas of cortical demineralization, vertebral body destruction and even collapse, and sclerotic new bone formation.	Rapid involvement of the intervertebral disks (loss of disk spaces and destruction of adjacent end plates), in contrast to the vertebral body involvement and preservation of disk spaces in metastatic disease.
Tuberculous **(Fig SP6-3)**	Irregular, poorly marginated bone destruction in a vertebral body, with narrowing of the adjacent intervertebral disk and extension of infection and bone destruction across the disk to involve the contiguous vertebral body.	Most commonly involves the anterior part of vertebral bodies in the thoracic and lumbar region. Often associated with a paravertebral abscess, an accumulation of purulent material that produces a soft-tissue mass about the vertebra. Unlike pyogenic infection, tuberculous osteomyelitis is rarely associated with periosteal reaction or bone sclerosis. In the untreated patient, progressive vertebral collapse and anterior wedging lead to the development of a characteristic sharp kyphotic angulation and gibbous deformity. Healed lesions may demonstrate mottled calcific deposits in a paravertebral abscess and moderate recalcification and sclerosis of the affected bones.
Brucellosis **(Fig SP6-4)**	In the less common central type of vertebral lesion, lytic destruction of the vertebral body leads to vertebral collapse with various degrees of wedging and often the development of a paraspinal abscess (overall pattern closely simulates that of tuberculous infection).	Primarily a disease of animals (cattle, swine, goats, sheep) that is transmitted to humans by the ingestion of infected dairy products or meat or through direct contact with animals, their carcasses, or their excreta. In the more common peripheral form, loss of cortical definition or frank erosions of the anterior and superior margins of the vertebral bodies and disk space narrowing is followed by reactive sclerosis and hypertrophic spur formation.
Fungal infections	Generally produce spinal involvement mimicking tuberculosis.	Infrequent manifestation of actinomycosis, blastomycosis, coccidioidomycosis, cryptococcosis, or aspergillosis. The diagnosis depends on biopsy and culture of the organism.
Fractures **(Fig SP6-5)**	Primarily anterior wedging of the superior end plate of a vertebral body. Severe compressive forces may drive the nucleus pulposus into the vertebral body, resulting in a burst fracture with the posterosuperior fragment often driven into the spinal canal. In patients who have jumped from great heights, compression fractures of the thoracolumbar junction are frequently associated with a fracture of the calcaneus.	Primarily involve the T11 to L4 region. In older patients it may be difficult to distinguish an acute spinal fracture from the vertebral compression that is frequently associated with osteoporosis. In acute trauma there is often evidence of cortical disruption, a paraspinal soft-tissue mass, or an ill-defined increase in density beneath the end plate of an involved vertebra, indicating bone impaction. In osteoporosis, vertebral compression is often associated with osteophytic spurs arising from the apposing margins of the involved and adjacent vertebral bodies. An acute spinal fracture may be difficult to distinguish from a pathologic fracture caused by metastases or multiple myeloma. (The presence of bone destruction, especially involving the cortex, indicates a pathologic fracture.)

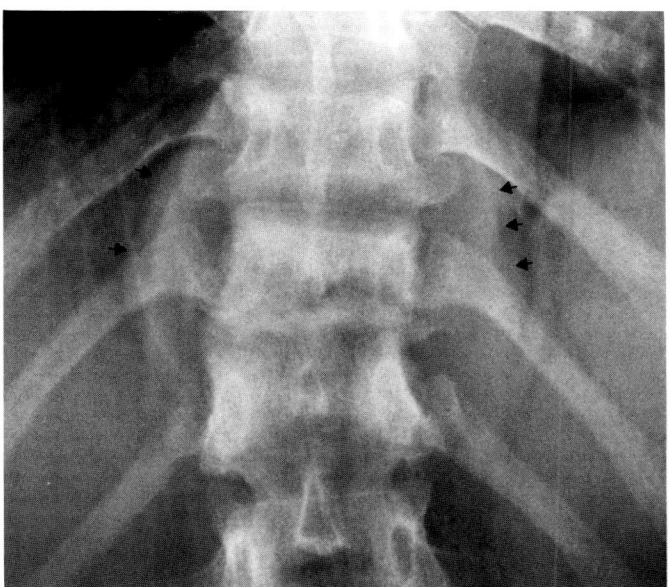
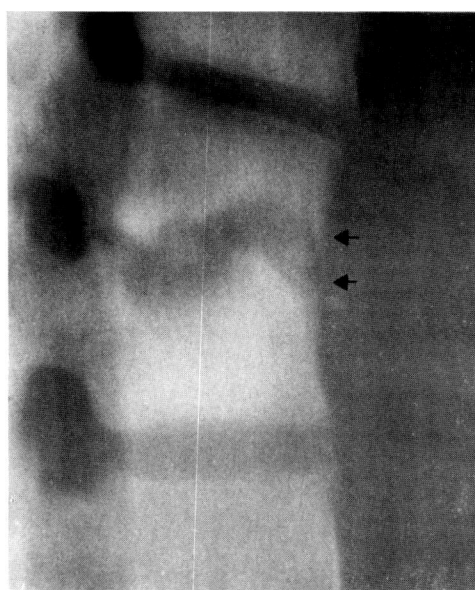

FIG SP6-4. Brucellosis. (A) Frontal plain film of the lower thoracic spine demonstrates loss of height of the T11 and T12 vertebral bodies with destruction of end plates and swelling of the paravertebral soft tissues (arrows). (B) A lateral tomogram of the lower thoracic spine demonstrates cortical destruction with sclerosis of the inferior end plate of T11 and the superior end plate of T12 (arrows). There is a mild degree of anterior wedging. The overall radiographic appearance is indistinguishable from that of tuberculous spondylitis.

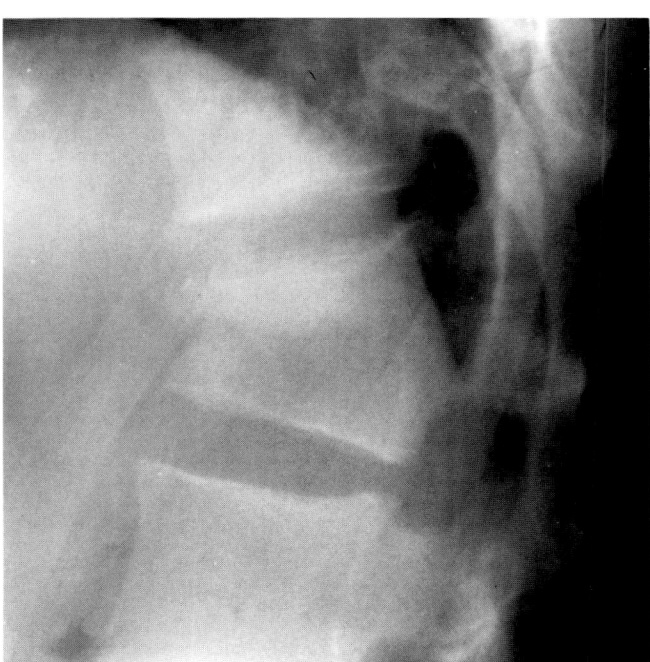

FIG SP6-5. Fracture. Characteristic anterior wedging of the superior end plate of the L1 vertebral body.

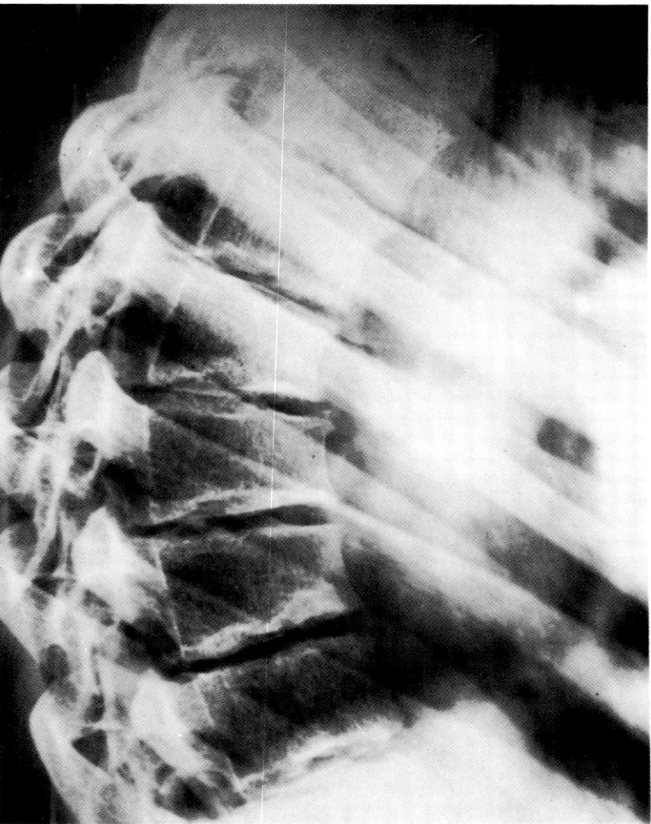

FIG SP6-6. Scheuermann's disease. Irregularity of the vertebral end plates and wedging of the vertebral bodies, which causes an arcuate kyphosis.[7]

Condition	Imaging Findings	Comments
Scheuermann's disease (vertebral epiphysitis) (Fig SP6-6)	Irregularity and loss of the sharp outline of the ringlike epiphyses along the upper and lower margins of vertebral bodies that is followed by fragmentation and sclerosis, causing the adjacent border of the vertebral body to become irregular. The affected vertebrae tend to become wedge shaped (they decrease in height anteriorly).	Occurs in both sexes between the ages of 12 and 17. Although the cause of this familial condition is unclear, possible contributing factors include circulatory disturbances, early disk degeneration, and faulty ossification. Wedging of vertebral bodies produces a dorsal kyphosis, which persists even after the disease has healed.
Eosinophilic granuloma (Fig SP6-7)	Spotty destruction in a vertebral body that proceeds to collapse. The vertebra assumes the shape of a thin flat disk (vertebra plana).	Most commonly occurs in children under age 10. The intervertebral disk spaces are preserved.
Morquio syndrome (Fig SP6-8)	Universal flattening of vertebral bodies (vertebrae planae).	Characteristic central anterior beaking in this form of mucopolysaccharidosis.
Spondyloepiphyseal dysplasia (Fig SP6-9)	Generalized flattening of lumbar vertebral bodies, often with a distinctive hump-shaped mound of bone on their superior and inferior surfaces.	Rare hereditary dwarfism that affects both the extremities and the vertebrae. Characteristic findings include flattening of the femoral capital epiphyses with early degenerative changes, a small pelvis, and a general delay in ossification of the skeleton.
Paget's disease	Archlike contour defects of the superior and inferior vertebral surfaces or a pathologic fracture.	Although there is typically enlargement of the vertebral body with increased trabeculation that is most prominent at the periphery, the weakened bone permits expansion of the nucleus pulposus and results in an increased incidence of pathologic fracture.
Sickle cell anemia (Fig SP6-10)	Localized steplike central depression of multiple vertebral end plates. There may also be biconcave indentations on the superior and inferior margins of the softened vertebral bodies due to expansile pressure of the adjacent intervertebral disks.	Probably caused by circulatory stasis and ischemia, which retard growth in the central portion of the vertebral cartilaginous growth plate while the periphery of the growth plate (with a different blood supply) continues to grow at a more normal rate.
Gaucher's disease	Localized steplike central depression of multiple vertebral end plates.	Probably caused by circulatory stasis and ischemia, which retard growth in the central portion of the vertebral cartilaginous growth plate while the periphery of the growth plate (with a different blood supply) continues to grow at a more normal rate. This inborn error of metabolism is characterized by the accumulation of abnormal quantities of complex lipids in the reticuloendothelial cells of the spleen, liver, and bone marrow.
Primary bone neoplasm	Various patterns of bone destruction and pathologic fracture.	Benign tumor (hemangioma, giant cell tumor, aneurysmal bone cyst); lymphoma; sarcoma; chordoma (sacrum).

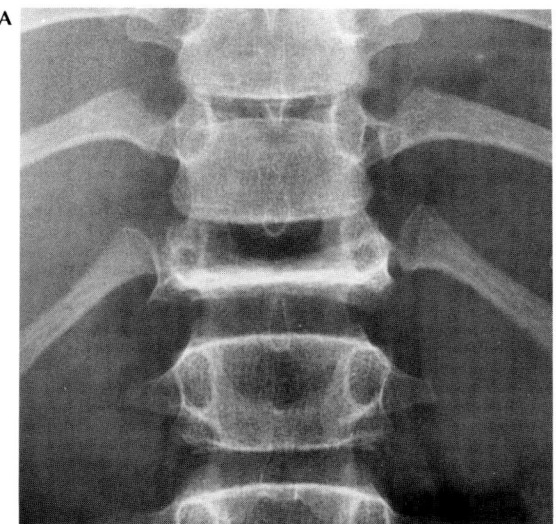

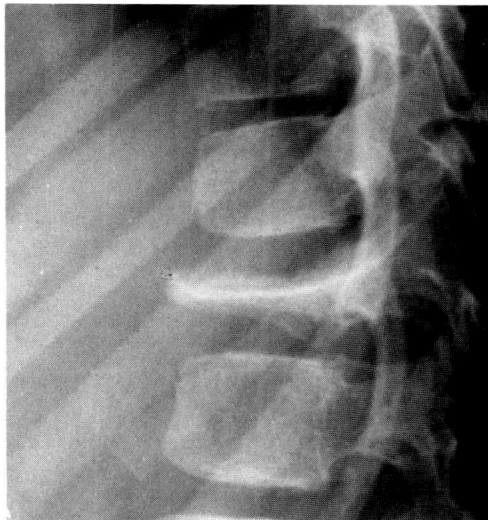

FIG SP6-7. Eosinophilic granuloma. (A) Frontal and (B) lateral views of the spine show complete collapse with flattening of the T12 vertebral body (vertebra plana).

FIG SP6-8. Morquio syndrome. Generalized flattening of vertebral bodies in the (A) cervical and (B) lumbar regions.

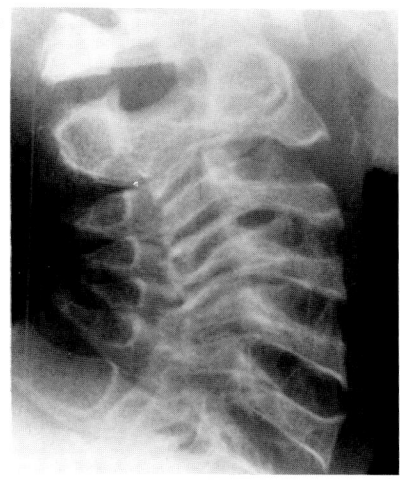

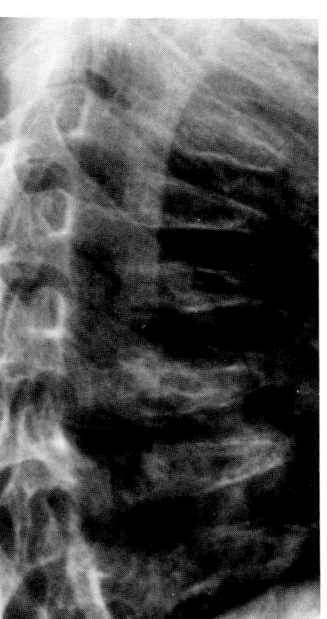

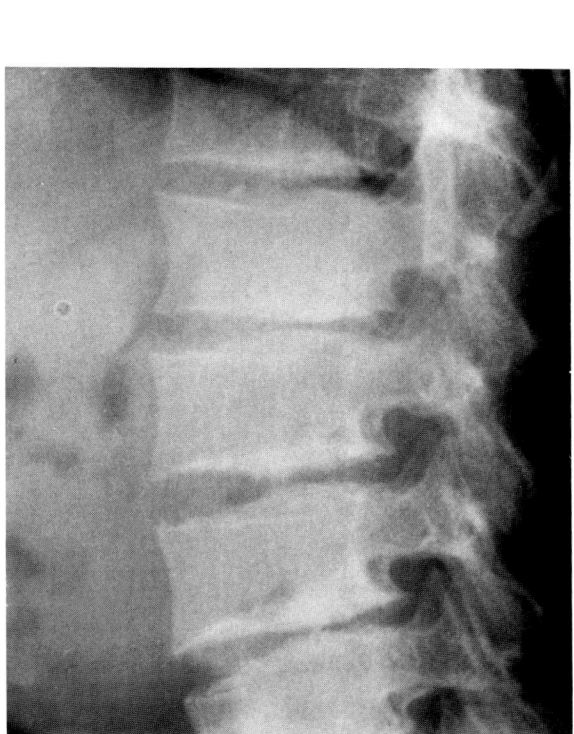

FIG SP6-9. Spondyloepiphyseal dysplasia. Generalized flattening of vertebral bodies (platyspondyly).

Condition	Imaging Findings	Comments
Osteogenesis imperfecta (Fig SP6-11)	Flattening of vertebral bodies, which are either biconcave or wedge shaped anteriorly.	Inherited generalized disorder of connective tissue causing thin, brittle bones. Severe kyphoscoliosis results from a combination of ligamentous laxity, osteoporosis, and posttraumatic deformities.
Convulsions (Fig SP6-12)	Multiple compression fractures, primarily involving the midthoracic vertebrae.	Tetanus (*Clostridium tetani*); tetany; hypoglycemia; shock therapy. Although the degree of compression may be substantial, the fractures infrequently cause pain and usually do not lead to neurologic sequelae.
Vanishing bone disease	Diffuse destruction of multiple vertebral bodies.	Rare condition that most often involves the pelvis, ribs, spine, and long bones. No sclerotic or periosteal reaction.
Amyloidosis	Loss of bone density and collapse of one or more vertebral bodies.	Rare manifestation caused by diffuse infiltration of the bone marrow by the amorphous protein. Generalized demineralization with collapse of vertebral bodies is usually a manifestation of underlying multiple myeloma.
Hydatid (echinococcal) cyst	Expanding lytic lesion causing a pathologic fracture.	Bone involvement occurs in about 1% of patients and most commonly affects the vertebral bodies, pelvis, and sacrum.
Traumatic ischemic necrosis (Kümmell's spondylitis)	Delayed posttraumatic reaction characterized by rarefaction of the vertebral body, intravertebral vacuum cleft, and vertebral collapse.	The existence of this condition is controversial. Most authorities believe that significant trauma to the spine occurred at the time of the initial injury in instances of alleged Kümmell's spondylitis.
Thanatophoric dwarfism	Extreme flattening of hypoplastic vertebral bodies.	An H or U configuration of the vertebral bodies can be seen on frontal projections.

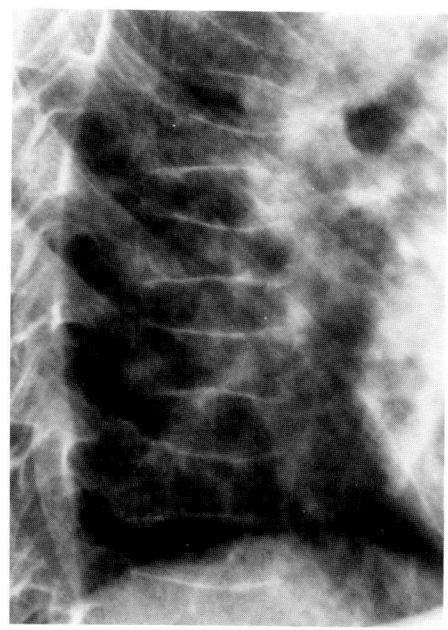
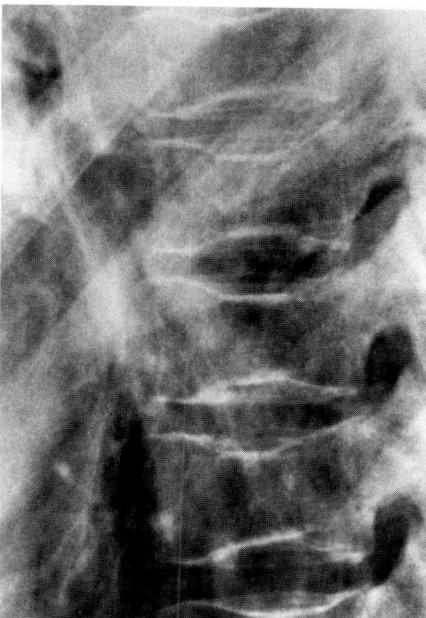

FIG SP6-10. Sickle cell anemia. (A) Biconcave indentations on both the superior and inferior margins of the soft vertebral bodies produce the characteristic "fish vertebrae." (B) Localized steplike central depressions of multiple vertebral end plates.

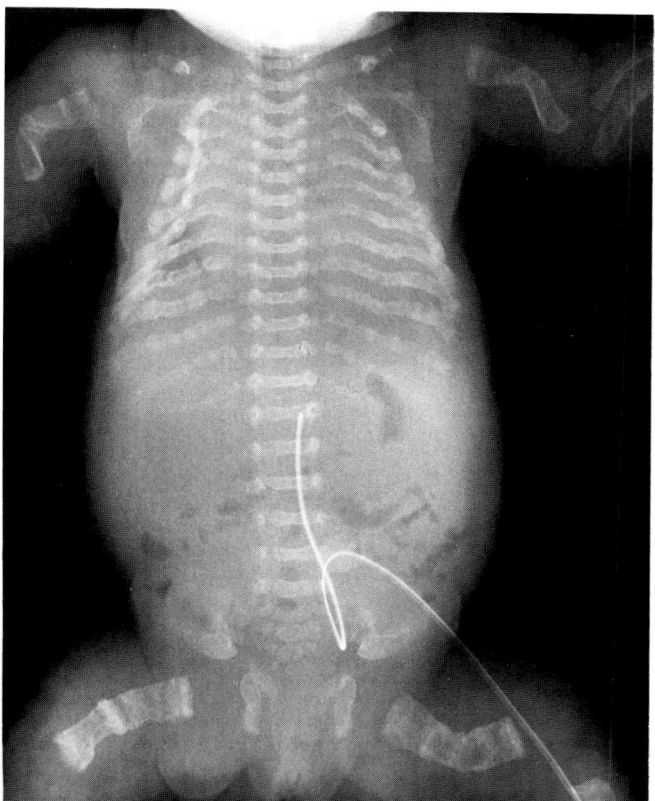

FIG SP6-11. Osteogenesis imperfecta. Generalized flattening of vertebral bodies associated with fractures of multiple ribs and long bones in an infant.

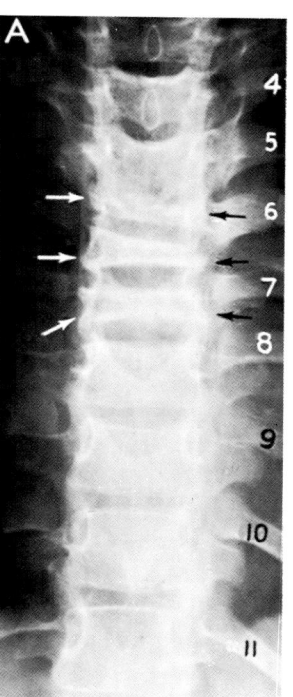
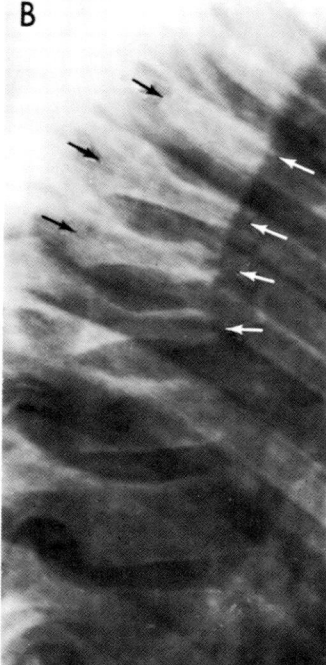

FIG SP6-12. Tetanus. (A) Frontal and (B) lateral projections show residual fractures and compression deformities of vertebral bodies (arrows).[8]

NARROWING OF THE INTERVERTEBRAL DISK SPACE
AND ADJACENT SCLEROSIS

Condition	Imaging Findings	Comments
Intervertebral osteochondrosis (degenerative disk disease) (Fig SP7-1)	Well-defined sclerosis of vertebral margins and characteristic "vacuum" phenomenon.	Degeneration of the nucleus pulposus and the cartilaginous end plate.
Infection (Figs SP7-2 to SP7-4)	Ill-defined vertebral margins and often a soft-tissue mass. Reactive sclerosis is common with pyogenic inflammation but infrequent with tuberculosis.	Depending on the site of disease, anterior extension of vertebral osteomyelitis may cause retropharyngeal abscess, mediastinitis, pericarditis, subdiaphragmatic abscess, psoas muscle abscess, or peritonitis. Posterior extension of inflammatory tissue can compress the spinal cord or produce meningitis if the infection penetrates the dura to enter the subarachnoid space.
Trauma	Well-defined sclerotic vertebral margins, soft-tissue mass, and evidence of fracture.	Disk injury and degeneration is the underlying mechanism.
Neuroarthropathy (Fig SP7-5)	Extensive sclerosis of the vertebrae associated with osteophytosis, fragmentation, and malalignment.	Caused by repetitive trauma in patients with loss of sensation and proprioception due to such conditions as diabetes, syphilis, syringomyelia, leprosy, and congenital insensitivity to pain.
Calcium pyrophosphate dihydrate (CPPD) crystal deposition disease	Ill- or well-defined sclerotic vertebral margins associated with fragmentation, subluxation, and calcification.	Degenerative process secondary to the deposition of calcium pyrophosphate dihydrate crystals in cartilaginous end plates and intervertebral disks.
Ochronosis (see Fig SP14-2)	Well-defined sclerotic vertebral margins with "vacuum" phenomena and pathognomonic diskal calcification.	Degenerative change resulting from the deposition of the black pigment of oxidized homogentisic acid in cartilaginous end plates and intervertebral disks.
Rheumatoid arthritis	Ill- or well-defined sclerotic vertebral margins associated with subluxations and apophyseal joint abnormalities.	Loss of the intervertebral disk space (usually in the cervical region) may reflect apophyseal joint instability with recurrent diskovertebral trauma or extension of inflammatory tissue from neighboring articulations.

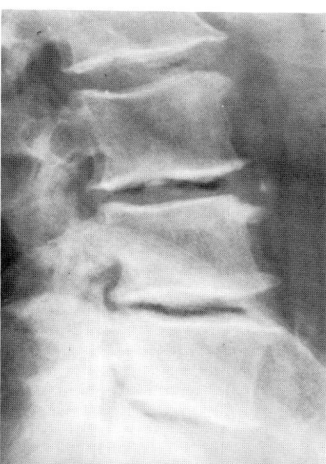

FIG SP7-1. Degenerative disk disease. Hypertrophic spurring, intervertebral disk space narrowing, and reactive sclerosis. Note the linear lucent collections (vacuum phenomenon) overlying several of the intervertebral disks.

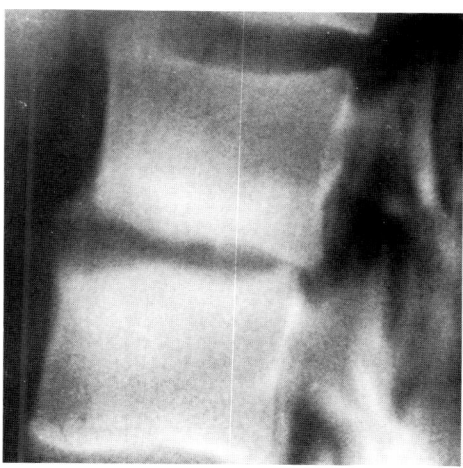

FIG SP7-2. Pyogenic vertebral osteomyelitis. Narrowing of the intervertebral disk space with irregularity of the end plates and reactive sclerosis.

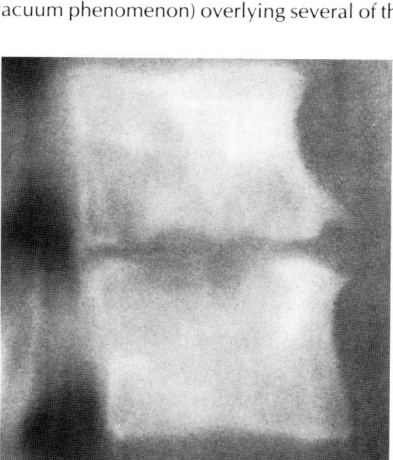

FIG SP7-3. *Pseudomonas* osteomyelitis. Tomogram shows the destructive process in L2 and L3, irregular narrowing of the intervertebral disk space, and reactive sclerosis.

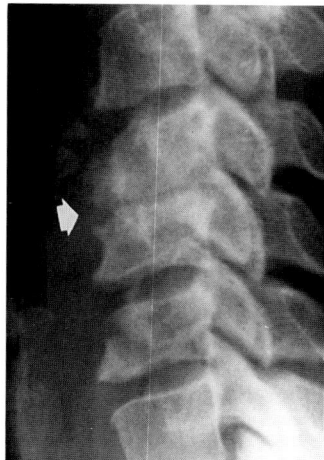

FIG SP7-4. Tuberculous osteomyelitis of the cervical spine. Narrowing of the intervertebral disk space (arrow) is accompanied by diffuse bone destruction involving the adjacent vertebrae. Note the lack of sclerotic reaction.

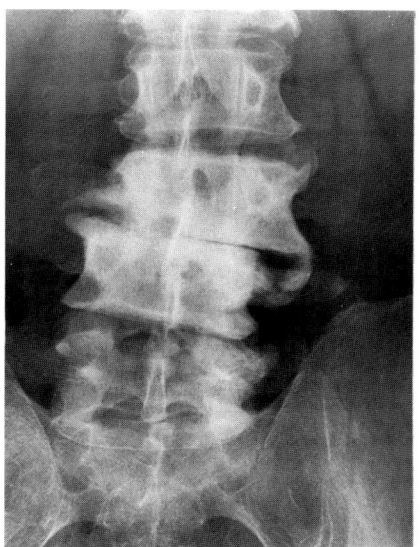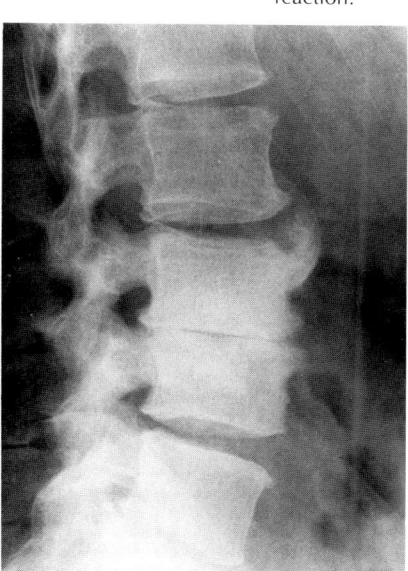

FIG SP7-5. Neuroarthropathy. (A) Frontal and (B) lateral views of the lumbosacral spine in a patient with tabes dorsalis show marked hypertrophic spurring with virtual obliteration of the intervertebral disk space between L3 and L4. Note the reactive sclerosis of the apposing end plates and the subluxation of the vertebral bodies seen on the frontal view.

A   B

LOCALIZED WIDENING OF THE INTERPEDICULAR DISTANCE

Condition	Comments
Intramedullary neoplasm of spinal cord	Large tumors can cause localized thinning and re-molding of the pedicles, most commonly at the L1 to L3 level. The most common cause is an ependymoma of the cord, especially of the conus or filum terminale. Also may occur with astrocytoma, oligodendroglioma, glioblastoma multiforme, and medulloblastoma.
Meningocele/ myelomeningocele (Fig SP8-1)	Large posterior spinal defect through which there is herniation of the meninges (meningocele) or of the meninges and a portion of the spinal cord or nerve roots (myelomeningocele). The posterior defect is marked by absence of the spinous processes and laminae and widening of the interpedicular distance, as well as a soft-tissue mass representing the herniation itself.
Diastematomyelia (Fig SP8-2)	Fusiform widening of the spinal canal with an increase in the interpedicular distance that extends over several segments is a characteristic finding in this rare malformation in which the spinal cord is split by a midline bony, cartilaginous, or fibrous spur extending posteriorly from a vertebral body. If the septum dividing the cord is ossified, it may appear on frontal views as a pathognomonic thin vertical bony plate lying in the middle of the neural canal. The condition most commonly occurs in the lower thoracic and upper lumbar regions and is often associated with a variety of skeletal and central nervous system anomalies.

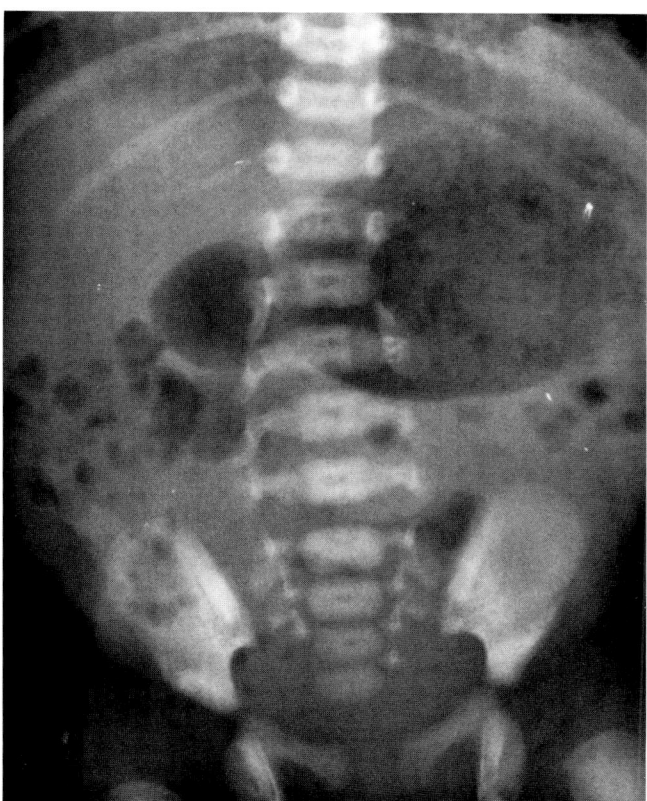

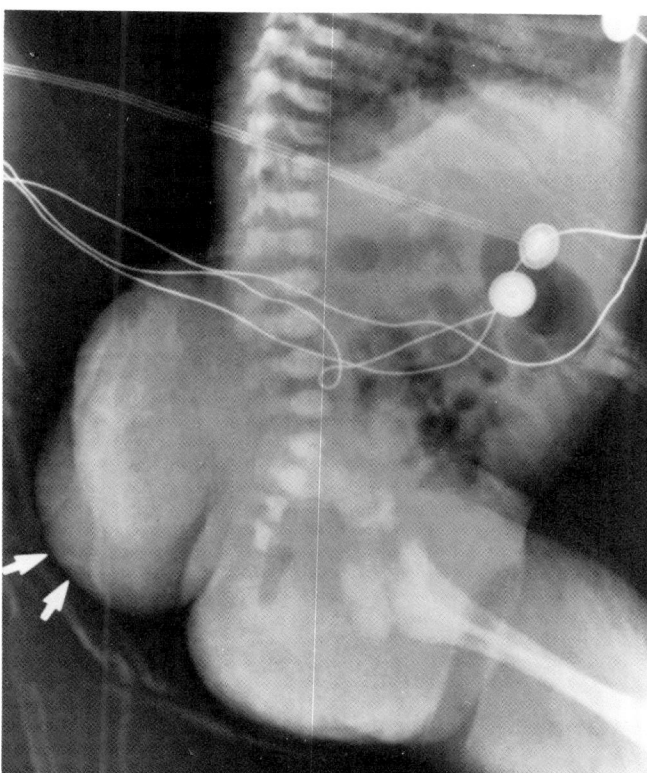

A

B

FIG SP8-1. Meningomyelocele. (A) Frontal view of the abdomen shows the markedly increased interpedicular distance of the lumbar vertebrae. (B) In another patient, a lateral view demonstrates the large soft-tissue mass (arrows) situated posterior to the spine. Note the absence of the posterior elements in the lower lumbar and sacral regions.

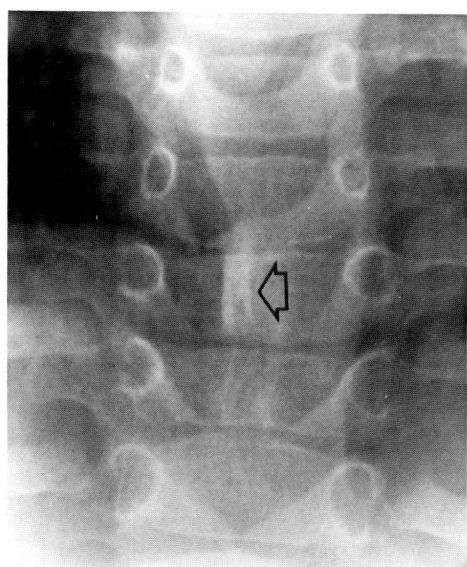

FIG SP8-2. Diastematomyelia. Note the pathognomonic ossified septum (arrow) lying in the midline of the neural canal.

ANTERIOR SCALLOPING OF A VERTEBRAL BODY

Condition	Comments
Lymphoma/chronic leukemia	Erosion of the anterior surfaces of upper lumbar and lower thoracic vertebral bodies is caused by direct neoplastic extension from adjacent lymph nodes. Other skeletal abnormalities include paravertebral soft-tissue masses, dense vertebral sclerosis (ivory vertebrae), and a mottled pattern of destruction and sclerosis with hematogenous spread that may simulate metastatic disease.
Other causes of lymphadenopathy	Metastases or inflammatory processes (especially tuberculosis).
Aortic aneurysm	Continuous pulsatile pressure can rarely cause erosions of the anterior aspect of one or more vertebral bodies. The concomitant demonstration of the calcified wall of the bulging aneurysm is virtually pathognomonic.

POSTERIOR SCALLOPING OF A VERTEBRAL BODY

Condition	Comments
Normal variant (physiologic scalloping)	Minimal to moderate posterior scalloping limited to the lumbar spine can be demonstrated in about half of normal adults. The appearance is identical to that of a mild degree of pathologic scalloping, but there is no associated pedicle abnormality or widening of the interpedicular distance.
Increased intraspinal pressure	Posterior scalloping most commonly occurs with local expanding lesions that are situated in the more caudal portion of the spinal canal, are relatively large and slow growing, and originate during the period of active growth and bone modeling. Generally reflects an intraspinal neoplasm (ependymoma, dermoid, lipoma, or neurofibroma). Intraspinal meningiomas rarely produce even minor bone changes because they are situated above the level of the conus and tend to produce cord symptoms while still relatively small. Other rare underlying causes include spinal cysts, syringomyelia and hydromyelia, and severe generalized communicating hydrocephalus.
Achondroplasia (Fig SP10-1)	Decreased endochondral bone formation causes the pedicles to be short and the interpedicular spaces to narrow progressively from above downward (opposite of normal), thus reducing the volume of the spinal canal. This is postulated to limit the normal posterior enlargement of the vertebral canal during the early growth period, with the result that the growing subarachnoid space must gain room for expansion through scalloping of the posterior aspects of the vertebral bodies.
Neurofibromatosis (Fig SP10-2)	Posterior scalloping may reflect an osseous dysplasia, weakness of the dura (permitting transmission of cerebrospinal fluid pulsations to the bone), or an associated thoracic meningocele.
Hereditary connective tissue disorders (dural ectasia)	Posterior scalloping is secondary to loss of the normal protection afforded the posterior surfaces of the vertebral bodies by an intact, strong dura. The underlying mesodermal dysplasia causes dural ectasia or weakness that permits transmission of cerebrospinal fluid pulsations to the bone. Occurs in such congenital syndromes as Ehlers-Danlos, Marfan's, and osteogenesis imperfecta tarda.

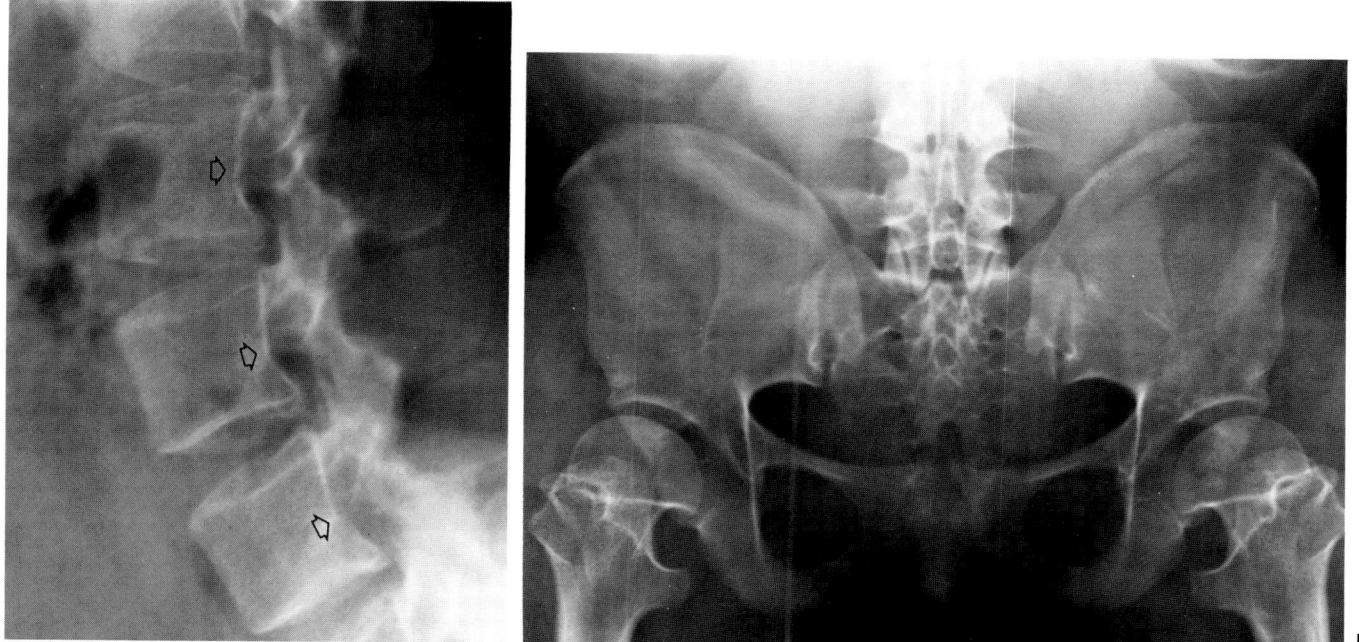

Fɪɢ SP10-1. Achondroplasia. (A) Posterior scalloping of multiple vertebral bodies (arrows). (B) Characteristic short, broad pelvis with small sacro-sciatic notch.

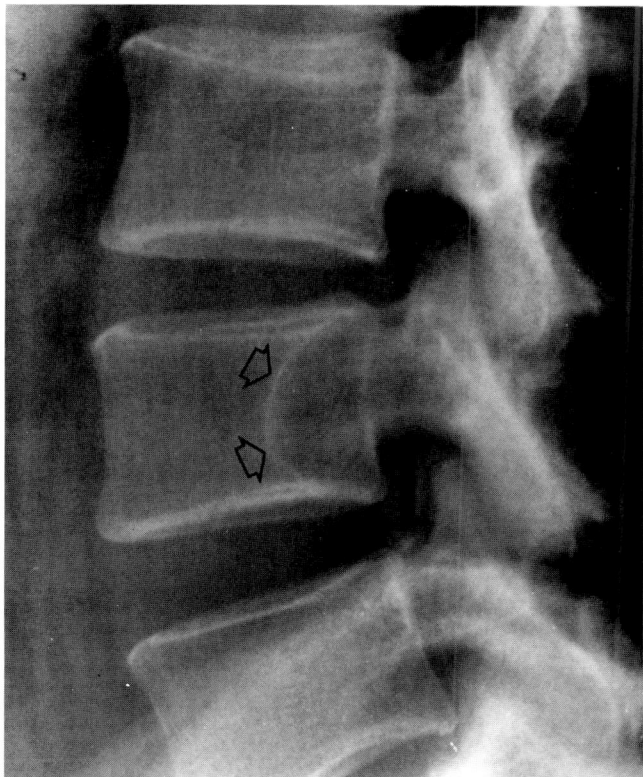

Fɪɢ SP10-2. Neurofibromatosis (arrows).

Condition	Comments
Mucopolysaccharidoses (Fig SP10-3)	Inborn disorders of mucopolysaccharide metabolism in Hurler's and Morquio's syndromes may produce abnormal vertebral bodies that are unable to resist the normal cerebrospinal fluid pulsations over their posterior surfaces (even though the dura is normal).
Acromegaly (Fig SP10-4)	Hypertrophy of soft tissue may produce posterior scalloping.

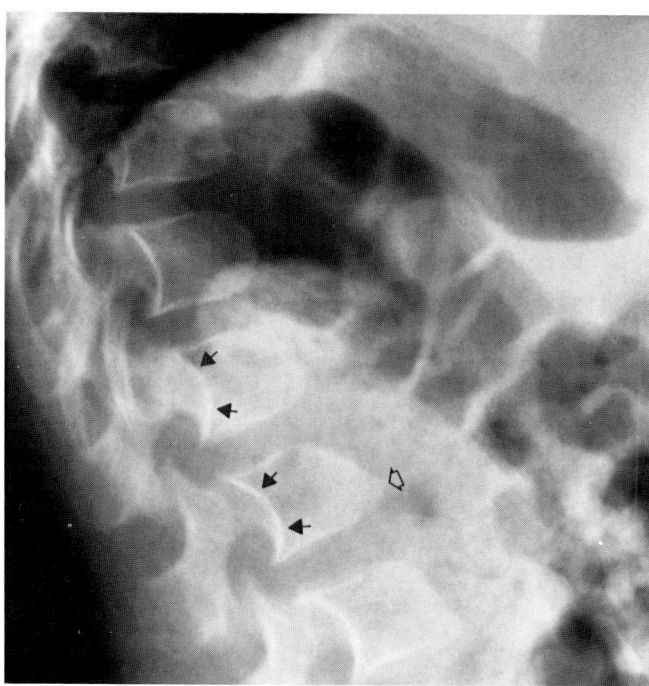

FIG SP10-3. Hurler's syndrome. In addition to the posterior scalloping (closed arrows), there is typical inferior beaking (open arrow) of the anterior margin of the vertebral body.

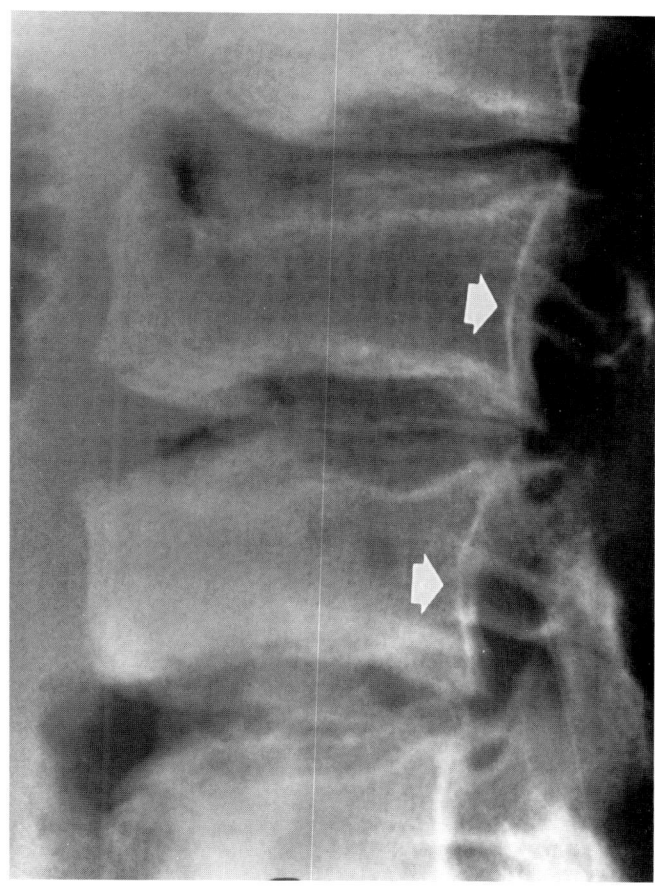

FIG SP10-4. Acromegaly. Posterior scalloping (arrows) associated with enlargement of vertebral bodies (especially in the anteroposterior dimension).

SQUARING OF ONE OR MORE VERTEBRAL BODIES

Condition	Comments
Ankylosing spondylitis (Fig SP11-1)	Erosive osteitis of the corners of the vertebral bodies produces a loss of the normal anterior concavity and a characteristic squared vertebral body. Spinal involvement initially involves the lower lumbar area and progresses upward to the dorsal and cervical regions. Characteristic bilateral and symmetric sacroiliitis and a ''bamboo'' spine (ossification in paravertebral tissues and longitudinal spinal ligaments combined with extensive lateral bony bridges, or syndesmophytes).
Paget's disease	Enlargement of affected vertebral bodies with increased trabeculation that is most prominent at the periphery of the bone and produces a rim of thickened cortex and a squared, picture-frame appearance. Dense sclerosis may produce an ivory vertebra.
Rheumatoid variants	Uncommon manifestation of rheumatoid arthritis, psoriatic arthritis, or Reiter's syndrome.
Down's syndrome (mongolism)	Manifestations include a decrease in the acetabular and iliac angles with hypoplasia and marked lateral flaring of the iliac wings, multiple manubrial ossification centers, the presence of 11 ribs, and shortening of the middle phalanx of the fifth finger.

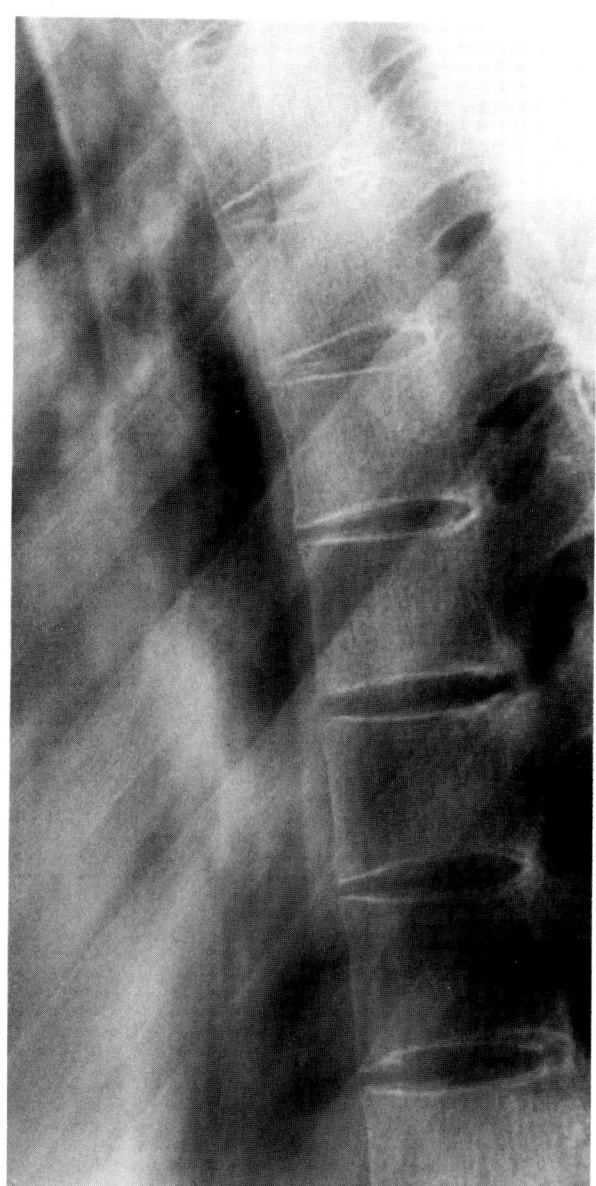

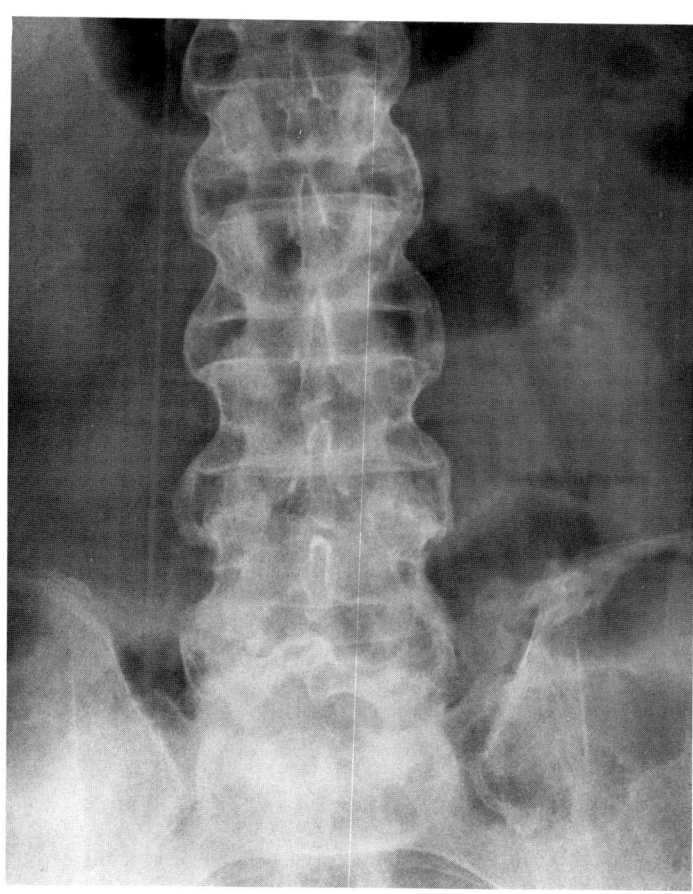

A   B

FIG SP11-1. Ankylosing spondylitis. (A) Characteristic squaring of thoracic vertebral bodies. (B) Extensive lateral bony bridges (syndesmophytes) connect all the lumbar vertebral bodies to produce a bamboo spine.

ENLARGED CERVICAL INTERVERTEBRAL FORAMEN

Condition	Comments
Neurofibroma **(Fig SP12-1)**	The most common cause of an enlarged cervical intervertebral foramen is the "dumbbell" type of neurofibroma (intradural and extradural components) that erodes the superior or inferior margins of the pedicles. Enlargement of an intervertebral foramen may also develop because of protrusion of a lateral intrathoracic meningocele in a patient with generalized neurofibromatosis.
Other spinal tumors	Rare manifestation of dermoid, lipoma, lymphoma, meningioma, and neuroblastoma.
Congenital absence of pedicle	Produces the radiographic appearance of an enlarged cervical intervertebral foramen.
Vertebral artery aneurysm or tortuosity **(Fig SP12-2)**	Erosion is caused by pulsatile flow as the vertebral artery passes through the foramina transversaria of the upper six cervical vertebrae between its origin from the subclavian artery and its entrance into the cranial vault through the foramen magnum.
Traumatic avulsion of nerve root **(Fig SP12-3)**	On myelography, a brachial root avulsion produces a pouchlike appearance of the root sleeve, which is blunted and distorted and extends for a variable distance into the intervertebral foramen. Nerve root avulsions can be readily differentiated from diverticula of the subarachnoid space, which have smooth, delicately rounded contours and exhibit the normal radiolucent outlines of intact nerve roots within the opaque, contrast-filled pocket.

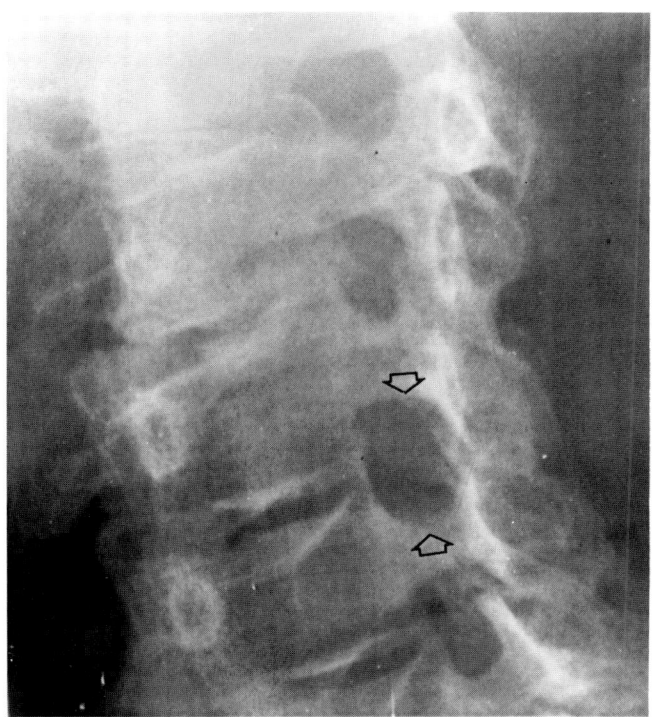

FIG SP12-1. Neurofibroma. Smooth widening (arrows) due to the contiguous mass, without evidence of bone destruction.

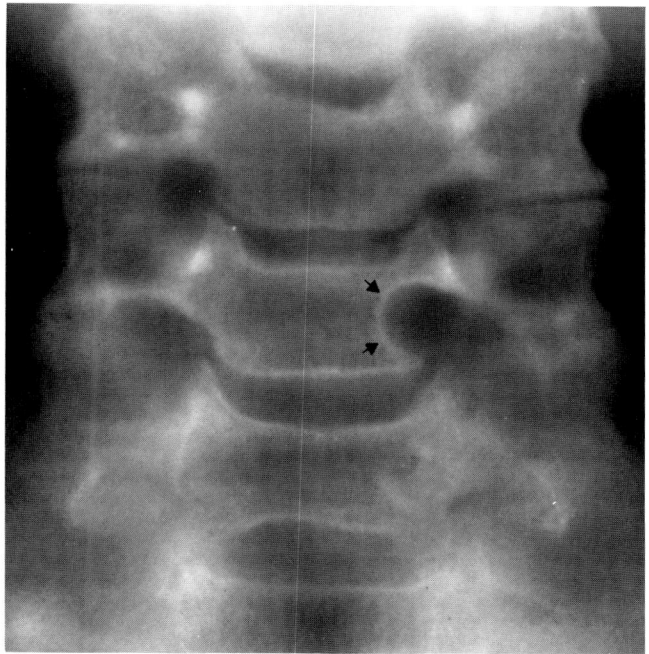

A

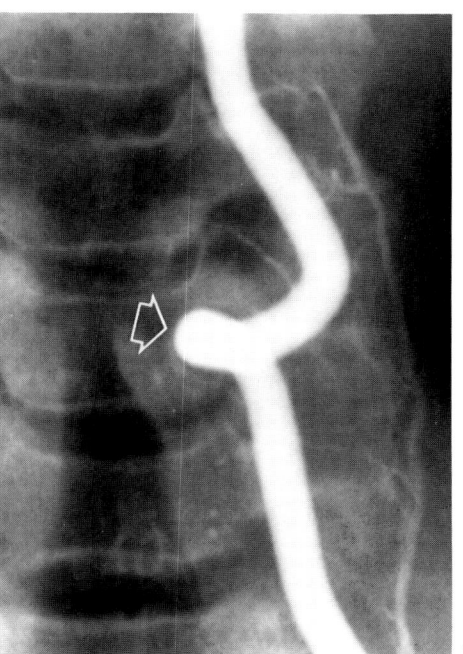

B

FIG SP12-2. Tortuous vertebral artery. (A) Frontal tomogram shows the enlarged foramen (arrows). (B) Arteriogram shows the tortuous vertebral artery (arrow) entering the enlarged foramen.

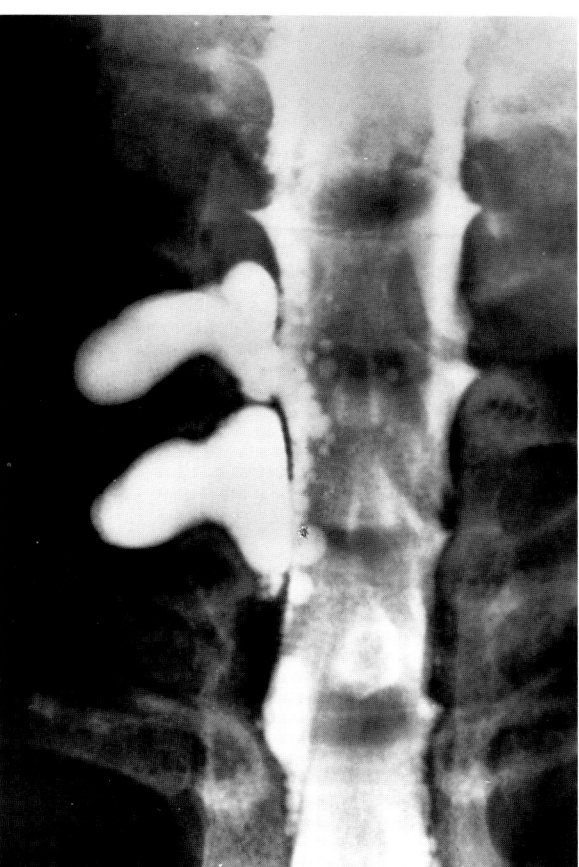

FIG SP12-3. Traumatic avulsion of nerve roots. Note the pouchlike appearance of the blunted nerve roots that extend into the cervical foramina.

ATLANTOAXIAL SUBLUXATION

Condition	Comments
Rheumatoid arthritis **(Fig SP13-1)**	Synovial inflammation causes weakening of the transverse ligaments. The odontoid process is often eroded, and the dens may be completely destroyed. Upward displacement of C2 may permit the dens to impinge on the upper cervical cord or medulla, producing acute neurologic symptoms requiring immediate traction or decompression. Atlantoaxial subluxation also occurs in juvenile rheumatoid arthritis.
Rheumatoid variants	Ankylosing spondylitis; psoriatic arthritis. Inflammatory changes of the synovial and adjacent ligamentous structures can lead to erosion of the dens.
Trauma	Almost always accompanied by a fracture of the odontoid process resulting from hyperflexion (dens and atlas displaced anteriorly) or hyperextension (posterior displacement). Isolated atlantoaxial subluxation (without fracture) indicates tearing of the transverse ligaments.
Congenital cervicobasilar anomaly	Absent anterior arch of the atlas; absent or separate odontoid process; atlanto-occipital fusion.
Retropharyngeal abscess (child)	Presumably causes laxity of the transverse ligaments due to the hyperemia associated with the inflammatory process.
Down's syndrome	Results from laxity of the spinal ligaments and has been reported in up to 20% of cases. Although usually mild and asymptomatic, a few patients develop symptoms ranging from discomfort in the neck to quadriparesis.
Morquio's syndrome	Hypoplasia of the dens in this condition predisposes to atlantoaxial subluxation with consequent damage to the spinal cord. This risk is so high that some authors recommend early prophylactic posterior cervical fusion for patients with this disease.

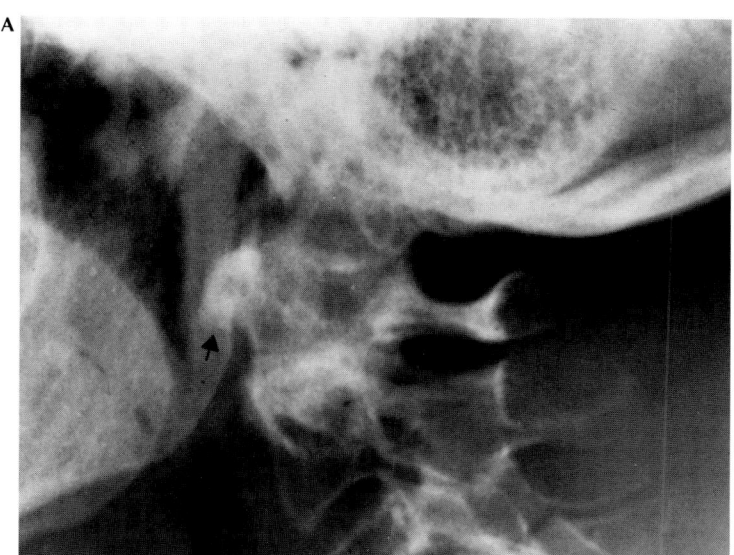

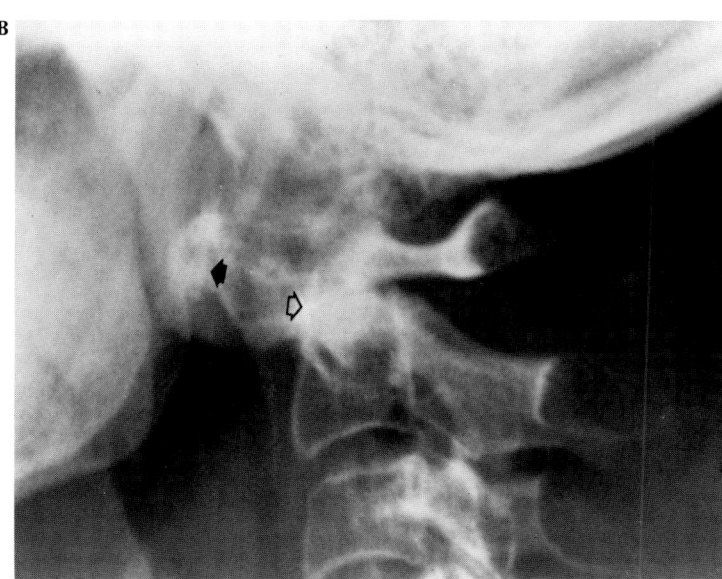

FIG SP13-1. **Rheumatoid arthritis.** (A) Routine lateral film of the cervical spine shows a normal relation between the anterior border of the odontoid process and the superior portion of the anterior arch of the atlas (arrow). (B) With flexion, there is wide separation between the anterior arch of the atlas (closed arrow) and the odontoid (open arrow).

CALCIFICATION OF INTERVERTEBRAL DISKS

Condition	Comments
Degenerative disk disease **(Fig SP14-1)**	Radiographic manifestations include osteophytosis, narrowing of intervertebral disk spaces with marginal sclerosis, and the vacuum phenomenon (linear lucent collection overlying one or more intervertebral disks).
Transient calcification in children	Unlike most other causes of intervertebral disk calcification, in children the cervical region is most commonly involved and there is a high frequency of associated clinical signs and symptoms. A self-limited condition requiring only conservative symptomatic treatment.
Posttraumatic	Associated findings of previous spinal injury.
Ochronosis **(Fig SP14-2)**	Dense laminated calcification of multiple intervertebral disks (beginning in the lumbar spine and extending to the dorsal and cervical regions) is virtually pathognomonic of this rare inborn error of metabolism in which deposition of the black pigment of oxidized homogentisic acid in cartilage and other connective tissue produces a distinctive form of degenerative arthritis. The intervertebral disk spaces are narrowed, the vertebral bodies are osteoporotic, and limitation of motion is common. Severe degenerative arthritis may develop in peripheral joints, especially the shoulders, hips, and knees (an infrequent manifestation of osteoarthritis, especially in young patients).
Ankylosing spondylitis **(Fig SP14-3)**	Central or eccentric, circular or linear calcific collections may appear in the intervertebral disks at single or multiple sites along the spinal column. Usually associated with apophyseal joint ankylosis at the same vertebral levels and adjacent syndesmophytes. The development of similar calcific deposits in other conditions affecting the vertebral column that are characterized by ankylosis (diffuse idiopathic skeletal hyperostosis, juvenile rheumatoid arthritis) suggests that immobilization of a segment of the spine may interfere with diskal nutrition and lead to degeneration and calcification.
Calcium pyrophosphate dihydrate (CPPD) crystal deposition disease	Calcification frequently affects the intervertebral disks and may be associated with back pain. The deposits involve the annulus fibrosis (not the nucleus pulposus, as in ochronosis). Disk space narrowing often occurs.

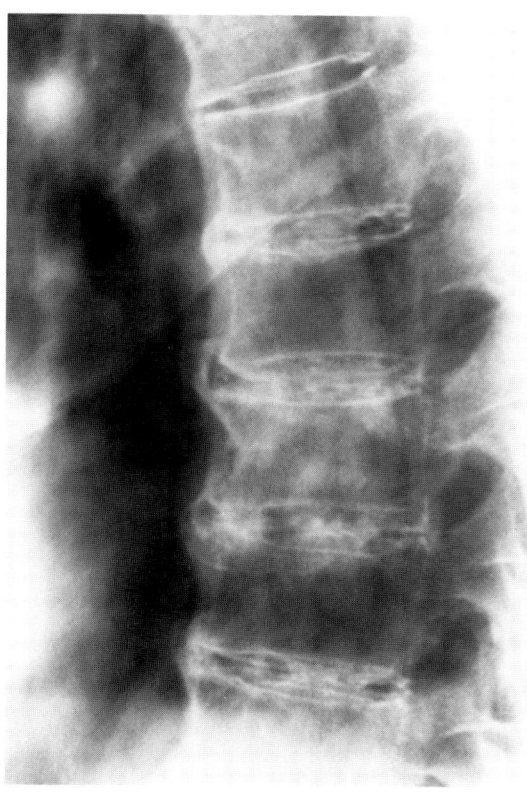

FIG SP14-1. **Degenerative disk disease.** Note the anterior osteophytes, narrowing of intervertebral disk spaces, and calcification in the anterior longitudinal ligament.

A

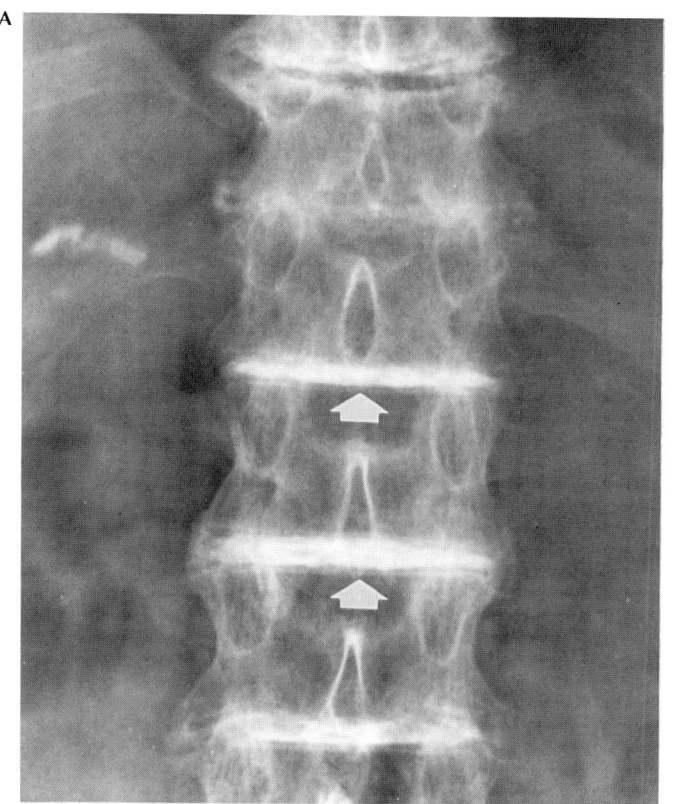

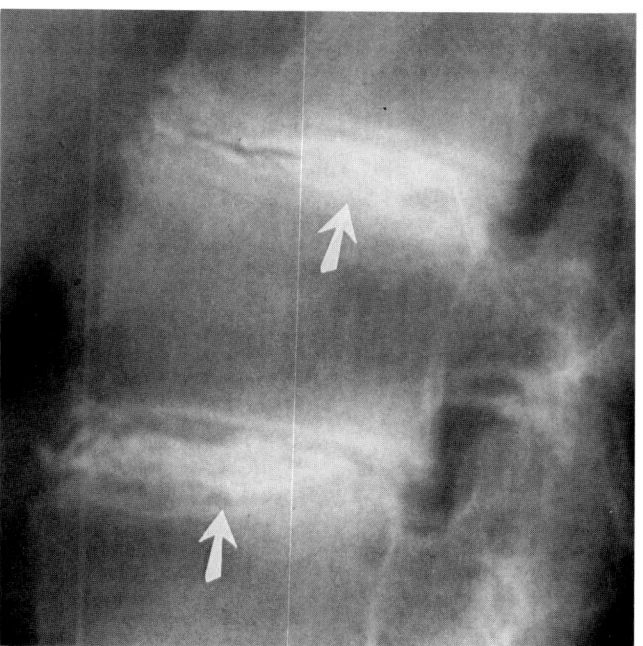

B

FIG SP14-2. **Ochronosis.** (A) Frontal and (B) lateral views of the lumbar spine in two different patients show dense laminated calcification of multiple intervertebral disks (arrows).

234

Condition	Comments
Hemochromatosis	Deposition of calcium pyrophosphate dihydrate crystals occurs in the outer fibers of the annulus fibrosis, as in CPPD. Other radiographic manifestations include diffuse osteoporosis of the spine associated with vertebral collapse and a peripheral arthropathy that most commonly involves the small joints of the hands (especially the second and third metacarpophalangeal joints).
Hypervitaminosis D	Calcification of the annulus fibrosis is an uncommon finding. More often causes generalized osteoporosis with extensive masses of soft-tissue calcification.

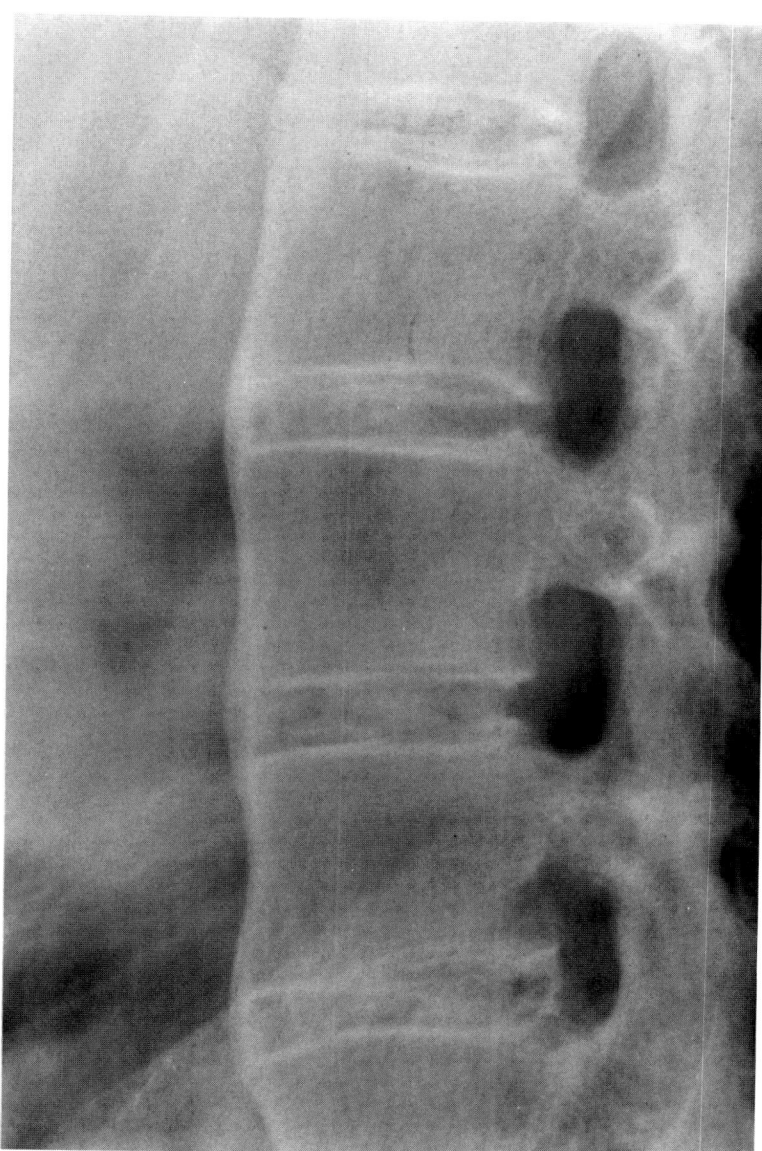

FIG SP14-3. **Ankylosing spondylitis.** Calcification of intervertebral disks is associated with squaring of vertebral bodies and dense calcification of the anterior longitudinal ligament.

BONE-WITHIN-A-BONE APPEARANCE

Condition	Comments
Normal neonate **(Fig SP15-1)**	Not uncommon appearance in infants 1 to 2 months of age caused by loss of bone density at the periphery of vertebral bodies (but with retention of their sharp cortical outlines). The bone subsequently assumes a normal density; thus this appearance probably reflects a normal stage in the transformation of the architecture of the neonatal vertebrae to that of later infancy.
Osteopetrosis **(Fig SP15-2)**	Miniature inset in each lumbar vertebral body is a typical manifestation of this rare hereditary bone abnormality characterized by a symmetric generalized increase in bone density and lack of tubulation.
Thorotrast administration **(Fig SP15-3)**	Radiographic densities of infantile vertebrae and pelvis (ghost vertebrae) in adult bones may be seen in adults who received intravenous Thorotrast during early childhood. The deposition of Thorotrast causes constant alpha radiation and temporary growth arrest, so that the size of the ghost vertebrae corresponds to the vertebral size at the time of injection. Most patients also have reticular or dense opacification of the liver, spleen, and lymph nodes.
Transverse growth lines **(growth arrest lines)** **(Fig SP15-4)**	Opaque transverse lines paralleling the superior and inferior margins of vertebral bodies. Underlying causes include chronic childhood diseases, malnutrition, and chemotherapy.

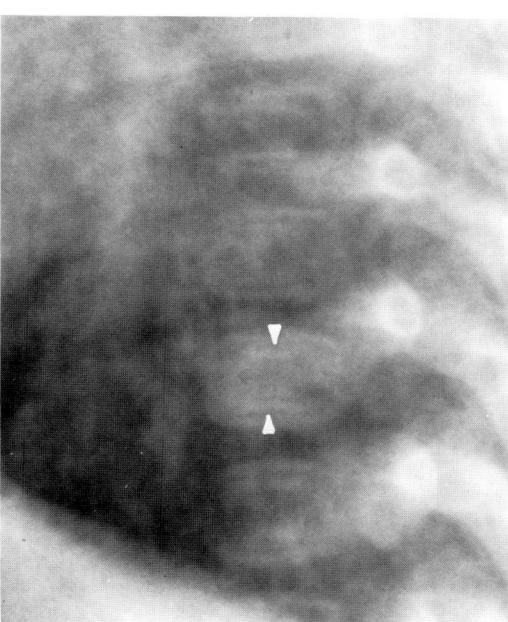

FIG SP15-1. Normal neonate. The arrowheads point to one example of the bone-within-a-bone appearance.

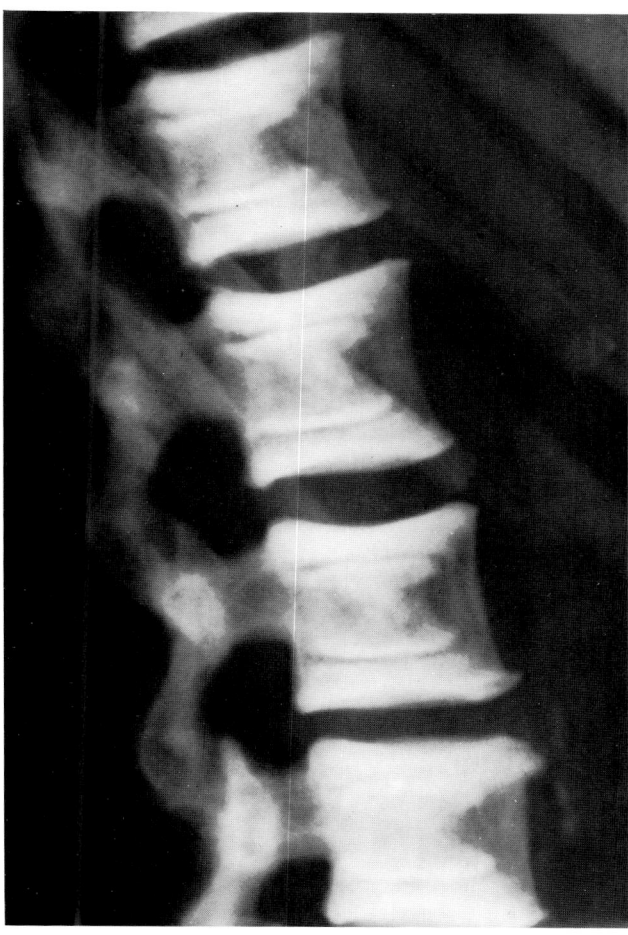

FIG SP15-2. Osteopetrosis. A miniature inset is seen in each lumbar vertebral body, giving it a bone-within-a-bone appearance. There is also sclerosis at the end plates.[7]

Condition	Comments
Heavy metal poisoning	Radiodense lines paralleling the superior and inferior margins of multiple vertebral bodies are an infrequent manifestation of lead or phosphorus poisoning.
Gaucher's disease	Initial collapse of an entire vertebral body with subsequent growth recovery peripherally may be associated with horizontal and vertical sclerosis, giving the bone-within-a-bone appearance.
Paget's disease	May involve one or multiple vertebrae. More commonly produces enlarged, coarsened trabeculae with condensation of bone most prominent along the contours of a vertebral body (picture frame) or uniform increase in osseous density of an enlarged vertebral body (ivory vertebra).
Sickle cell anemia	Rare manifestation. More commonly generalized osteoporosis, localized steplike central depressions, and characteristic biconcave indentations on both the superior and inferior margins of softened vertebral bodies (fish vertebrae).
Hypervitaminosis D	The margins of the vertebral bodies are outlined by dense bands of bone that are exaggerated by adjacent radiolucent zones. The central, normal-appearing bone may simulate the bone-within-a-bone appearance.

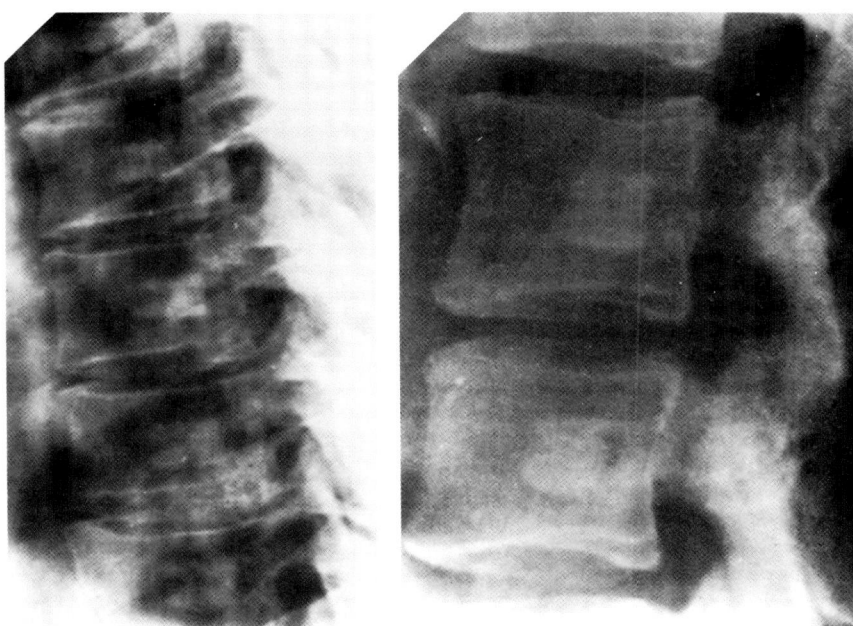

FIG SP15-3. Thorotrast. Two examples of persistence of radiographic densities of infantile vertebrae in adult bones of patients who received intravenous Thorotrast during early childhood.[9]

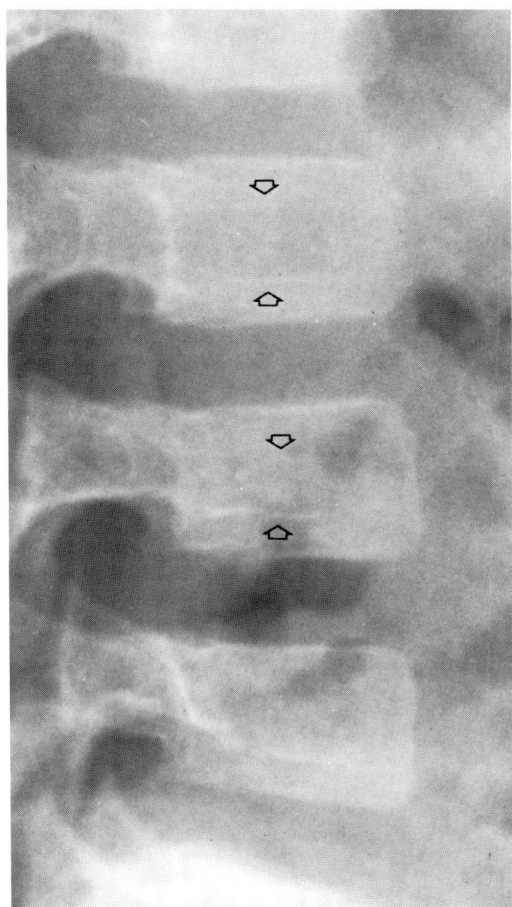

FIG SP15-4. Transverse growth lines. Opaque lines paralleling the superior and inferior margins of the vertebral body (arrows) in a child with severe chronic illness.

BEAKED, NOTCHED, OR HOOKED VERTEBRAE
IN A CHILD

Condition	Imaging Findings	Comments
Normal variant	Variable pattern of vertebral notching.	Vertebral notching can be seen in infants who are presumably normal. This incidental finding is probably secondary to subclinical hyperflexion trauma or to the exaggerated thoracolumbar kyphosis that is seen in all young infants who are unable to remain erect in the sitting position because of normal muscular immaturity.
Mucopolysaccharidoses		Genetically determined disorders of mucopolysaccharide metabolism that result in a broad spectrum of skeletal, visceral, and mental abnormalities.
Hurler's syndrome (gargoylism) (Fig SP16-1)	Inferior beaking. The centrum of the second lumbar vertebra is usually hypoplastic and displaced posteriorly, giving rise to an accentuated kyphosis, or gibbous, deformity.	Other radiographic manifestations include swelling of the central portions of long bones (due to cortical thickening or widening of the medullary canal), "canoe-paddle" ribs, and J-shaped sella (shallow, elongated sella with a long anterior recess extending under the anterior clinoid processes).
Morquio's syndrome (Fig SP16-2)	Generalized flattening of the vertebral bodies with central anterior beaking. There is often hypoplasia and posterior displacement of L1 or L2, resulting in a sharp, angular kyphosis.	Other radiographic manifestations include tapering of long bones (less marked than in Hurler's syndrome) and flaring, fragmentation, and flattening of the femoral heads combined with irregular deformity of the acetabula (often results in subluxations at the hip).
Cretinism (hypothyroidism)	Inferior or central beaking.	Radiographic manifestations include delay in appearance and subsequent growth of ossification centers, epiphyseal dysgenesis (fragmented epiphyses with multiple foci of ossification), retarded bone age, increased thickness of the cranial vault, and widened sutures with delayed closure.
Achondroplasia (Fig SP16-3)	Central anterior wedging of vertebral bodies. Progressive narrowing of the interpedicular distances from above downward (opposite of normal) and scalloping of the posterior aspects of the vertebral bodies.	Radiographic manifestations include symmetric shortening of all long bones, ball-and-socket epiphyses, trident hand, and a characteristic short, broad pelvis with short and square ilia and decreased acetabular angles.
Down's syndrome (mongolism)	Variable pattern of vertebral notching.	Radiographic manifestations include a decrease in the acetabular and iliac angles with hypoplasia and marked lateral flaring of the iliac wings, squaring of vertebral bodies, multiple manubrial ossification centers, the presence of only 11 ribs, and shortening of the middle phalanx of the fifth finger.

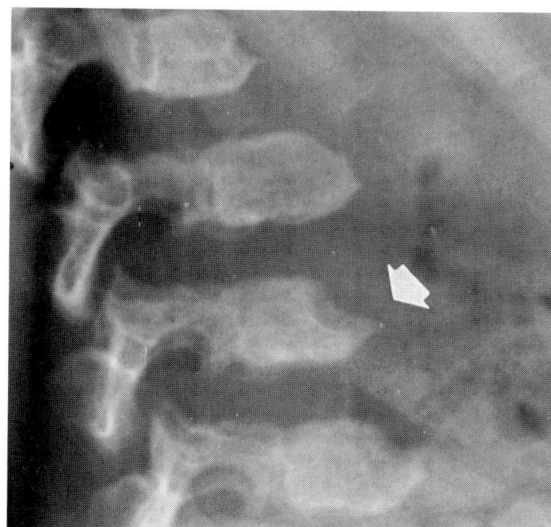

FIG SP16-1. Hurler's syndrome. Typical inferior beaking (arrow) of the anterior margin of a vertebral body.

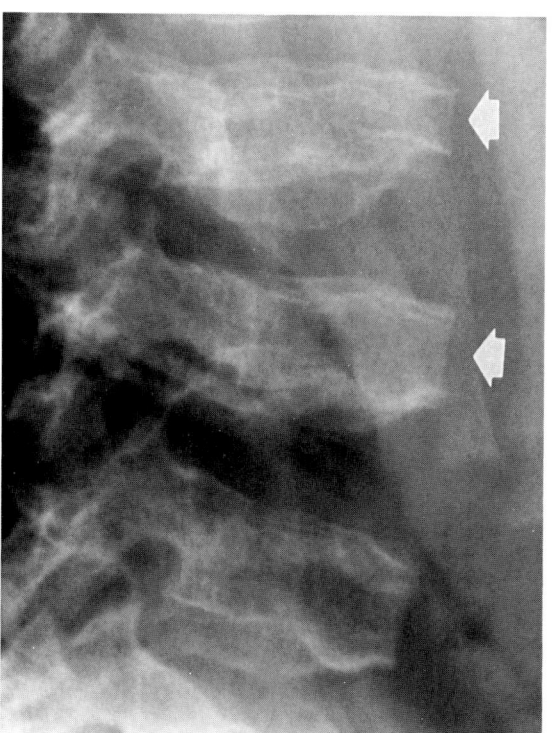

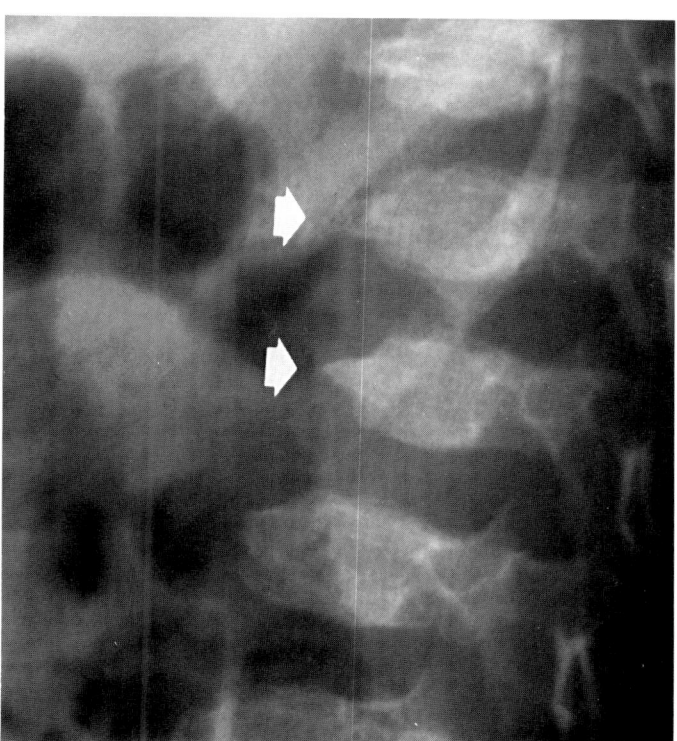

A   B

FIG SP16-2. Morquio's syndrome. (A and B) Two examples of universal flattening of the vertebral bodies with central anterior beaking (arrows).

Condition	Imaging Findings	Comments
Neuromuscular disease with generalized hypotonia	Variable pattern of vertebral notching.	Niemann-Pick disease, phenylketonuria, Werdnig-Hoffmann disease, mental retardation. Probably related to an exaggerated kyphotic curvature of the thoracic spine.
Trauma	Variable pattern of vertebral notching.	Hyperflexion-compression spinal injuries. Repeated hyperflexion of the spine is postulated to be the underlying cause of vertebral notching in battered children.

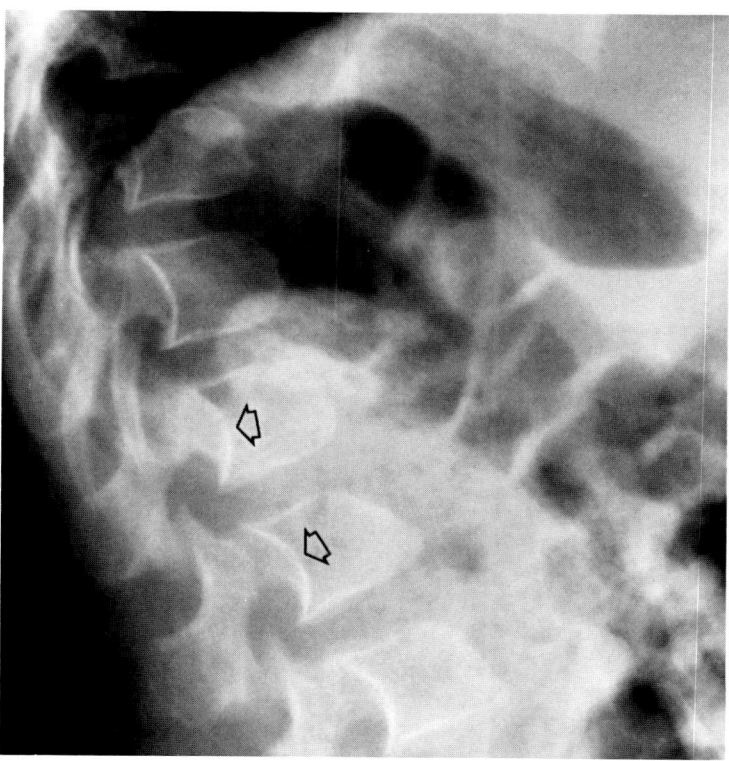

FIG SP16-3. **Achondroplasia.** Central anterior wedging of several vertebral bodies. Note the characteristic posterior scalloping (arrows).

SACROILIAC JOINT ABNORMALITY

Condition	Comments
Bilateral, symmetric distribution **Ankylosing spondylitis** **(Fig SP17-1)**	Sacroiliac joints are the initial site of involvement. Early findings include blurring of articular margins, irregular widening of the joints, and patchy sclerosis. This generally progresses to narrowing of the joint spaces and may lead to complete fibrosis and bony ankylosis. Dense reactive sclerosis often occurs, though it may become less prominent as the joint spaces become obliterated.
Inflammatory bowel disease **(Fig SP17-2)**	Appearance identical in all respects to that of classic ankylosing spondylitis. Underlying conditions include ulcerative colitis, Crohn's disease, and Whipple's disease.
Hyperparathyroidism/ renal osteodystrophy	Subchondral resorption of bone (predominantly in the ilia) leads to irregularity of the osseous surface, adjacent sclerosis, and widening of the interosseous joint space. Articular space narrowing and bony fusion do not occur.
Osteitis condensans ilii **(Fig SP17-3)**	Triangular zone of dense sclerosis along the inferior aspect of the ilia. The surfaces are well defined, the sacrum is normal, and the sacroiliac joint spaces are preserved. The condition probably represents a reaction to the increased stress to which the sacroiliac region is subjected during pregnancy and delivery (a similar type of sclerotic reaction, osteitis pubis, may occur in the pubic bones adjacent to the symphysis in women who have borne children).
Osteoarthritis	After age 40, most patients have some narrowing of the sacroiliac joint spaces, which may involve the entire articulations or appear as focal areas of abnormality at the inferior aspect of the joints. In comparison with ankylosing spondylitis, sacroiliac joint disease in osteoarthritis occurs in older patients, is often associated with prominent osteophytosis (especially at the anterosuperior and anteroinferior limits of the articular cavity) and prominent subchondral sclerosis, does not show erosions, and rarely demonstrates intra-articular bony ankylosis (though periarticular bridging osteophytes are common). Degenerative joint disease also may have a bilateral and asymmetric or a unilateral distribution.
Gout	Irregularity and sclerosis of articular margins are common (may reflect osteoarthritis in older patients). Large cystic areas of erosion in the subchondral bone of the ilia and sacrum are uncommon. Sacroiliac joint changes occur more frequently with early onset disease and tend to have a left-sided predominance. As with degenerative joint disease, sacroiliac joint involvement in gouty arthritis may be bilateral and asymmetric or unilateral.

(continued page 246)

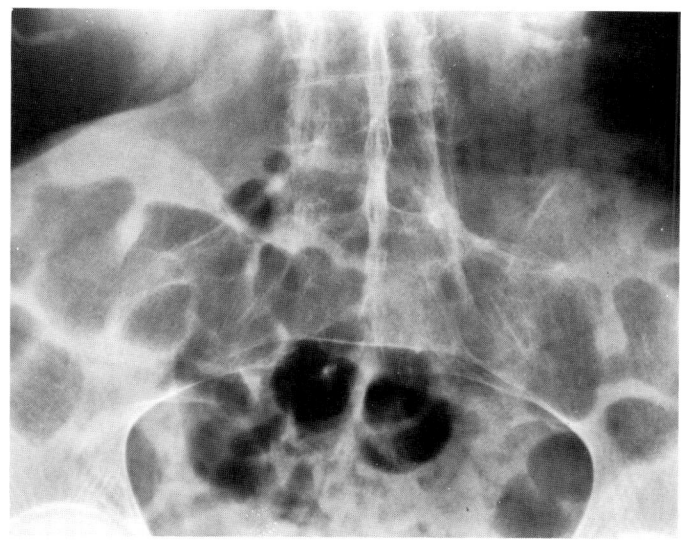

FIG SP17-1. **Ankylosing spondylitis.** Bilateral, symmetric obliteration of the sacroiliac joints.

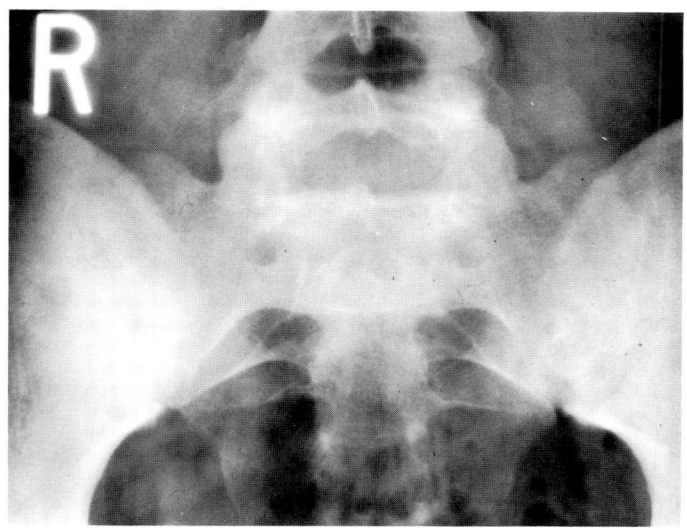

FIG SP17-2. **Inflammatory bowel disease.** Bilateral, symmetric involvement of the sacroiliac joints in a patient with ulcerative colitis.

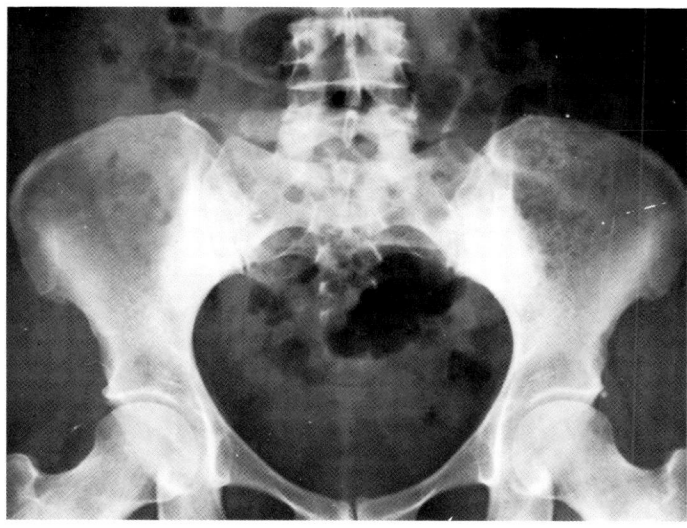

FIG SP17-3. **Osteitis condensans ilii.** There is sharply demarcated sclerosis of the ilia adjacent to the sacroiliac joints. The sacrum is not affected, and the margins of the sacroiliac joints are sharp and without destruction. The sclerosis that overlies the sacral wing is actually in the ilium, where it curves posteriorly behind the sacrum.[4]

Condition	Comments
Multicentric reticulohistiocytosis	Erosions and joint space narrowing leading to bony ankylosis, but no subchondral sclerosis.
Bilateral, asymmetric distribution **Psoriatic arthritis** **(Fig SP17-4)**	Bilateral, asymmetric distribution is probably most common, though bilateral, symmetric abnormalities are frequent and even unilateral involvement may occur. The radiographic changes include erosions and sclerosis, predominantly affecting the ilium, and widening of the articular space. Although joint space narrowing and bony ankylosis can occur, this is much less frequent than in classic ankylosing spondylitis. A prominent finding may be blurring and eburnation of apposing sacral and iliac surfaces above the true joint in the region of the interosseous ligament.
Reiter's syndrome **(Fig SP17-5)**	Bilateral, asymmetric distribution is probably most common, though bilateral, symmetric abnormalities are frequent and unilateral sacroiliac joint abnormalities may infrequently occur (especially early in the disease process). Sacroiliac joint changes are common in Reiter's syndrome, eventually developing in about 50% of patients. Osseous erosions primarily involve the iliac surface and adjacent sclerosis varies from mild to severe. Early joint space widening may later be replaced by narrowing. Although intra-articular bony ankylosis may eventually appear, it occurs much less frequently than in ankylosing spondylitis. A prominent finding may be blurring and eburnation of apposing sacral and iliac surfaces above the true joint in the region of the interosseous ligament.
Rheumatoid arthritis **(Fig SP17-6)**	Relatively uncommon manifestation that usually produces minor subchondral erosions, mild or absent sclerosis, and either no or only focal intra-articular bony ankylosis. Infrequently has a unilateral distribution.
Familial Mediterranean fever **(Fig SP17-7)**	Initially, widening of the articular space with loss of normal cortical definition primarily involving the ilium. Eventually, sclerosis with or without erosions and even bony ankylosis. Involvement may also be bilateral and symmetric or even unilateral.
Relapsing polychondritis	Joint space narrowing, erosion, and eburnation. Involvement may also be bilateral and symmetric or even unilateral.

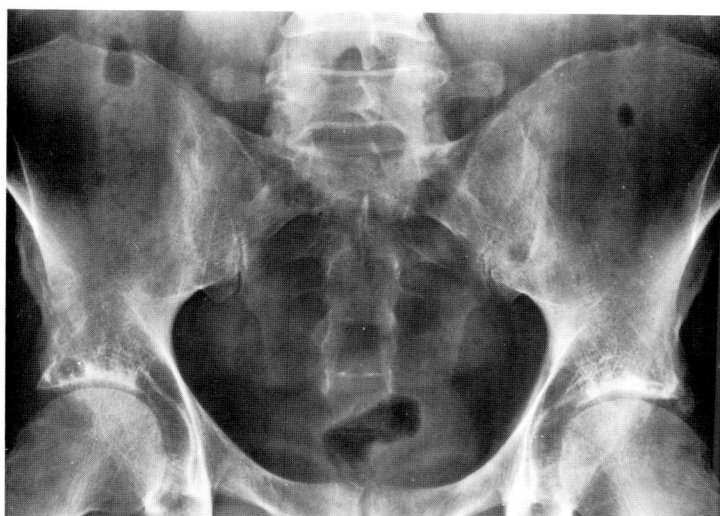

FIG SP17-4. Psoriatic arthritis. Bilateral, though somewhat asymmetric, narrowing of the sacroiliac joints.

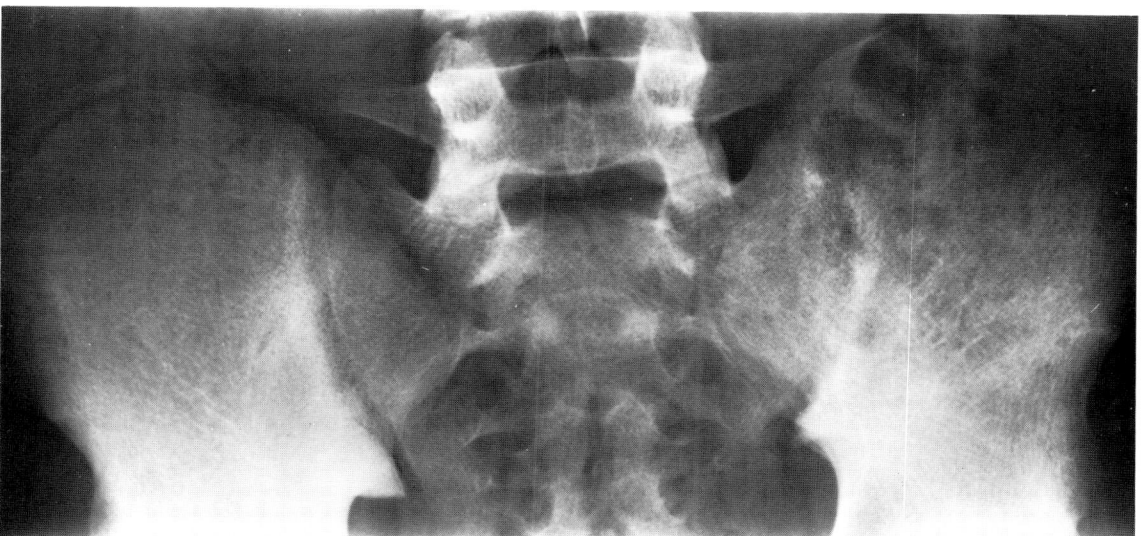

FIG SP17-5. Reiter's syndrome. Bilateral, though asymmetric, sclerosis and narrowing of the sacroiliac joints with reactive sclerosis.

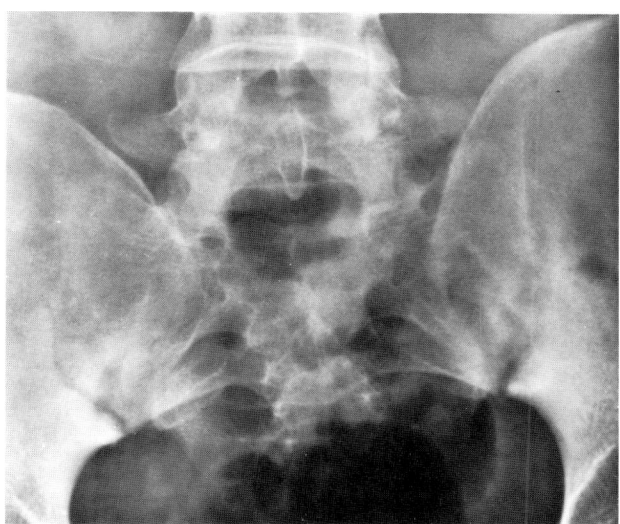

FIG SP17-6. Rheumatoid arthritis. Bilateral, though asymmetric, sclerosis and narrowing of the sacroiliac joints.

Condition	Comments
Unilateral distribution **Infection** **(Fig SP17-8)**	By far the most common cause of unilateral sacroiliac involvement. May be related to bacterial, mycobacterial, or fungal agents and is relatively common in drug abusers.
Paralysis	Cartilage atrophy accompanying paralysis or disuse produces diffuse joint space narrowing with surrounding osteoporosis and may even lead to intra-articular osseous fusion (perhaps related to chronic low-grade inflammation).
Osteoarthritis	May occur in conjunction with degenerative joint disease involving the contralateral hip.

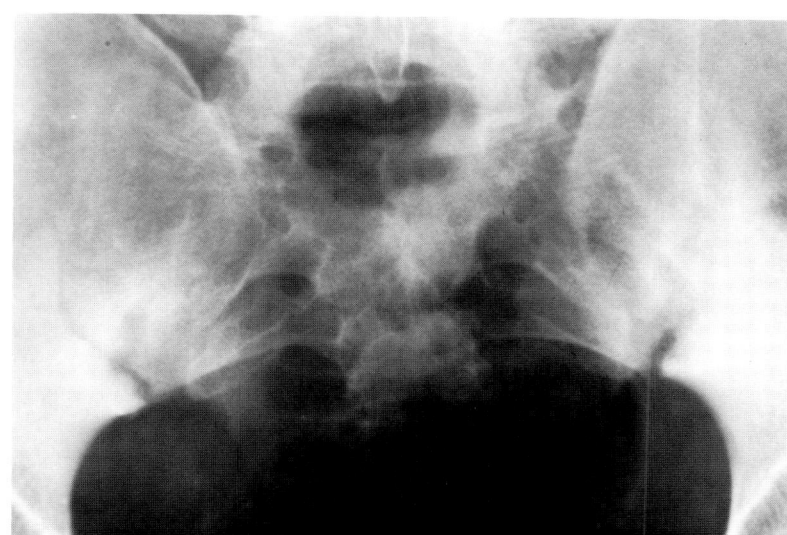

FIG SP17-7. Familial Mediterranean fever. Bilateral, though asymmetric, narrowing, erosive changes, and reactive sclerosis about the sacroiliac joints.

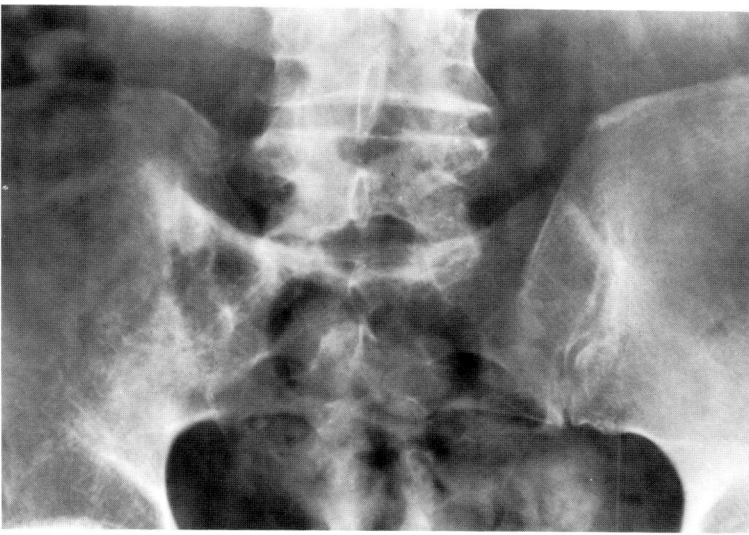

FIG SP17-8. Healed tuberculosis. Obliteration of the right sacroiliac joint. The left sacroiliac joint remains intact.

INTRAMEDULLARY LESION ON MYELOGRAPHY
(WIDENING OF THE SPINAL CORD)*

Condition	Imaging Findings	Comments
Primary intramedullary neoplasm (Fig SP18-1)	Fusiform widening of the spinal cord, often with localized thinning and remolding of the pedicles.	About two thirds are ependymomas, particularly of the conus and filum terminale. Other intramedullary tumors include astrocytoma, glioblastoma, hemangioblastoma, lipoma, dermoid, epidermoid, teratoma, and metastases.
Syringomyelia/hydromyelia (Fig SP18-2)	Fusiform widening of the spinal cord that is indistinguishable from an intramedullary tumor. In patients with hydromyelia who undergo air myelography in the semierect or erect position, fluid in the dilated central canal migrates caudally and permits the apparently enlarged cord to collapse (collapsing-cord sign), indicating the presence of a cystic lesion rather than a solid intramedullary neoplasm.	Syringomyelia is an intraspinal cystic cavity that may extend over many segments and is independent of, but may be connected with, the central canal. When the cavity is a distended central canal, the condition is termed hydromyelia. Usually associated with the Arnold-Chiari I malformation. CT shows low-density fluid in a syrinx (some intramedullary gliomas may also have low density, though they have a serrated border unlike the smooth margin of a syrinx). A delayed CT scan obtained hours after a myelogram permits filling of the syrinx cavity by direct connection from the subarachnoid space or by diffusion of contrast material across the spinal cord. MRI may be able to detect cavities in normal-sized or diminished spinal cords.
Diastematomyelia (Fig SP18-3)	Fusiform widening of the spinal canal with increased interpedicular distance extending over several segments. The contrast material is split around a round or oval midline defect representing the septum (septum and two hemicords about it can be well demonstrated by CT).	Rare malformation in which the spinal cord is split by a midline bony, cartilaginous, or fibrous spur extending posteriorly from a vertebral body. Most commonly occurs in the lower thoracic and upper lumbar regions and is often associated with a variety of skeletal and central nervous system anomalies. If the septum dividing the cord is ossified, it may appear on frontal views as a pathognomonic vertical, thin bony plate lying in the midline of the neural canal.
Arteriovenous malformation/angioma (Fig SP18-4)	Focal mass or, more commonly, multiple parallel or serpiginous filling defects representing dilated, tortuous vessels.	May vary in size from a few insignificant vessels to huge intertwined masses of abnormal vasculature reaching from one end of the spinal cord to the other. MRI demonstrates serpiginous areas of signal void representing vascular structures containing rapidly flowing blood. The lesion may have a markedly heterogeneous appearance because of the presence of old hemorrhage and calcification.
Metastasis	Fusiform or irregular widening of the cord (or no enlargement).	Uncommon manifestation that may result from spread of a primary central nervous system (CNS) neoplasm by means of cerebrospinal fluid pathways or from hematogenous spread of non-CNS primary tumors.

*Pattern: Fusiform widening of the spinal cord with symmetric narrowing of the surrounding contrast-filled subarachnoid space. Complete obstruction causes an abrupt concave termination of the contrast column, which appears similar in all radiographic projections.

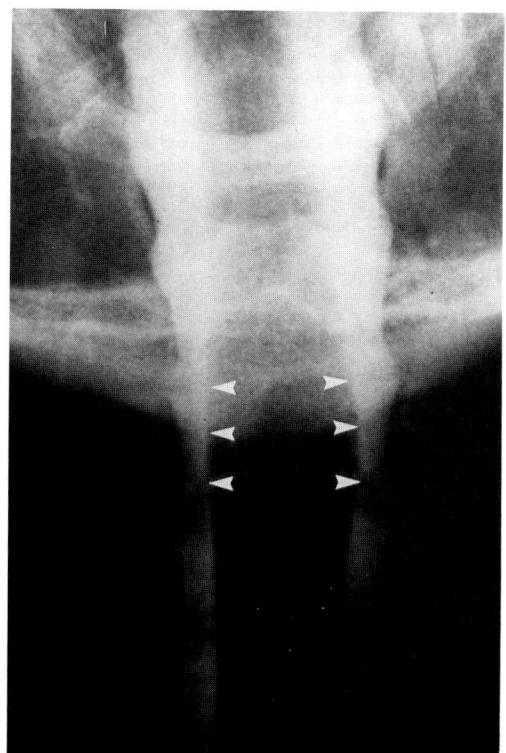

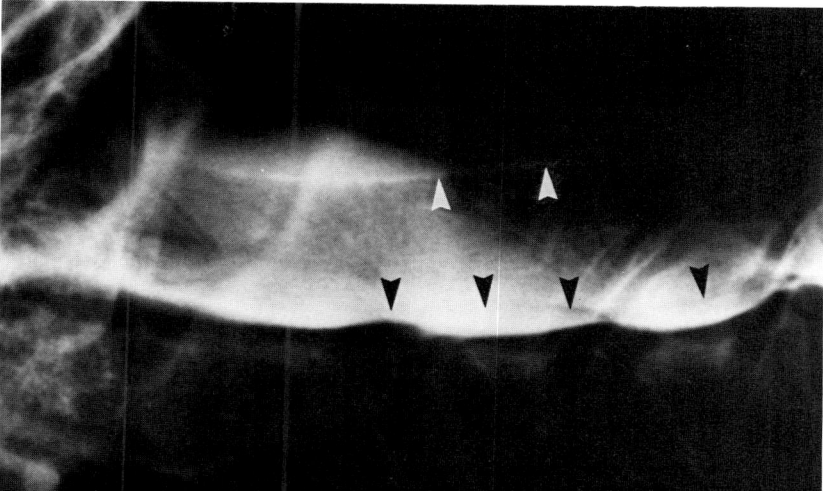

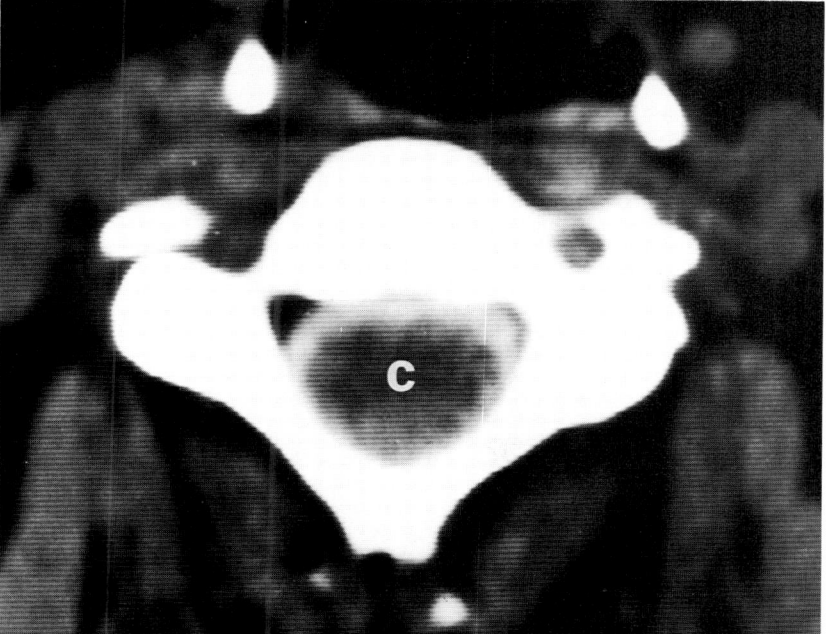

FIG SP18-1. Intramedullary tumor (cervical cord astrocytoma). (A) Frontal and (B) lateral views from a myelogram show enlargement of the cervical cord (arrowheads). It is important to demonstrate the cervical cord enlargement in both planes to exclude an extradural lesion, such as cervical spondylosis, that may simulate an intramedullary process. (C) CT scan confirms the enlargement of the spinal cord (C).

Condition	Imaging Findings	Comments
Hematoma/contusion	Intramedullary lesion.	Intramedullary bleeding may be related to trauma, neoplasm, or vascular malformation.
Granulomatous lesion	Intramedullary lesion.	Very rare manifestation of tuberculosis or sarcoidosis.
Infection	Intramedullary lesion.	Isolated infection is rare (usually spread from vertebral infection, trauma, lumbar puncture, or via a congenital skin sinus).
Neurenteric cyst	Intramedullary lesion.	May be associated with developmental vertebral anomalies and tethering of the cord.

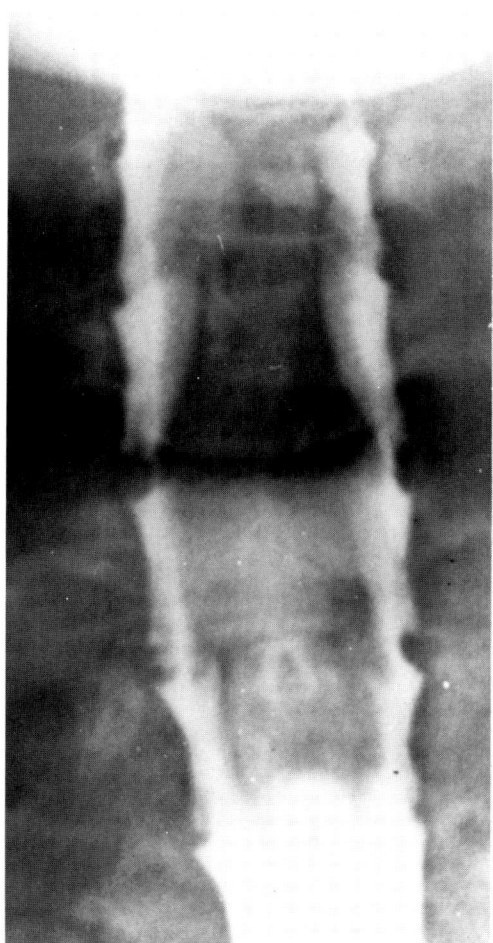

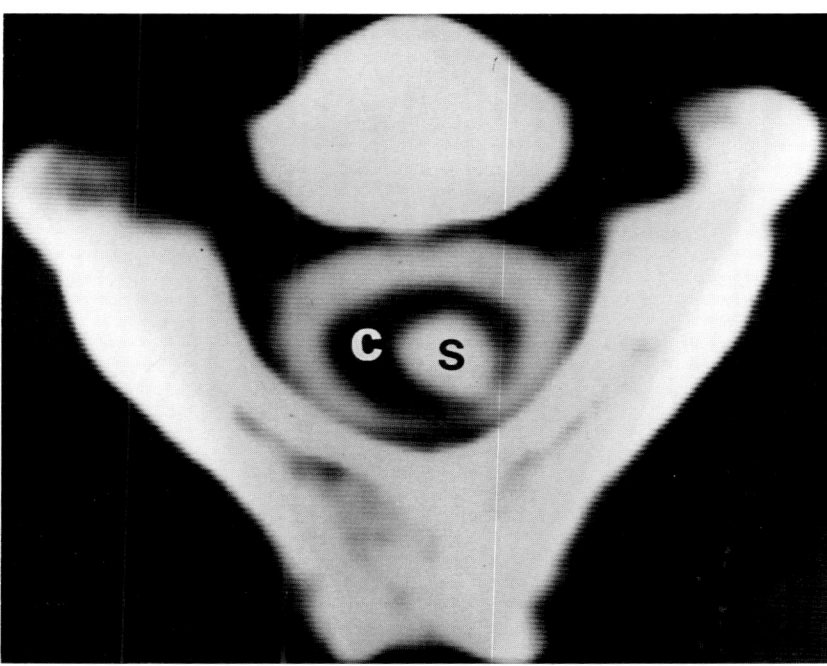

FIG SP18-2. **Syringomyelia/hydromyelia.** (A) Fusiform widening of the spinal cord in syringomyelia. (B) Hydromyelia. CT scan after the subarachnoid injection of metrizamide shows enlargement of the cervical spinal cord (C) with the high-density contrast material filling the central cavity (S).

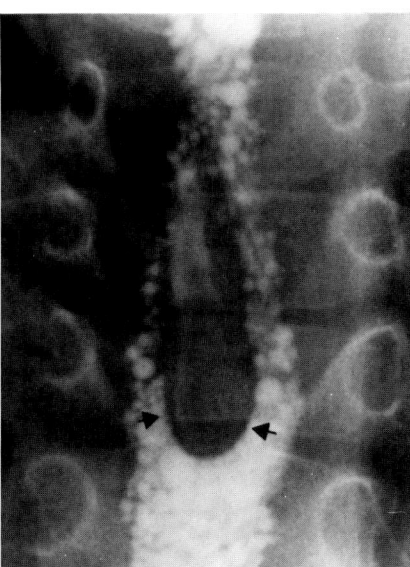

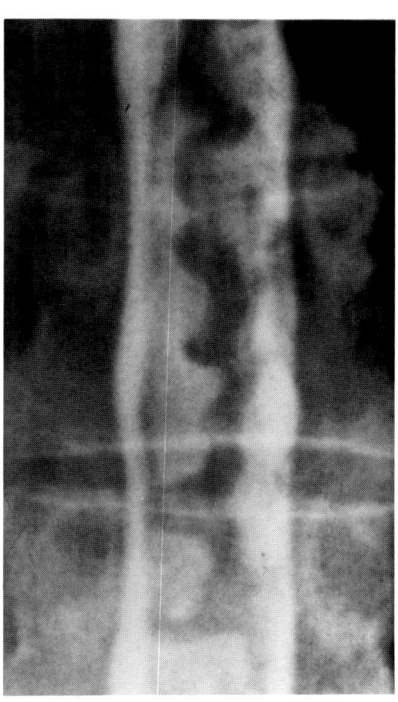

FIG SP18-3. **Diastematomyelia.** Splitting of the contrast material around an oval midline defect (arrows), which represents the septum.

FIG SP18-4. **Arteriovenous malformation.** Serpiginous filling defect representing dilated, tortuous vessels.

INTRADURAL, EXTRAMEDULLARY LESION
ON MYELOGRAPHY*

Condition	Imaging Findings	Comments
Meningioma **(Fig SP19-1)**	Intradural, extramedullary mass.	Typically occurs in middle-aged or elderly females. About 80% are located in the thoracic portion of the spinal canal, while most of the remainder are situated in the region of the foramen magnum.
Neurofibroma **(Fig SP19-2)**	Intradural, extramedullary mass.	More evenly distributed along the course of the spinal canal than are meningiomas; there is no age or sex predominance. Because of their very slow growth and (in about 30%) their location partially or completely in the extradural space, neurofibromas tend to erode the bony margins of the spinal canal (especially the inner borders of the pedicles and the posterior margins of the vertebral bodies).
Metastases ("seeding") **(Fig SP19-3)**	Multiple spherical lesions (1 mm to 2 cm) that generally arise on individual nerve roots and thus do not usually displace the cord.	Multiple metastases, which tend to attach to the lower lumbar and sacral roots by spreading from primary intracerebral tumors, are becoming more common since primary tumors are now better controlled with radiation and chemotherapy. The most common brain tumors giving rise to spinal metastases are medulloblastoma and pinealoma. Occasional metastases from glioblastoma multiforme and ependymoma.
Other tumors **(Fig SP19-4)**	Intradural, extramedullary lesion.	Dermoid; epidermoid; lipoma.
Arachnoiditis **(Fig SP19-5)**	Thickened and tortuous nerve roots that appear fixed in position. Associated epidural and peridural inflammatory changes may lead to irregular constriction of the thecal sac with obliteration of nerve-root sheaths.	Chronic inflammation in the dural sac that causes the normal gentle netlike pattern of the arachnoid to become dense and thickened with crisscrossing arachnoid septa producing pockets and cysts. The most frequent cause is the introduction of foreign substances (antibiotics, radiopaque contrast media, spinal anesthetics). Trauma and chronic infection may cause similar changes. Lumbar puncture may be painful, and in severe cases a "dry tap" may be obtained because of obliteration of the thecal sac.
Arachnoid cyst	Intradural, extramedullary lesion.	Usually posterior, may extend over several vertebral segments, primarily involves the thoracic region, and may be multiple. CT shows the cerebrospinal fluid density of the cyst.

*Pattern: Spinal cord appears to be displaced and compressed against the opposite wall, causing narrowing of the contralateral subarachnoid space with widening of the space on the ipsilateral side.

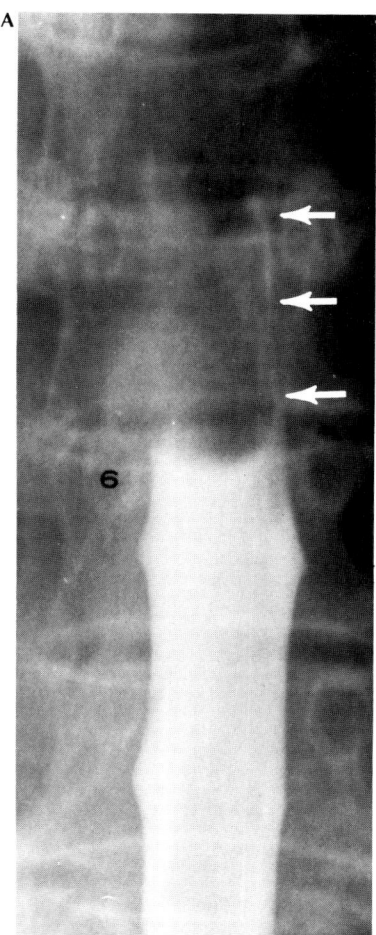

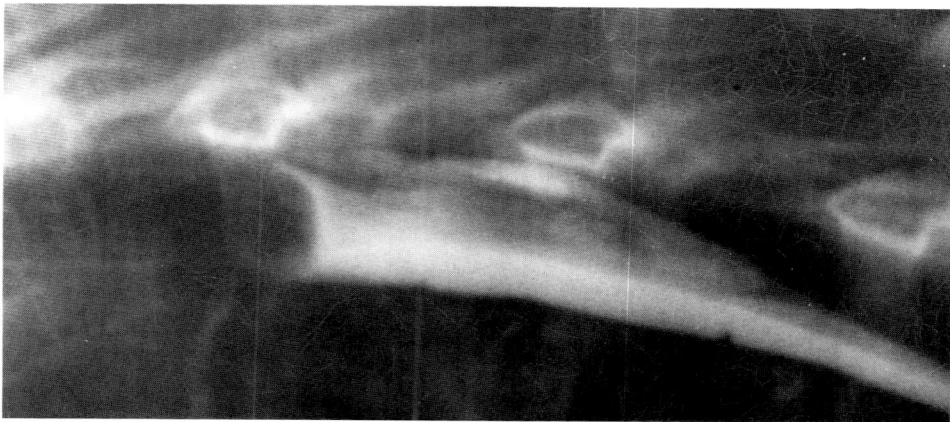

FIG SP19-1. Meningioma. (A) Frontal view shows the spinal cord displaced to the right (reader's right) at the level of T6. At the upper margin of T6, the lower edge of the tumor produces a cuplike defect in the contrast column. A thin layer of contrast material ascends along the right lateral aspect of the tumor (arrows). (B) Cross-table lateral view shows that the tumor arises anteriorly and displaces the spinal cord posteriorly. Note the characteristic cupping of the upper margin of the subarachnoid contrast column.[10]

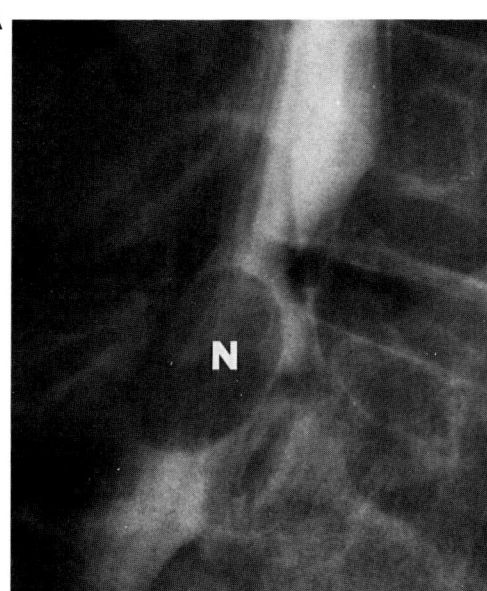

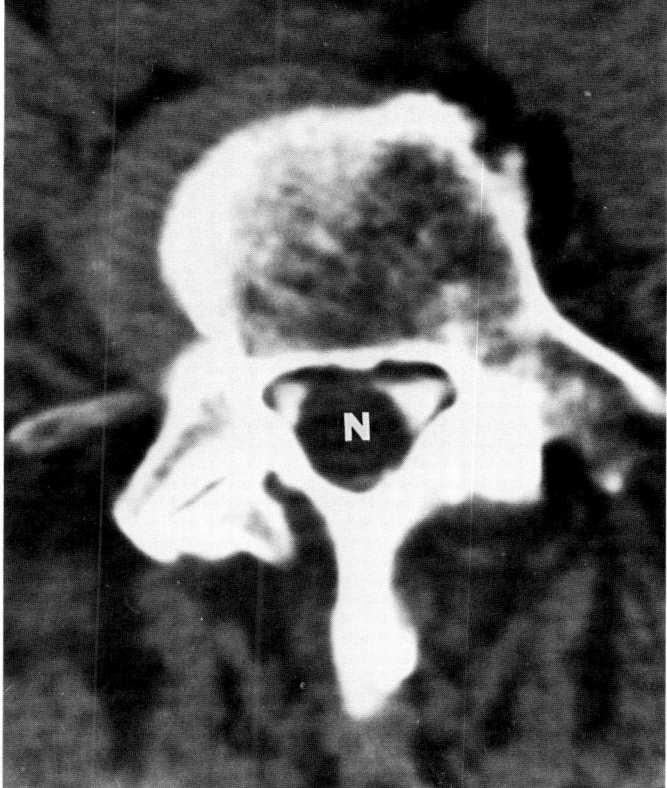

FIG SP19-2. Neurofibroma. (A) Oblique film from a myelogram shows a well-demarcated lesion (N) in the lower lumbar thecal sac. (B) A CT scan confirms that the neurofibroma (N) is intradural. Because the spinal cord ended at T12, the mass must represent an extramedullary, intradural process.

Condition	Imaging Findings	Comments
Vascular malformation/ angioma (Fig SP19-6)	Focal mass or, more commonly, multiple parallel or serpiginous filling defects representing dilated, tortuous vessels.	May vary in size from a few insignificant vessels to huge intertwined masses of abnormal vasculature reaching from one end of the spinal cord to the other.
Subdural abscess	Intradural, extramedullary lesion.	Rare occurrence that represents infection of the subdural space by direct extension, spinal puncture, or, more commonly, hematogenous spread from a distant focus.

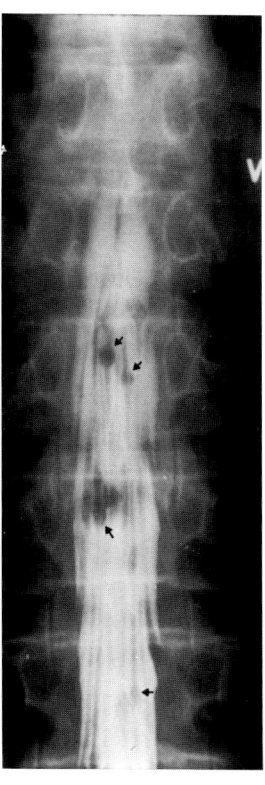

FIG SP19-3. Metastases. Multiple small lesions (arrows) arising from nerve roots.

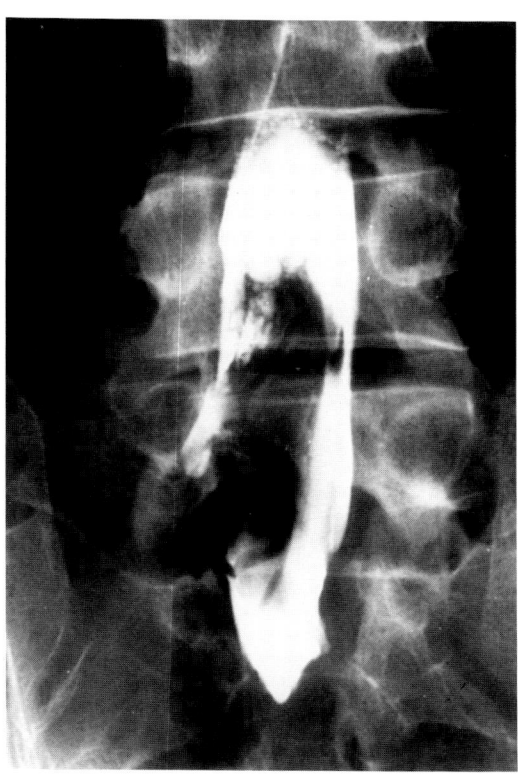

FIG SP19-4. Lipoma. Intradural, extramedullary mass with extradural extension.

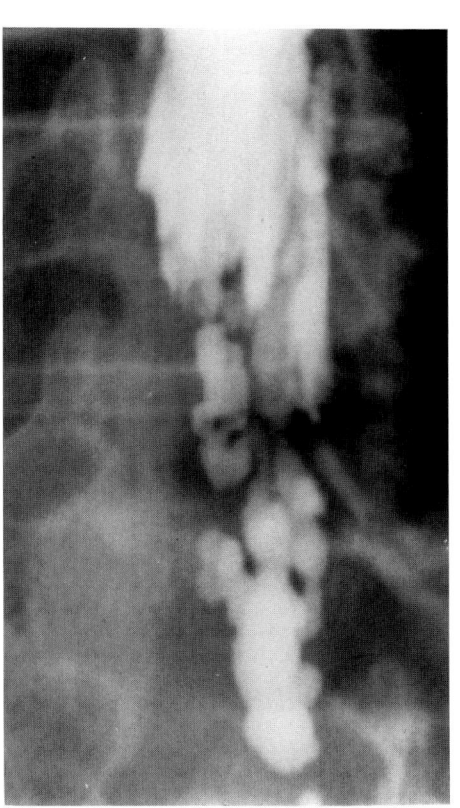

FIG SP19-5. Arachnoiditis. Collections of subarachnoid myelographic contrast material in irregular pockets that are separated by the radiolucent shadows of thickened nerve roots and arachnoid septa.

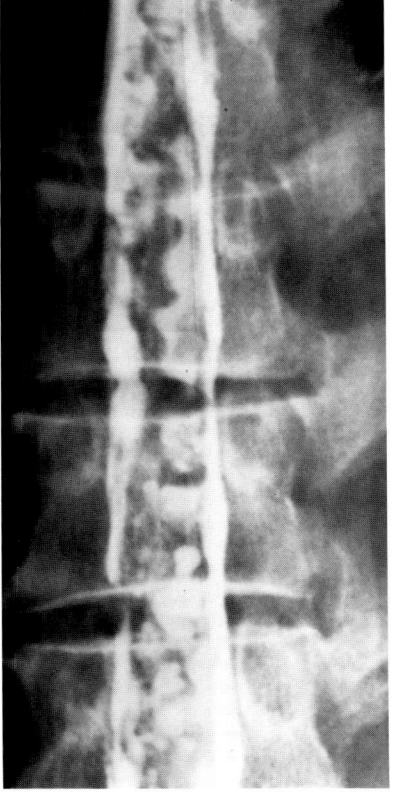

FIG SP19-6. Arteriovenous malformation. Multiple serpiginous filling defects representing dilated, tortuous vessels.

EXTRADURAL LESION ON MYELOGRAPHY*

Condition	Imaging Findings	Comments
Herniated disk (Fig SP20-1)	Smooth extradural defect at the anterior or lateral portion of the contrast column at the level of an intervertebral disk space. There is often amputation of the nerve root at the disk space and incomplete filling of the nerve-root sheath.	Protrusion of a lumbar intervertebral disk is the major cause of severe acute, chronic, or recurrent low back and leg pain. Most frequently occurs at the L4-L5 and L5-S1 levels.
Osteophyte (Fig SP20-2)	Bony spurs arising from the posterior margins of the vertebral bodies can cause anterior compression of the contrast column at the level of an intervertebral disk space.	Multiple irregularities on the ventral aspect of the radiopaque column frequently occur in patients with osteoarthritis of the spine. To produce symptoms, the spurs must be sufficiently large to obliterate the ventral subarachnoid space and reach the anterior surface of the spinal cord.
Thickening of ligamentum flavum	Extradural impression on the dorsal aspect of the subarachnoid space.	Thickening of the dorsolateral structures that connect the laminae of successive vertebrae represents a degenerative process with resulting fibrosis. Although rarely of any significance in itself, ligamentous thickening can impede the posterior displacement of the dural sac by a large ventral mass (eg, a herniated intervertebral disk) and thus contribute to further nerve root compression.
Metastases (Fig SP20-3)	Asymmetric extradural defect with a smooth or lobular margin. May extend along the spinal canal for a variable distance. There is usually evidence of bone destruction.	Hematogenous metastases to the bodies or pedicles of one or several vertebrae may be caused by almost any malignant neoplasm of epithelial origin (about two thirds are secondary to carcinomas of the lung or breast). As the metastasis enlarges, it breaks through the bony cortex and spreads into the spinal canal, compressing and displacing the thecal sac.
Lymphoma	Extradural defect that is typically longer, smoother, and more often circumferential than carcinomatous metastases.	Lymphoma usually involves the extradural soft tissues without producing recognizable changes in the adjacent vertebral bodies.
Vertebral neoplasm with intraspinal extension	Smooth or irregular extradural defect associated with vertebral destruction.	Myeloma; chordoma; sarcoma; hemangioma.

*Pattern: Extrinsic displacement of the entire thecal sac and its contents that causes the distance between the lateral margin of the sac and the medial margin of the pedicle to be widened on the side of the mass and narrowed on the opposite side. The margins of the sac remain smooth unless the lesion has invaded through the dura to produce a concomitant intradural component. Large masses compress the subarachnoid space on the side of the lesion and displace the spinal cord away from the mass.

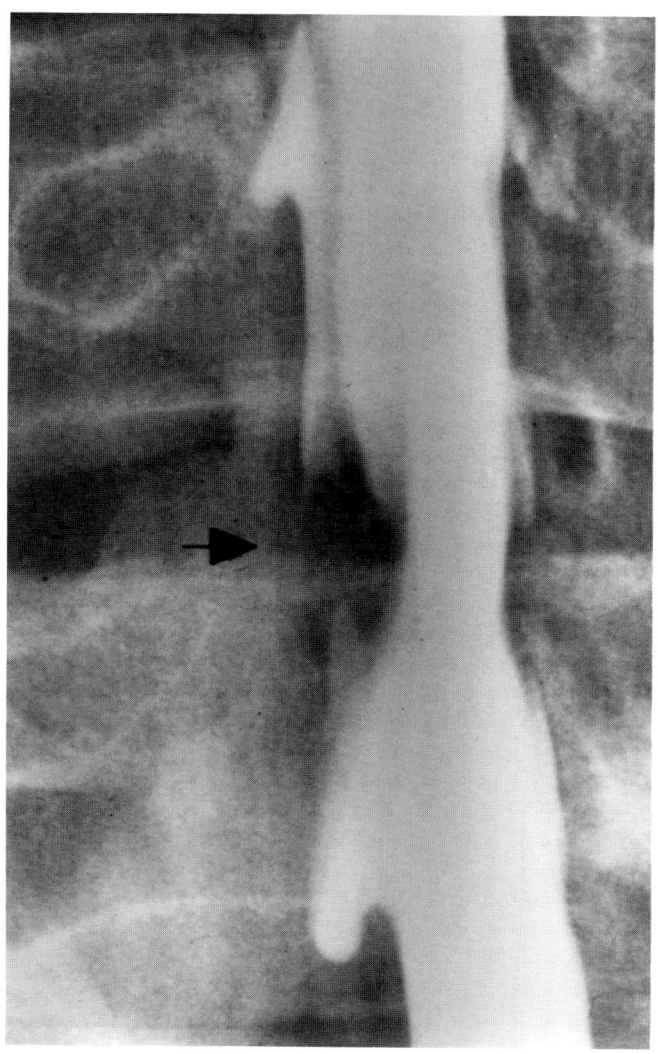

FIG SP20-1. Lumbar disk herniation. Extradural lesion at the level of the intervertebral disk space. Note the amputation of the nerve root by the disk compression (arrow).

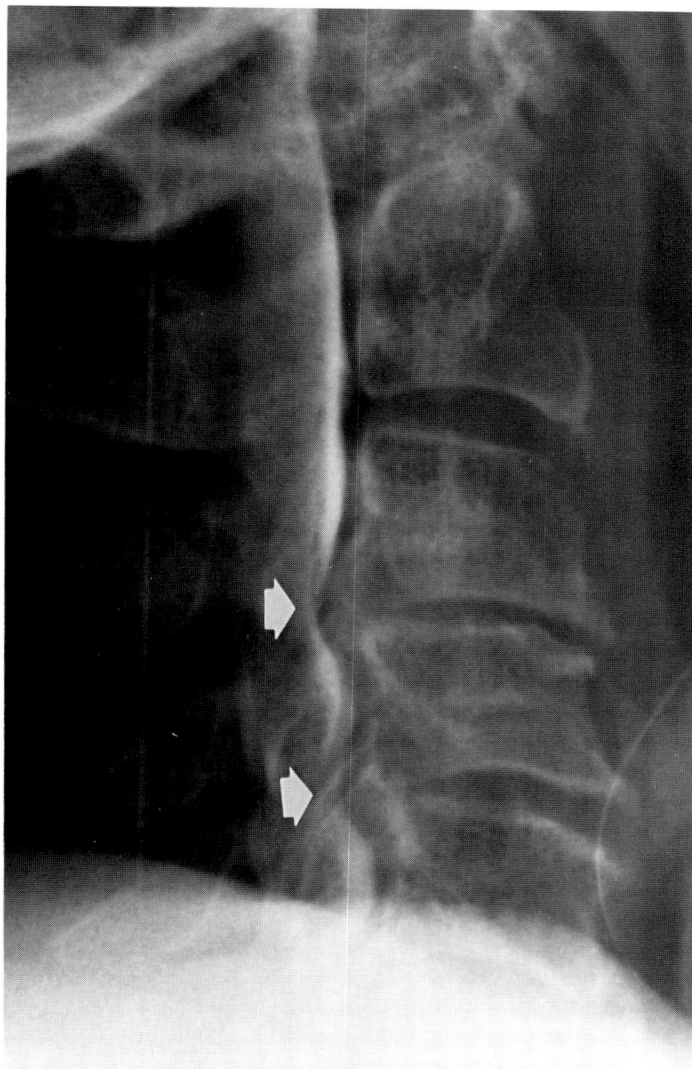

FIG SP20-2. Osteophyte. Posterior spurs cause impingement on the contrast column (arrows).

Condition	Imaging Findings	Comments
Benign extradural tumor	Extradural lesion that may be associated with vertebral erosion resulting from local pressure by the tumor.	Neuroma; meningioma; lipoma; fibroma; dermoid; epidermoid. Extradural neuromas frequently extend through and enlarge one or more intervertebral foramina and may be contiguous with a large mass in the paraspinal region. Extradural meningiomas are much less common but may produce local erosion of vertebral pedicles, laminae, or bodies. Lipomas are often associated with spina bifida or other anomalies of the vertebral column.
Fracture or dislocation	Extradural lesion.	Displaced and comminuted fragments of vertebral bodies or neural arches, lacerated ligaments, and hematoma may all contribute to the extradural mass.
Hematoma (Fig SP20-4)	Extradural lesion.	Posttraumatic or spontaneous (defect in blood coagulation due to anticoagulant therapy or a bleeding diathesis).
Scar tissue	Extradural lesion.	Usually a sequela of disk surgery.
Epidural abscess	Extradural lesion that is often associated with vertebral destruction.	Most commonly the result of extension of vertebral osteomyelitis. An epidural infection may occasionally follow spinal or pelvic surgery, trauma, or even lumbar puncture. The initial site of infection is usually the posterior epidural space, where the loose fatty tissue permits the development of rapid inflammatory change.
Arachnoid cyst	Extradural lesion that is usually posterior and occasionally multiple.	An extradural arachnoid cyst is frequently accompanied by dysraphism. It fills slowly or not at all and usually causes a partial or complete block of contrast flow. The cerebrospinal fluid density of the cyst can be shown by CT.
Paget's disease	Extradural defect mimicking the extension of tumor from a vertebral body.	The combination of flattening of a vertebral body, proliferation of uncalcified osteoid tissue on all sides, and enlargement of the pedicles may constrict the vertebral canal and intervertebral foramina, resulting in compression of the spinal cord and nerve roots.

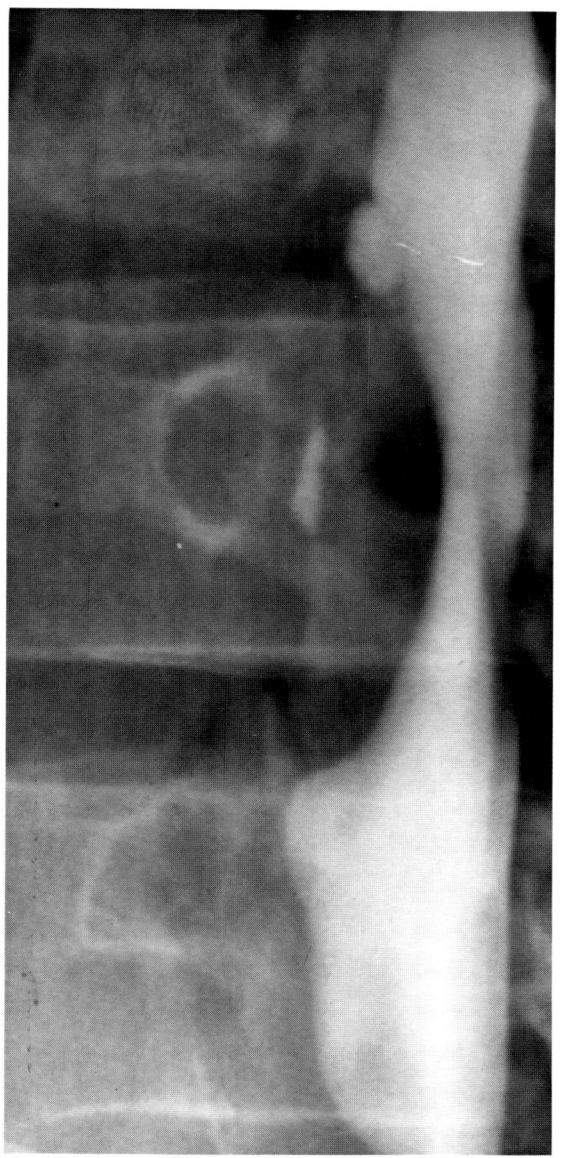

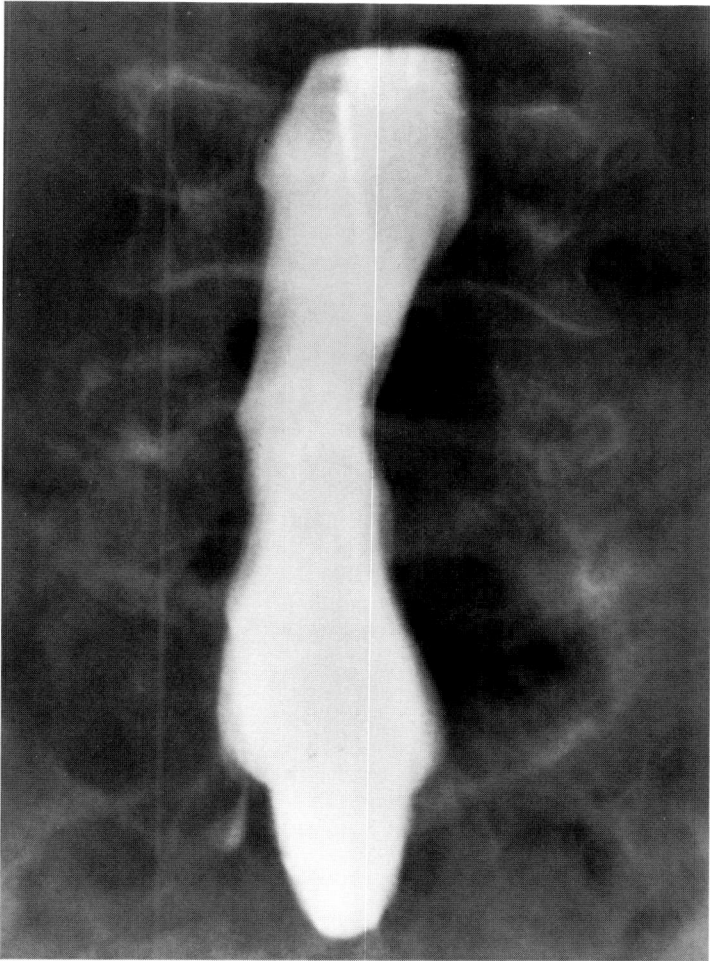

FIG SP20-4. **Postoperative hematoma** producing a broad extradural defect.

FIG SP20-3. **Metastasis** from carcinoma of the lung. Broad extradural defect.

SPINAL CORD TUMORS ON MAGNETIC RESONANCE IMAGING

Condition	Imaging Findings	Comments
Intramedullary Ependymoma (Fig SP21-1)	Isointense or hypointense fusiform widening of the spinal cord on T_1-weighted images. Increased signal, often with a multinodular appearance, on T_2-weighted images. Generally intense, homogeneous, and sharply marginated focal contrast enhancement.	Boundaries of the tumor are difficult to define on T_1-weighted images unless they are outlined by syrinx cavities capping the upper and lower poles of the tumor. On T_2-weighted images, it is difficult to distinguish the tumor from surrounding edema.
Astrocytoma (Fig SP21-2)	Widening of the spinal cord that is isointense on T_1-weighted images and hyperintense on T_2-weighted images. Tendency to more patchy and irregular contrast enhancement consistent with a more diffusely infiltrating tumor.	Although different patterns of contrast enhancement have been reported in some ependymomas and astrocytomas, they cannot be reliably differentiated by MRI.
Hemangioblastoma (Fig SP21-3)	Irregular and diffuse widening of the cord with cystic components and heterogeneous signal intensity. Intense enhancement of the highly vascular tumor nidus.	Dilated posterior pial venous plexus draining the tumor nodule may produce serpentine flow voids (simulating an arteriovenous malformation) on the dorsal aspect of the cord. The association of a strongly enhancing tumor nodule within a cystic intramedullary mass is very suggestive of hemangioblastoma.
Metastasis (Fig SP21-4)	Single or multiple masses producing fusiform or irregular widening of the cord (or no cord enlargement at all) that is hypointense on T_1-weighted images and hyperintense on T_2-weighted images. Generally marked contrast enhancement.	May develop from primary CNS neoplasms via CSF pathways or hematogenous spread from non-CNS primary tumors. After contrast injection, the enhancing tumor nodule (often smaller than the area of cord enlargement) can be distinguished from surrounding edema.

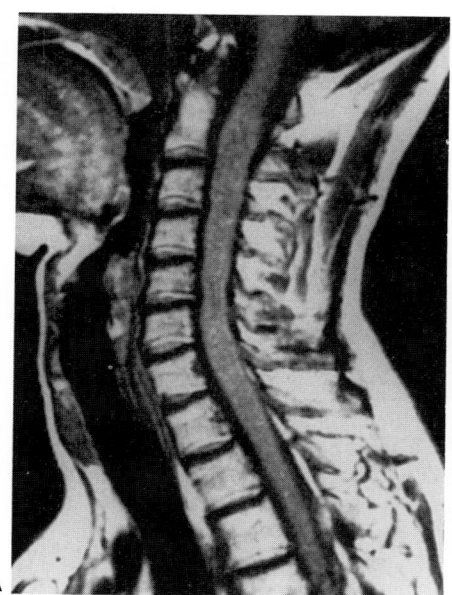
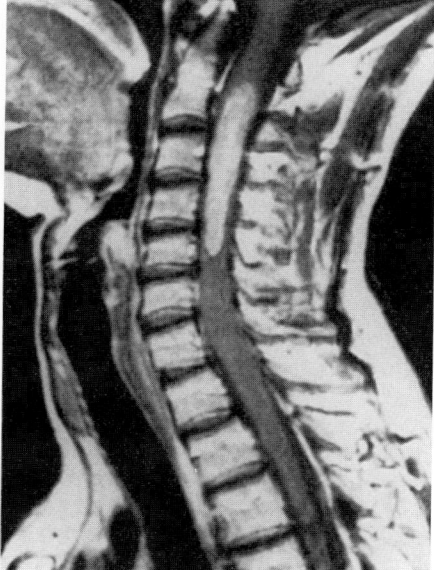

A

B

FIG SP21-1. **Ependymoma.** (A) Nonenhanced sagittal T_1-weighted image shows widening of the cervical cord from C1 to T2, suggesting intramedullary tumor. (B) Postcontrast scan shows a well-defined oval area of enhancement extending from C2 to C5.[11]

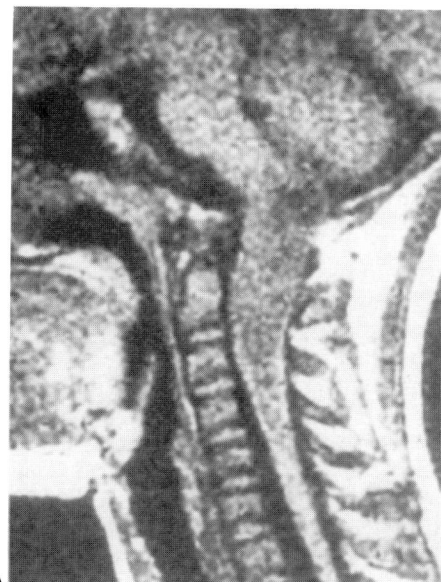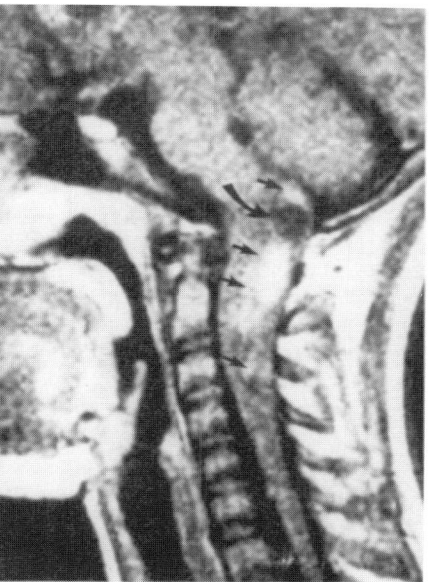

Fig SP21-2. Low-grade astrocytoma. (A) Non-enhanced sagittal T₁-weighted image shows widening of the upper cervical spinal cord with a relatively low signal intensity area extending into the medulla. (B) Postcontrast scan shows irregular areas of contrast enhancement (straight arrows) especially along the posterior aspect of the cord. A hypointense, presumably cystic component is seen posteriorly (curved arrow) at the junction of the upper cervical cord and medulla.[11]

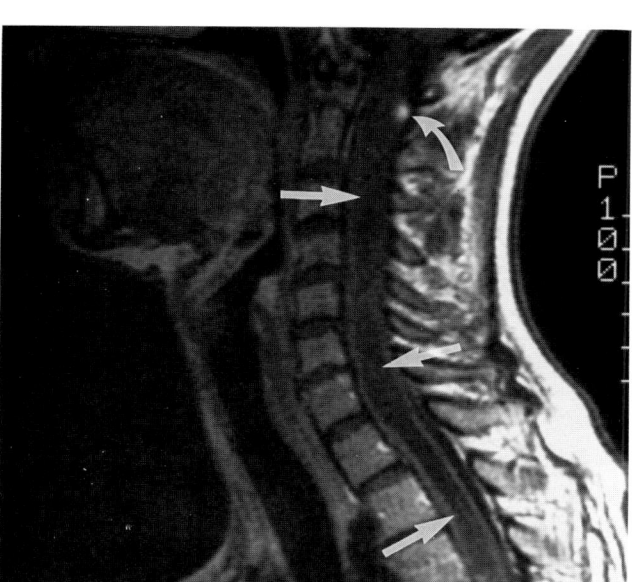

Fig SP21-3. Hemangioblastoma. Postcontrast sagittal scan in a patient with von Hippel–Lindau disease demonstrates intramedullary expansion of the spinal cord by a long syrinx cavity that extends from C1 to at least T4 (arrows). The lower extent of the syrinx is not included on this image. A homogeneously enhancing tiny nodule is identified within the posterior aspect of the spinal cord at the first cervical interspace (curved arrow).[12]

Condition	Imaging Findings	Comments
Intradural extramedullary Meningioma (Fig SP21-5)	Generally isointense on T_1-weighted images and only slightly hyperintense on T_2-weighted images. Immediate and uniform contrast enhancement.	Typically occurs in the thoracic region (80%) in middle-aged or elderly women. Like meningiomas in the head, spinal tumors tend to maintain a signal intensity similar to that of cord parenchyma.
Neurofibroma (Fig SP21-6)	Smooth, sharply marginated mass that tends to be relatively isointense to the spinal cord on all sequences. Variable pattern of contrast enhancement depending on internal architecture of the tumor.	In contrast to meningiomas, neurofibromas have no sex predilection and are more evenly distributed along the course of the spinal canal. They may have a characteristic extradural component that extends through the neural foramen into the paraspinal tissues (dumbbell tumor). Neurofibromas have a more variable MR appearance than meningiomas because of their propensity to undergo cystic degeneration and central necrosis, which makes them hypointense on T_1-weighted images and hyperintense on T_2-weighted images.
Metastasis ("seeding") (Fig SP21-7)	Multiple focal nodular masses that show intense contrast enhancement.	Unless large, these tumor deposits generally are not visualized on noncontrast scans. Other patterns include enhancement of a thin leptomeningeal veil that diffusely coats the spinal cord or nerve roots and a homogeneous increase in signal within the subarachnoid space.

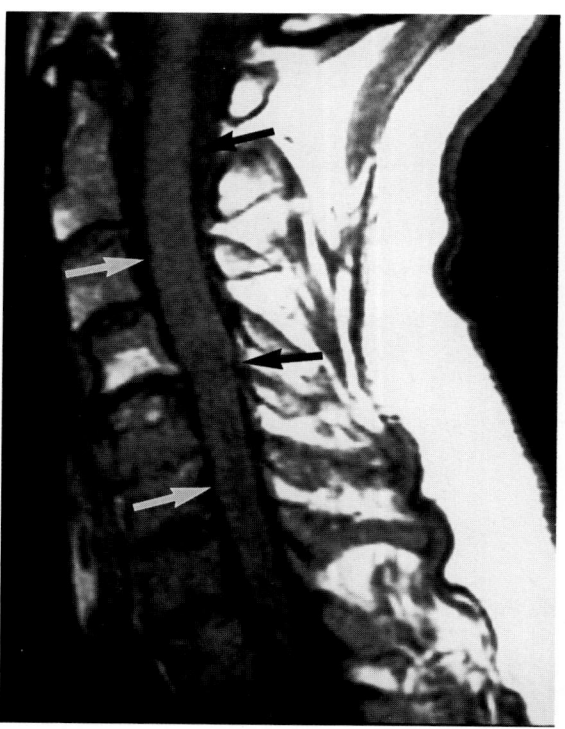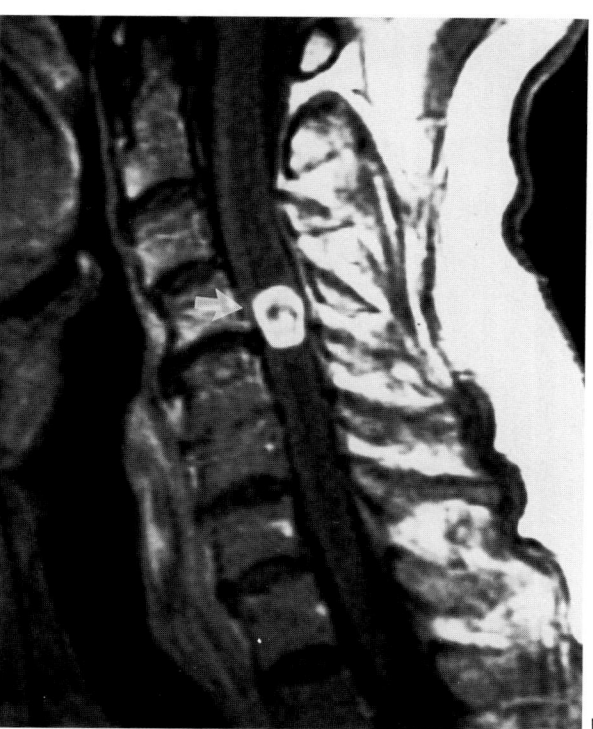

FIG SP21-4. Metastasis. (A) Nonenhanced sagittal T_1-weighted image shows nonspecific intramedullary expansion of a long segment of the cervical spinal cord (arrows). (B) Postcontrast scan shows intense enhancement of a partially necrotic mass at the C4 level (arrow). The intramedullary expansion of the cord above and below this level was attributed to cord edema.[12]

Condition	Imaging Findings	Comments
Lipoma (Fig SP21-8)	Well-circumscribed mass that is hyperintense to cord parenchyma on T_1-weighted images.	Uncommon lesion that can occur anywhere in the spinal canal and has no age or sex predilection. The characteristic bright signal on T_1-weighted images can be confused with contrast enhancement if only post-contrast studies are obtained, thus leading to the erroneous diagnosis of meningioma or neurofibroma.

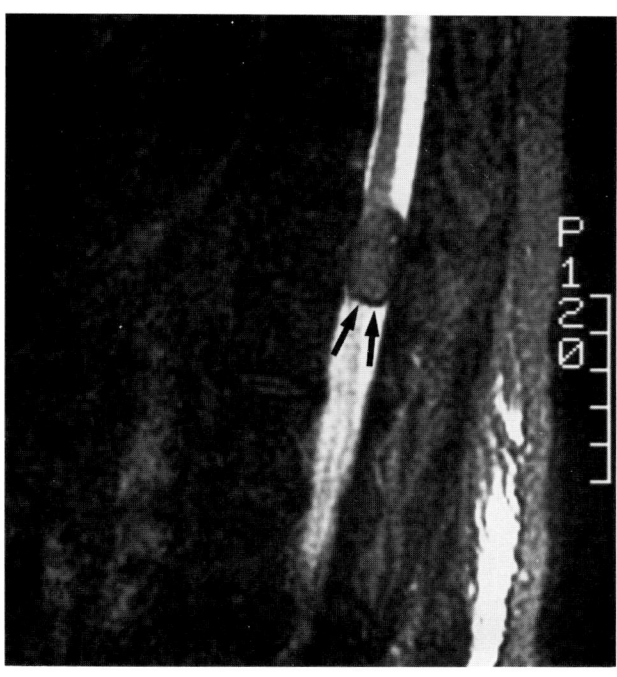

FIG SP21-5. Meningioma. Sagittal T_2-weighted image shows a well-circumscribed intradural extramedullary mass at the T10 level. The linear area of signal loss at the periphery of the mass (arrows) represented calcifications.[12]

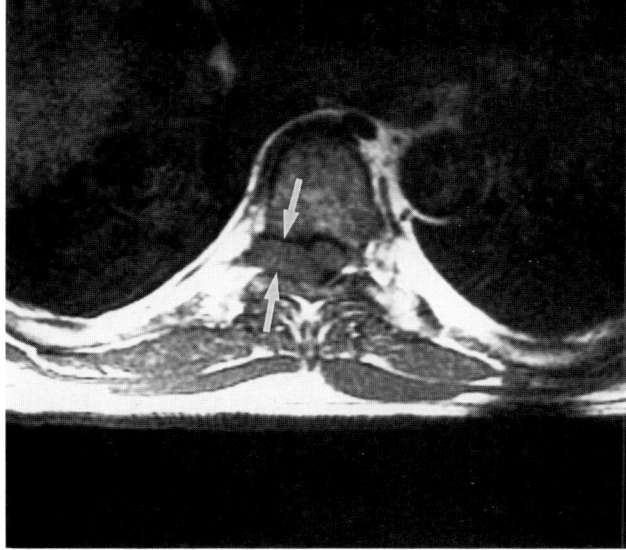

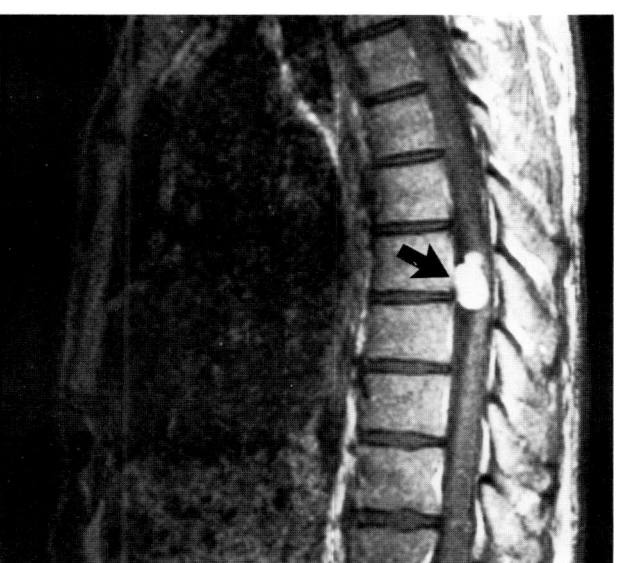

A   B

FIG SP21-6. Neurofibroma. (A) Axial T_1-weighted image demonstrates an oval, right-sided intraspinal mass that extends through an expanded T8 neural foramen (arrows). (B) Postcontrast midline sagittal scan in another patient shows a slightly lobulated, homogeneously enhancing intradural extramedullary mass (arrow).[12]

Condition	Imaging Findings	Comments
Extradural Metastasis (Fig SP21-9)	Mass that is hypointense on T_1-weighted images and of increased signal intensity on T_2-weighted images.	The most common primary tumors to metastasize to the spine are lung and breast carcinoma, followed by prostate carcinoma. Epidural metastases almost always occur in association with osseous metastases, in which the bright signal of marrow in the vertebral body is replaced by low-signal tumor on T_1-weighted images. Contrast studies may mask metastases by increasing the signal of osseous metastases, so that they appear isointense to normal marrow on T_1-weighted scans.
Lymphoma	Mass that is hypointense on T_1-weighted images and of increased signal intensity on T_2-weighted images.	Bulky soft-tissue mass insinuating itself into foramina, extending over multiple segments, and producing less skeletal involvement than expected for lesion size.
Vertebral neoplasm with intraspinal extension	Mass that is hypointense on T_1-weighted images and of increased signal intensity on T_2-weighted images.	Myeloma; chordoma; sarcoma.
Hemangioma	Lesion within the vertebral body that tends to be of high signal intensity on both T_1- and T_2-weighted images.	Although usually an incidental finding of little clinical significance, hemangiomas occasionally expand and break through the cortex to cause a myelopathic or radiculopathic syndrome. Hemangiomas can be differentiated from relatively common interosseous islands of fat because they maintain their high signal intensity on T_2-weighted images.

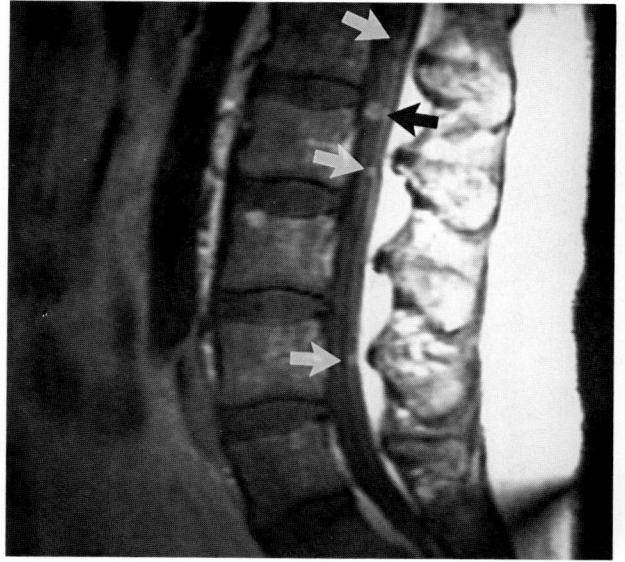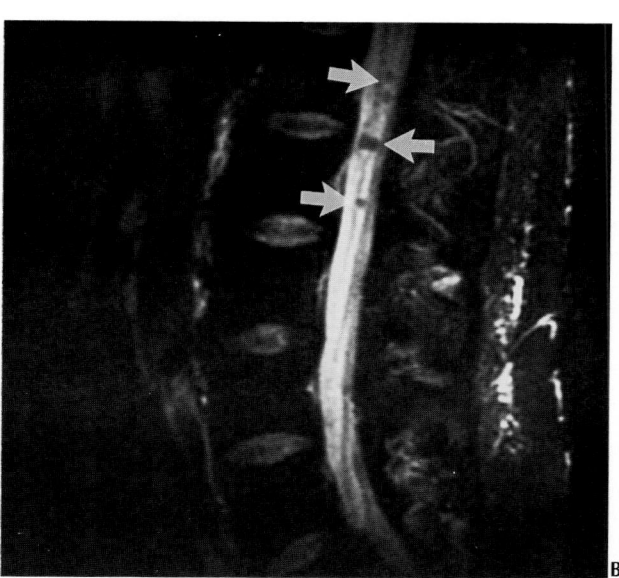

FIG SP21-7. **Metastatic seeding.** (A) Sagittal T_1-weighted image shows multiple high-intensity nodules (arrows) involving the nerve roots of the cauda equina in this patient with metastatic melanoma. The high intensity could represent either contrast enhancement or the paramagnetic effect of melanin. (B) The nodules also can be identified on a T_2-weighted scan (arrows).[12]

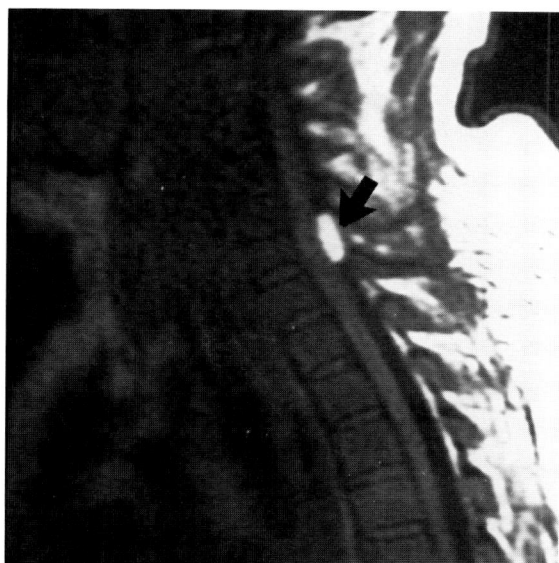

Fig SP21-8. Lipoma. A well-circumscribed, oval intraspinal mass is seen at C6 posteriorly on this sagittal T_1-weighted scan (arrow). It is characterized by increased signal, similar to the paraspinal and subcutaneous fat. This lipoma was an incidental finding in a neurologically normal patient.[12]

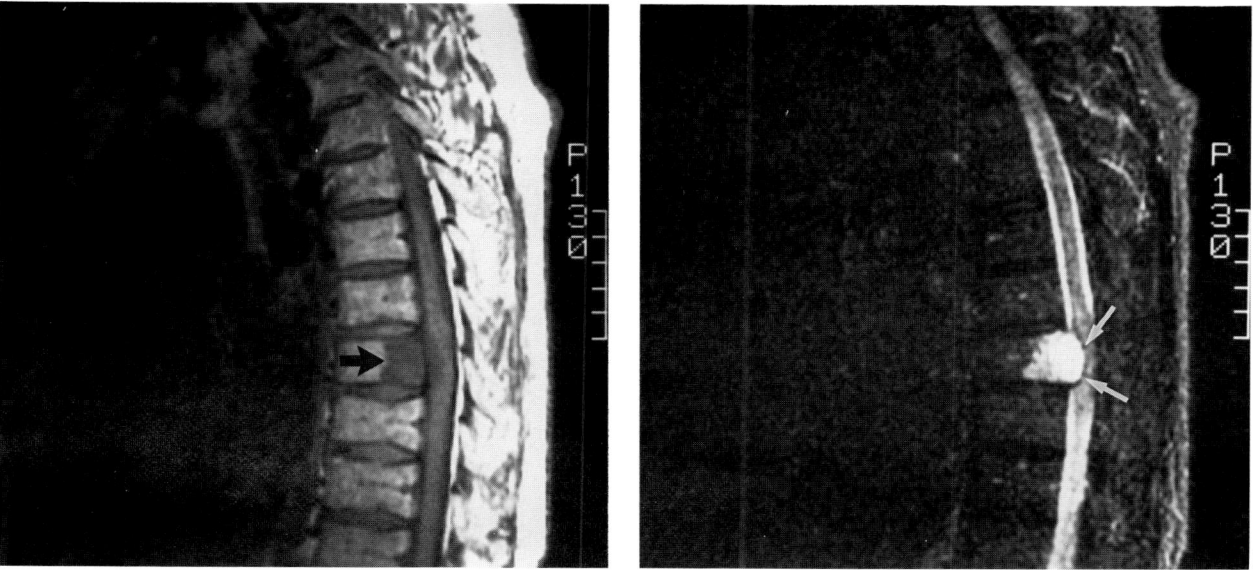

Fig SP21-9. Metastasis. (A) A T9 bony metastasis from known cranial chordoma is seen as a loss of the normal marrow fat on this T_1-weighted scan in a patient with a thoracic myelopathy (arrow). (B) An associated epidural soft tissue component is seen to better advantage with T2 weighting (arrows), resulting in spinal canal narrowing and compression of the thoracic spinal cord.[12]

NONNEOPLASTIC LESIONS OF VERTEBRAL BODIES ON MAGNETIC RESONANCE IMAGING

Condition	Imaging Findings	Comments
Degenerative disk disease		Marrow signal intensity abnormalities have been reported in up to 50% of intervertebral levels showing degenerative disk changes.
Type I **(Fig SP22-1)**	Decreased signal intensity on T_1-weighted images and increased signal intensity on T_2-weighted images.	Associated with local replacement of normal cellular marrow with vascularized fibrous tissue. Tends to convert to type II lesions over time.
Type II **(Fig SP22-2)**	Increased signal intensity on T_1-weighted images and slightly increased signal intensity on T_2-weighted images.	Associated with local fatty replacement of marrow. Type I and II changes are thought to represent a continuum in the response of adjacent marrow to degenerative disk disease.
Type III **(Fig SP22-3)**	Decreased signal intensity on both T_1- and T_2-weighted images.	Least common pattern that probably represents bone sclerosis or fibrosis adjacent to the end plate.
Schmorl's node **(Fig SP22-4)**	Continuous with the disk and of identical signal intensity.	Superior or inferior displacement of disk material through a cartilaginous and osseous end plate. Large lesions must be differentiated from metastases or infection on the basis of their sharp margins, low intensity of their rims, and association with narrowed disk spaces.
Compression fracture **Subacute** **(Fig SP22-5)**	Decreased signal intensity on T_1-weighted images and increased signal intensity on T_2-weighted images.	Cannot reliably differentiate between simple osteoporotic and pathologic fractures on the basis of signal intensity alone. Findings that suggest neoplasm include a large soft-tissue mass, destruction of bone cortex, and involvement of multiple levels. One clear indication of metastases is the presence of another lesion with similar signal characteristics at a nonfractured vertebral level.
Chronic (healed) **(Fig SP22-5)**	Signal intensity varies with the underlying cause.	In simple osteoporotic disease, the signal intensity of the marrow generally returns to normal on all sequences. Pathologic fractures secondary to metastatic disease usually are hypointense to marrow on T_1-weighted images and hyperintense on T_2-weighted images.

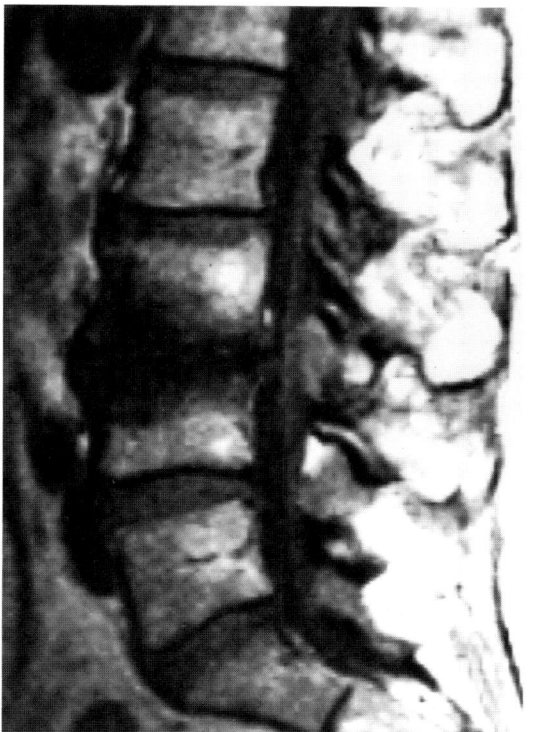
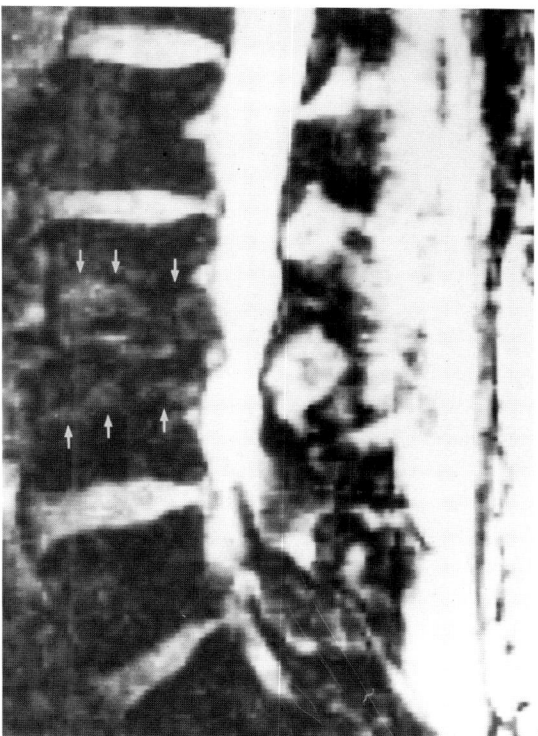

FIG SP22-1. Degenerative disk disease (type I changes). (A) Sagittal T_1-weighted image shows a broad area of decreased signal intensity adjacent to the L3-4 disk. (B) Gradient echo image shows mildly increased signal intensity (arrows) in the corresponding area.[11]

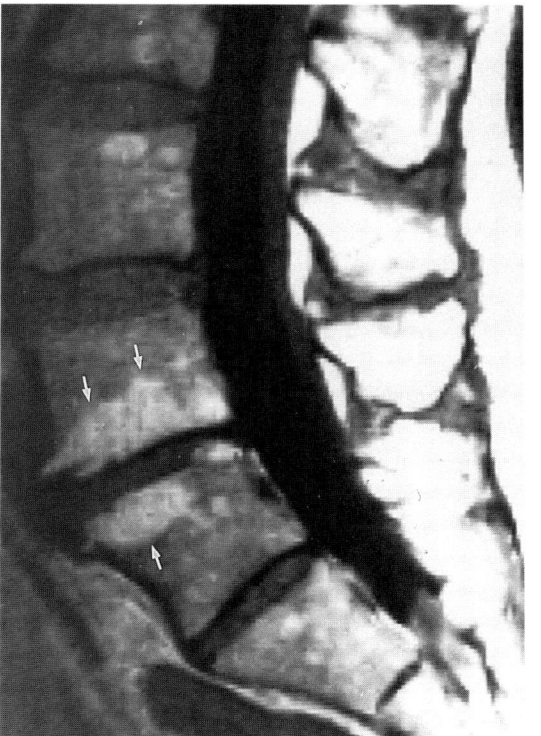
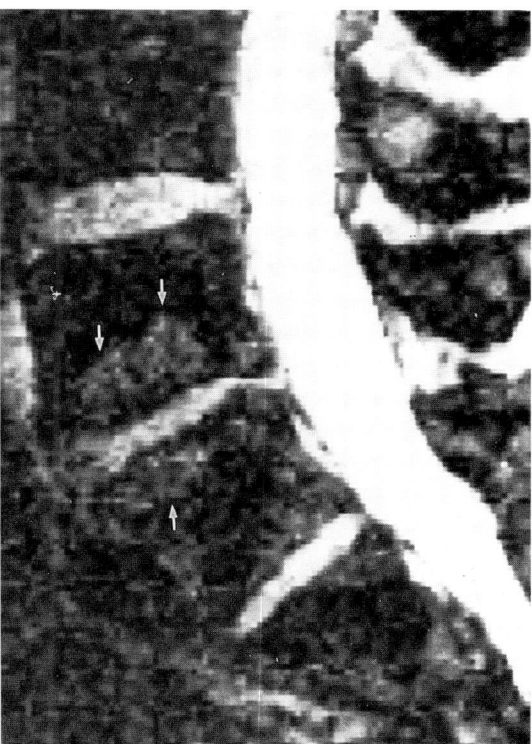

FIG SP22-2. Degenerative disk disease (type II changes). (A) Sagittal T_1-weighted image shows a sharply marginated area of increased signal intensity (arrows) adjacent to a narrowed disk space. (B) On the T_2-weighted image, this area has a slightly increased signal intensity.[13]

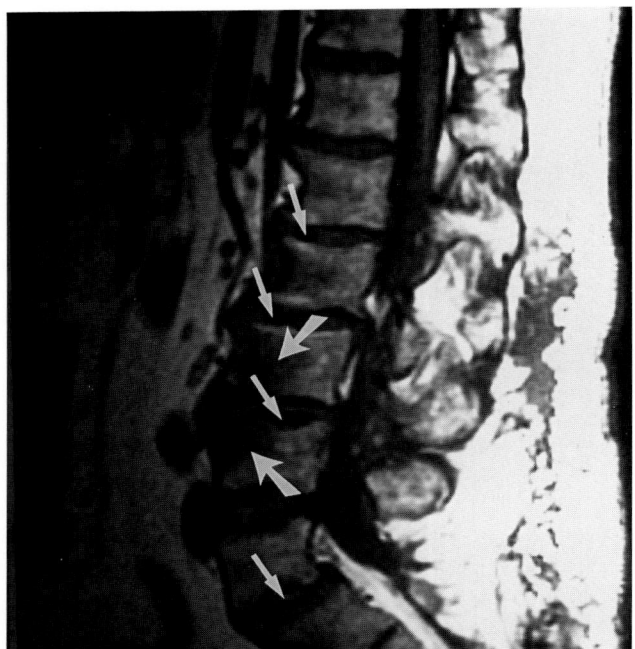

A

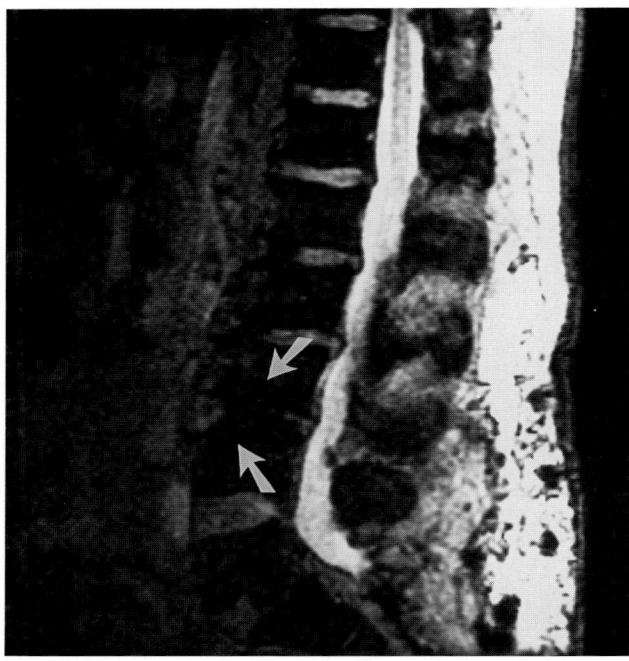

B

FIG SP22-3. **Degenerative disk disease (type III changes).** (A) Sagittal T$_1$-weighted image shows ill-defined zones of decreased signal intensity within the end plates adjacent to the L3-4 intervertebral disk (thick arrows). (Thin arrows indicate lumbar interspaces.) (B) On the T$_2$-weighted image, these end plates become isointense with normal marrow (arrows).[12]

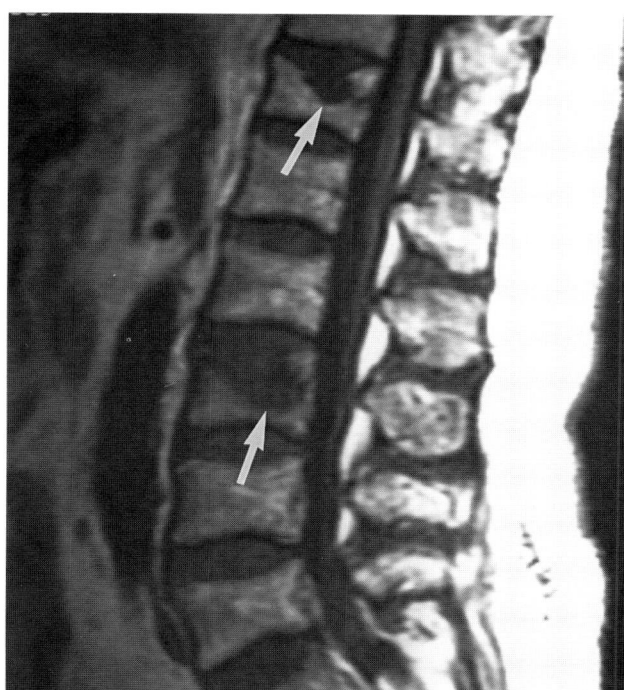

FIG SP22-4. Schmorl's nodes. Central herniation of disk material through the superior end plates of T12 and L3 (arrows).[12]

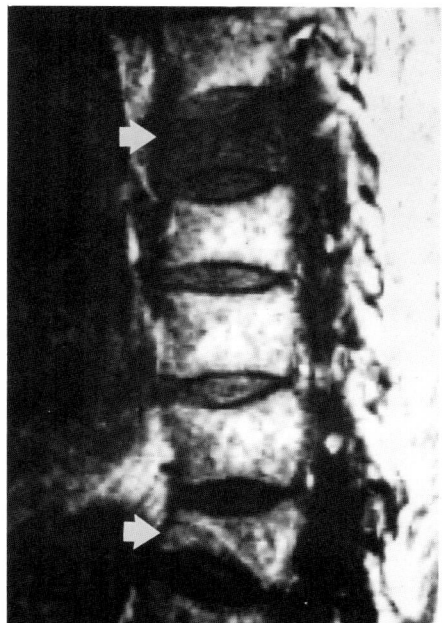

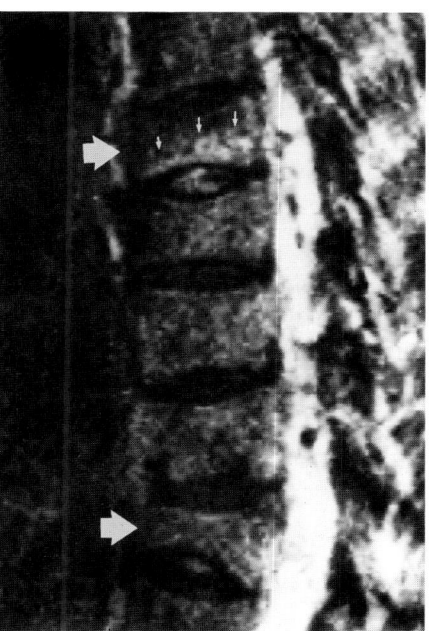

FIG SP22-5. Compression fractures (subacute and chronic). Sagittal (A) T_1-weighted and (B) T_2-weighted images show anterior compression deformities (wedging) of the T7 and T11 vertebral bodies (large arrows). The signal intensity of the marrow is normal at T11, indicating a healed chronic compression fracture. At T7, the signal intensity of the marrow is decreased on the T_1-weighted image and slightly increased on the T_2-weighted image in a linear, heterogeneous fashion (small arrows, B), consistent with a subacute compression fracture.[13]

Condition	Imaging Findings	Comments
Infection **(Fig SP22-6)**	Involved marrow shows decreased signal intensity on T_1-weighted images and increased signal intensity on T_2-weighted images.	Generally associated with a narrowed disk that on T_2-weighted images has increased signal intensity, unlike the decreased signal intensity seen with disk degeneration.
Radiation therapy **(Fig SP22-7)**	On T_1-weighted images, characteristic high signal intensity involving multiple contiguous vertebral bodies.	Areas of abnormal signal intensity reflect progressive fatty degeneration of bone marrow in a region corresponding to the radiation port.
Focal fatty infiltration	Focal area or areas of increased signal intensity on T_1-weighted images. On T_2-weighted images, the area(s) have signal intensity equal to or slightly higher than normal bone marrow (but substantially less than CSF).	Common phenomenon in both sexes after age 30. Must not be confused with metastases.

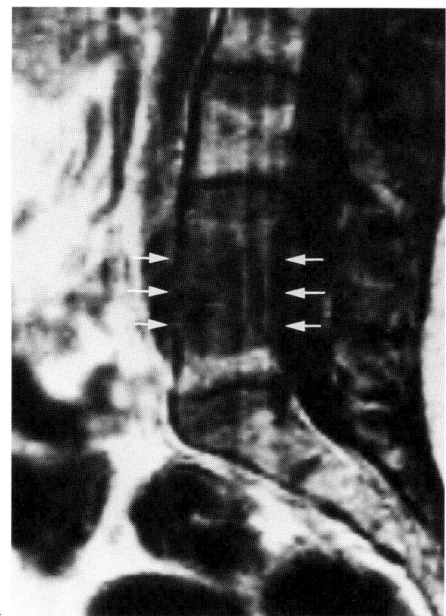
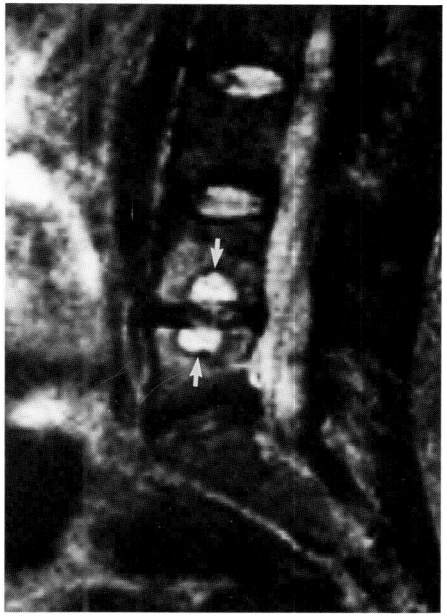

Fig SP22-6. Infection. (A) Sagittal T_1-weighted image shows a large area of decreased signal intensity involving both sides of the L4-5 disk space. The boundaries between the disks and the end plates are obliterated (arrows). (B) T_2-weighted image shows sharply marginated areas of increased signal intensity (arrows) adjacent to the disk, which shows mottled, irregular signal characteristics.[13]

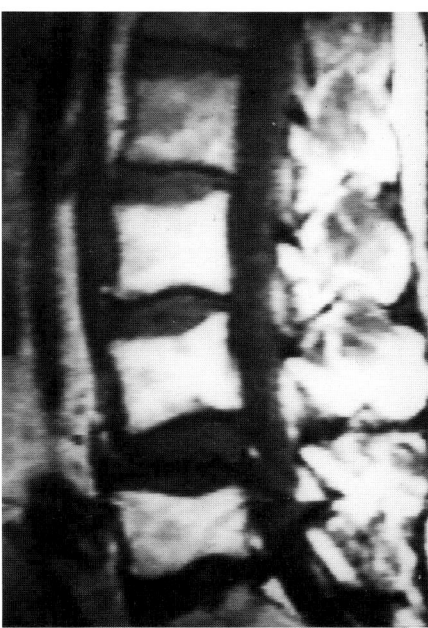

Fig SP22-7. Radiation therapy. Axial T_1-weighted image in a patient after radiation therapy for a plasmacytoma of L4 shows the typically increased signal intensity from L2, L3, L4, and the inferior aspect of L1, consistent with fatty replacement of bone marrow in a distribution corresponding to the radiation therapy port.[13]

NEOPLASTIC LESIONS OF VERTEBRAE ON MAGNETIC RESONANCE IMAGING

Condition	Imaging Findings	Comments
Hemangioma **(Fig SP23-1)**	Increased signal intensity on both T_1- and T_2-weighted images.	Benign vascular tumor that is usually an incidental finding. MRI can show paravertebral and epidural extension of tumor, which lacks adipose tissue and thus appears isointense on T_1-weighted images.
Osteochondroma	Heterogeneous appearance with the cartilaginous components of increased signal intensity on T_2-weighted images, whereas the osteoid or calcified portions have low signal intensity.	Primarily involves the posterior elements, especially the spinous processes. Rapid growth is an ominous sign. Factors favoring a benign lesion include cortical margins that are contiguous with the adjacent bone, well-defined lobular surfaces, lack of adjacent bone involvement, and a thin cartilaginous cap (usually less than 1 cm).
Osteoid osteoma	Heterogeneous appearance with the calcification within the nidus and the surrounding bony sclerosis having low signal intensity on all sequences, whereas the noncalcified portion of the nidus itself has increased signal intensity on T_2-weighted images.	Intense enhancement of the highly vascular nidus, which not only helps to localize the nidus but also aids in differentiating the lesion from a nonenhancing process such as a Brodie's abscess.
Osteoblastoma **(Fig SP23-2)**	High signal intensity on T_2-weighted images. Intense contrast enhancement.	May have an inhomogeneous appearance if there is hemorrhage or calcification.
Aneurysmal bone cyst **(Fig SP23-3)**	Expansile lesion of the posterior elements, often with internal septations and lobulations, that frequently has a thin, well-defined rim of low signal intensity.	A characteristic appearance is multiple fluid-fluid levels that can have varying signal intensities on the basis of hemorrhage of different ages within the large anastomosing blood-filled cavernous spaces of the lesion.
Giant cell tumor **(Fig SP23-4)**	Expansile lesion of low signal intensity on T_1-weighted images and increased signal intensity on T_2-weighted images.	Unenhanced scans show tumor displacing normal bright marrow fat, whereas contrast enhancement can separate tumor from adjacent normal structures.

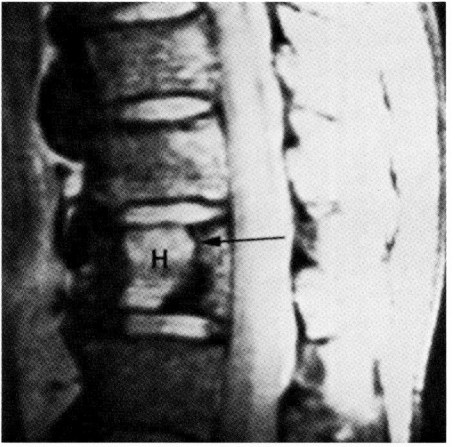

FIG SP23-1. Hemangioma. Sagittal proton-density image shows a high-signal lesion (H) within a lower thoracic vertebral body. The lesion is well defined, and a discrete cortical margin is evident posteriorly (arrow).[17]

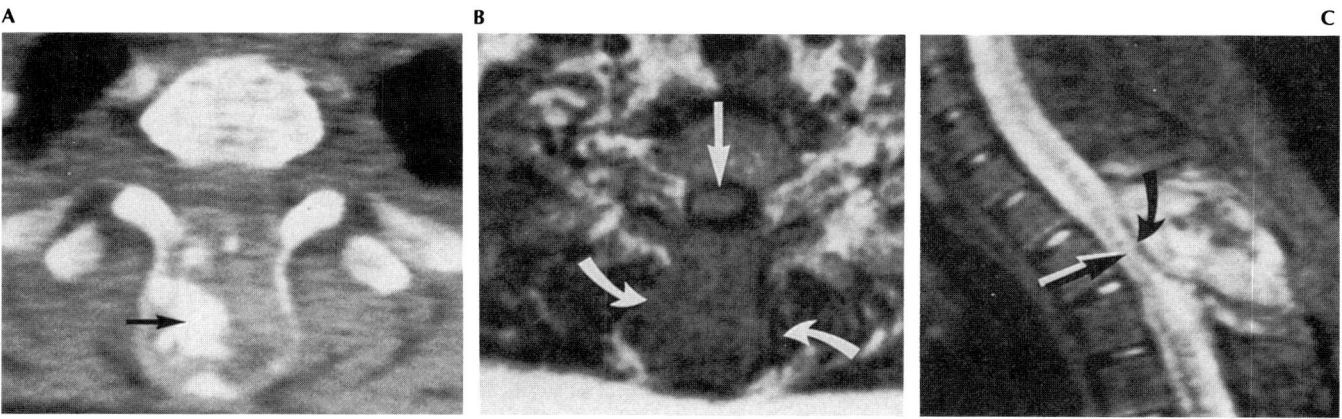

FIG SP23-2. **Osteoblastoma.** (A) Axial CT scan shows an expanded spinous process of T2 with internal amorphous calcifications (arrow). The anterior extent of the tumor and its relationship with the cord cannot be established. (B) Axial T_1-weighted and (C) midline sagittal T_2-weighted images show the cord (straight arrows) and its relationship with the tumor (curved arrows in B). Note the partial obliteration of the posterior subarachnoid space (curved arrow in C) on the sagittal image.[18]

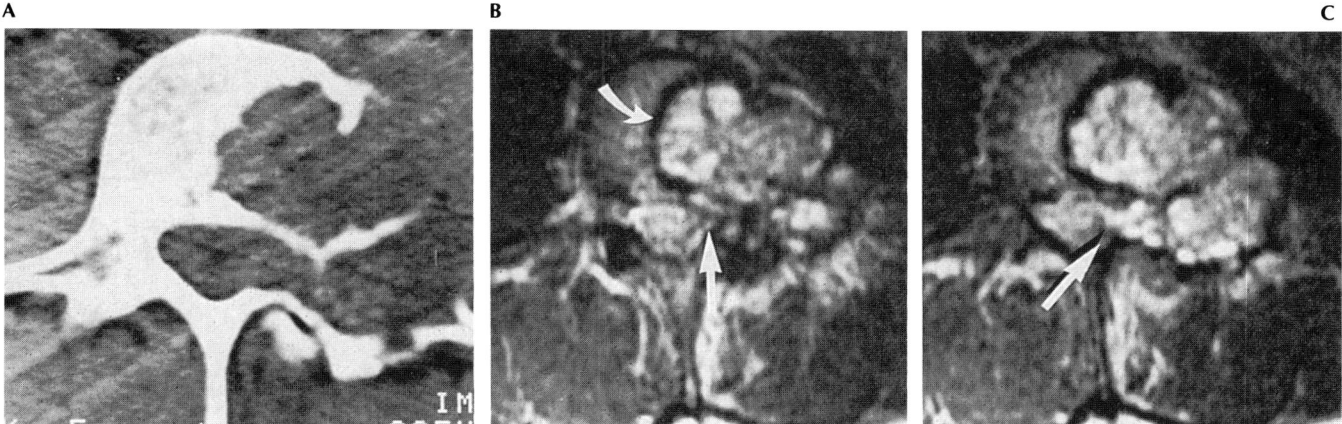

FIG SP23-3. **Aneurysmal bone cyst.** (A) Axial CT scan shows osseous extension of the tumor but cannot evaluate possible spinal canal invasion. (B) Axial T_2-weighted image shows the relationship between the tumor and the thecal sac (straight arrows). Note the bubbly appearance of the tumor, with small cysts of different signal intensity. (C) Left parasagittal proton-density image shows the superior extension of the tumor into the spinal canal (straight arrows). Note the band of decreased signal intensity (curved arrow in B) between the tumor and vertebral body, representing the rim of sclerosis.[18]

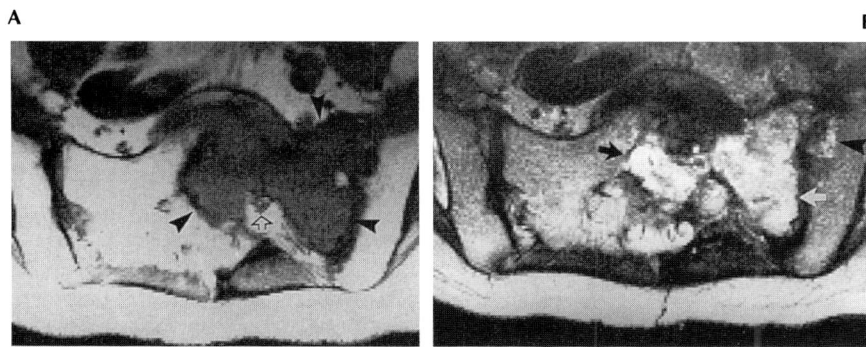

FIG SP23-4. **Giant cell tumor.** (A) Axial T_1-weighted image shows tumor (arrowheads) replacing normal marrow fat in the left sacral ala and body of S1. Tumor surrounds the neural canal containing the first left ventral sacral nerve root (arrow). (B) On the T_2-weighted image, the tumor (arrows) is inhomogeneous and of intermediate signal intensity. Note the tumor extension (arrowhead) across the left sacroiliac joint.[19]

Condition	Imaging Findings	Comments
Sacrococcygeal teratoma (Fig SP23-5)	Pelvic mass adjacent to the coccyx that often contains cystic components and has variable intensity patterns. After injection of contrast material, solid portions of the tumor enhance.	Rare childhood tumor arising from multipotential cells of Hensen's node that migrate to lie within the coccyx. Cystic components generally have low signal intensity on T_1-weighted images and are of increased signal intensity on T_2-weighted images, though they may have different intensities if they contain hemorrhage.
Eosinophilic granuloma (Fig SP23-6)	Lytic process, frequently with vertebral collapse, that has decreased signal intensity on T_1-weighted images and increased signal intensity on T_2-weighted images.	MRI can well delineate any spinal cord compression resulting from vertebral collapse or an associated epidural hematoma. The lesion may be difficult to differentiate from metastatic disease.
Chordoma (Fig SP23-7)	Isointense or hypointense to spinal cord on T_1-weighted images. High signal intensity on T_2-weighted images.	Frequently has internal septations and a surrounding capsule of low signal intensity. May contain areas of hemorrhage and cystic change. Although CT is superior for showing bone destruction or calcification, MRI better shows any epidural disease.
Primary malignant tumors (Fig SP23-8)	Destructive lesions that have decreased signal intensity on T_1-weighted images and increased signal intensity on T_2-weighted images.	Osteosarcoma, chondrosarcoma, Ewing's sarcoma. Leukemia and lymphoma can present an identical appearance, as can metastatic carcinoma.

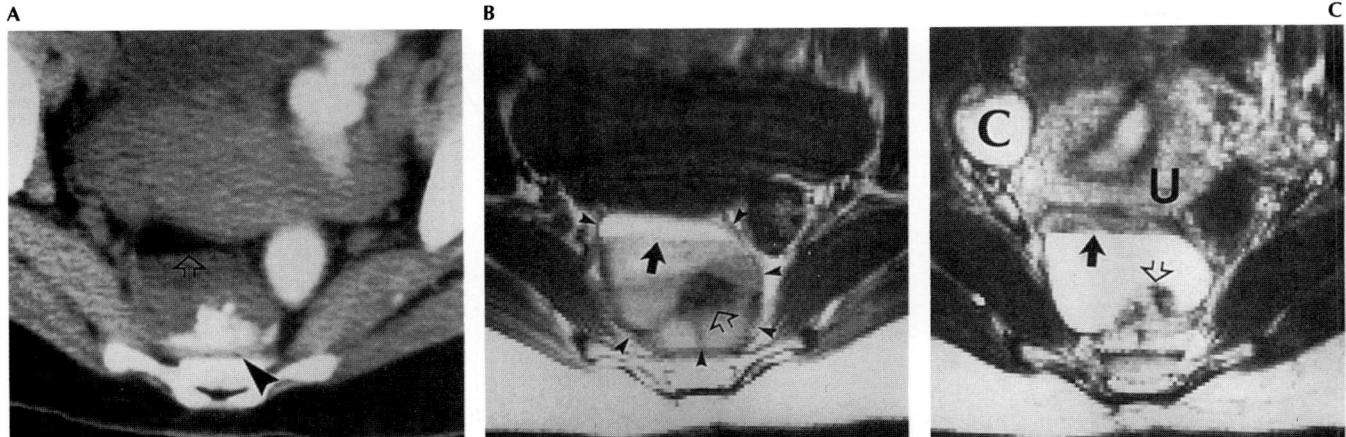

FIG SP23-5. Sacral teratoma. (A) CT scan shows a presacral mass without evidence of sacral erosion. Note the posterior calcification (arrowhead) and fat-fluid level (arrow) in the lesion. (B) Axial T_1-weighted MR scan shows the presacral mass (arrowheads). The high-intensity fat (solid arrow) is layering on the lower-intensity fluid in the lesion. The low intensity area posteriorly (open arrow) represents calcification. (C) On the T_2-weighted image, the signal intensities have reversed at the fat-fluid interface (solid arrow). The posterior calcification (open arrow) remains of low intensity. C = ovarian cyst; U = uterus.[19]

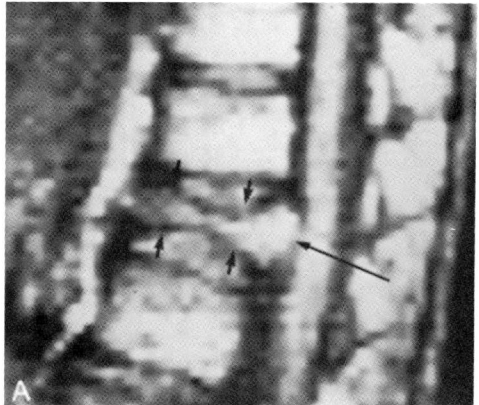 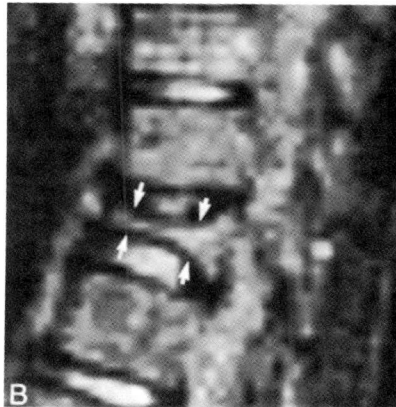

FIG SP23-6. Eosinophilic granuloma. (A) T₁-weighted and (B) proton-density sagittal images demonstrate compression deformity (vertebra plana) of the T11 vertebral body (short arrows). Soft tissue (long arrow) also projects posteriorly into the ventral epidural space. The intervertebral disks are not involved.[17]

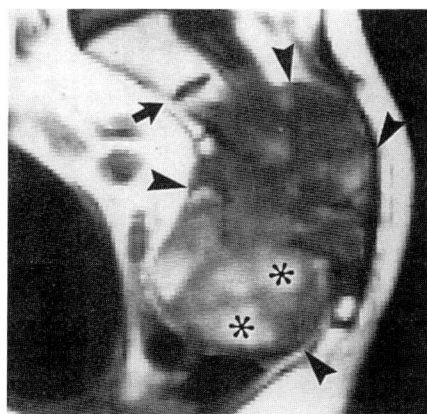

FIG SP23-7. Chordoma. Sagittal T₁-weighted scan shows an extensive neoplasm (arrowheads) with obliteration of the sacral canal and presacral and postsacral extension. Note preservation of the S1-S2 disk (arrow), which indicates potential for radical resection. High-intensity areas in the neoplasm (asterisks) represented areas of hemorrhage.[19]

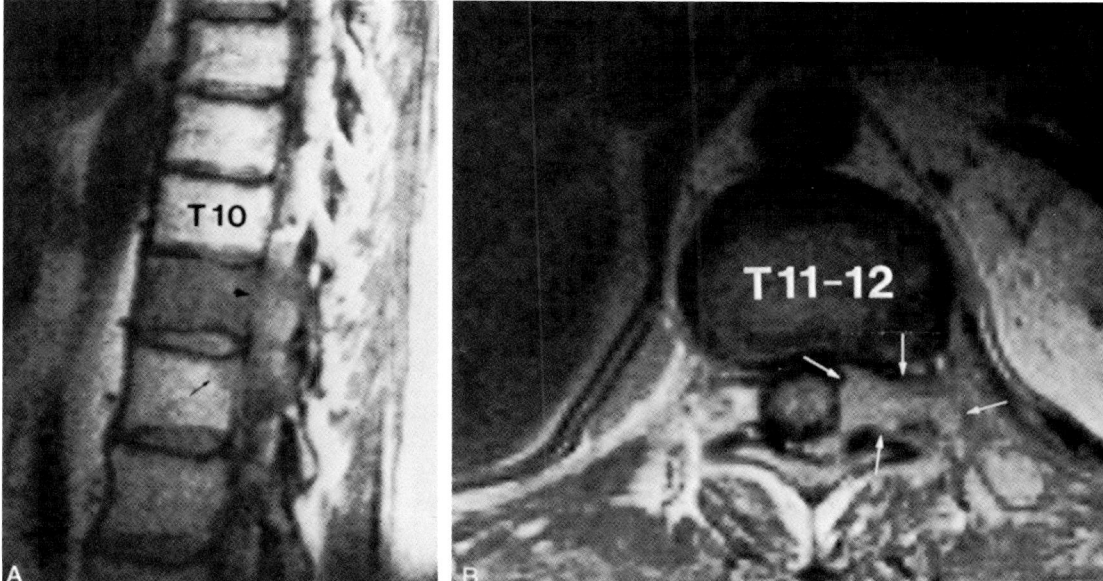

FIG SP23-8. Lymphoma. (A) Parasagittal T₁-weighted image shows tumor replacement of much of the normal marrow of the T11 vertebral body. The tumor has broken through the cortex posteriorly (arrowhead) to displace the high-signal epidural fat. Note that the posterosuperior portion of T12 has decreased signal intensity consistent with tumor involvement (small arrow). (B) Axial T₁-weighted scan through the T11-T12 foramen shows tumor infiltration (arrows) into the left epidural space, compressing the left side of the thecal sac and filling the left neural foramen.[17]

POSTOPERATIVE LUMBAR REGION OF SPINE ON MAGNETIC RESONANCE IMAGING

Condition	Imaging Findings	Comments
Herniated disk (Fig SP24-1)	Hypointense or isointense to disk (on T_1-weighted images) and contiguous with it. No contrast enhancement.	May show some delayed enhancement 30 to 60 minutes after injection, though not to the same degree as a scar. The perimeter of a disk may enhance because of the development of vascular granulation tissue surrounding it.
Epidural fibrosis (scar) (Fig SP24-2)	Hypointense or isointense to disk on T_1-weighted images. Often linear and extending above or below level of disk. Conforms to epidural space, and tends to retract thecal sac. Intense contrast enhancement.	Enhancing scar occasionally may obscure tiny disk fragments or cause underestimation of disk size. Must not be confused with normal epidural venous plexus and dorsal root ganglia that also show contrast enhancement. Distinction of postoperative scar from recurrent herniated disk is critical because second operation of scar generally leads to a poor surgical result, as opposed to removal of a reherniated disk.
Arachnoiditis (Fig SP24-3)	Centrally clumped (intradural pseudomass) or peripheral adherent nerve roots (empty thecal sac). Mild contrast enhancement.	Best detected on T_2-weighted images because of high contrast between hyperintense CSF and low-intensity signal of the nerves. Extensive clumping of nerves may make it difficult to determine where the spinal cord ends and the cauda equina begins.
Infection	Mass that is hypointense on T_1-weighted images and of increased signal intensity on T_2-weighted images.	Because of its high soft-tissue sensitivity, MRI can detect changes in the disk, adjacent end plates, and bone marrow, whereas plain radiographs and radionuclide scans are still negative.
Hematoma	Usually an epidural mass containing material that has varying signal characteristics depending on the stage of its hemorrhagic contents.	Patient generally presents with a neurologic deficit in the immediate postoperative period.

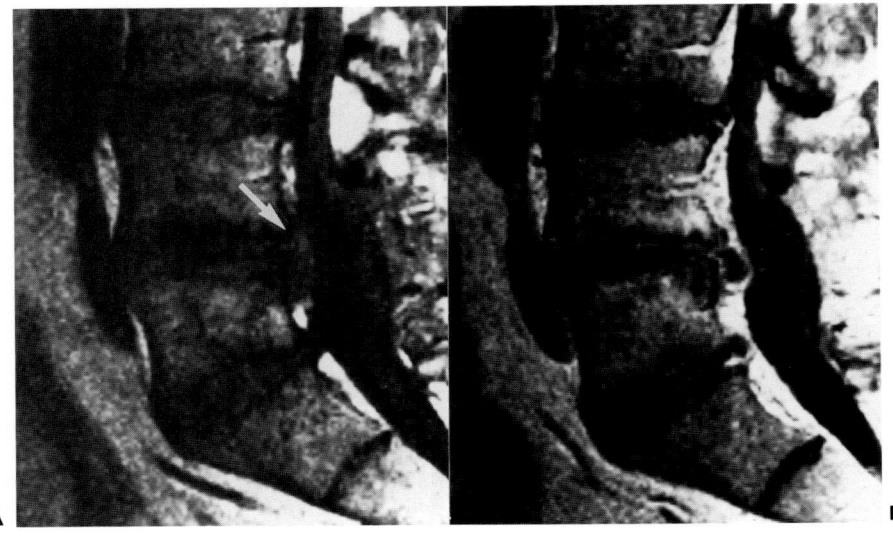

A   B

FiG SP24-1. Herniated disk. (A) Sagittal T_1-weighted precontrast image shows a very ill-defined anterior epidural soft-tissue mass at the L4-L5 level (arrow), with slight mass effect on the anterior thecal sac. Differentiation of scar from disk is not possible. (B) Repeat scan after intravenous injection of contrast material clearly defines the central nonenhancing herniation surrounded by enhancing scar tissue.[14]

Condition	Imaging Findings	Comments
Pseudomeningocele	Well-circumscribed mass posterior to the thecal sac that is of CSF density (hypointense on T_1-weighted images and hyperintense on T_2-weighted images).	Usually does not produce symptoms until weeks or months after surgery. Caused by a small dural tear at the time of surgery that allows progressive herniation of the arachnoid membrane or produces a CSF leak into adjacent soft tissues.

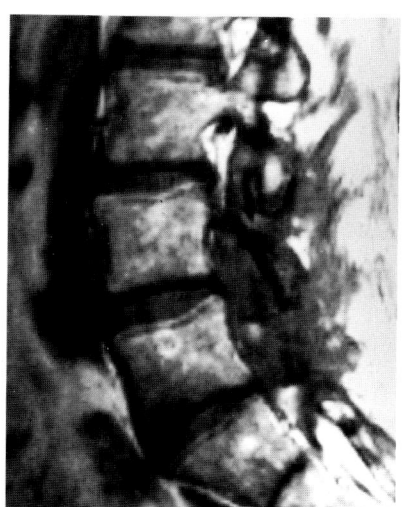
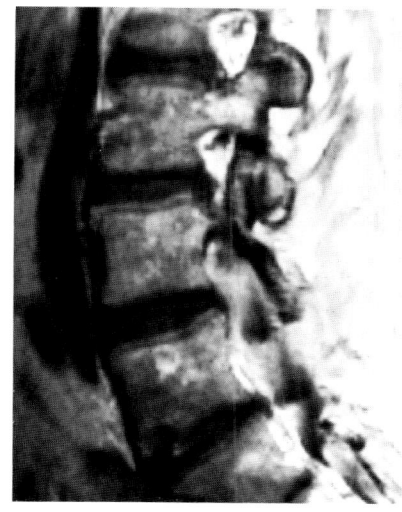

FIG SP24-2. Epidural scar. (A) Sagittal T_1-weighted precontrast image shows a large amount of abnormal tissue within the epidural space at the L4-L5 through L5-S1 levels. (B) Repeat scan after intravenous injection of contrast material demonstrates diffuse and intense enhancement throughout the epidural tissue, consistent with scar.[14]

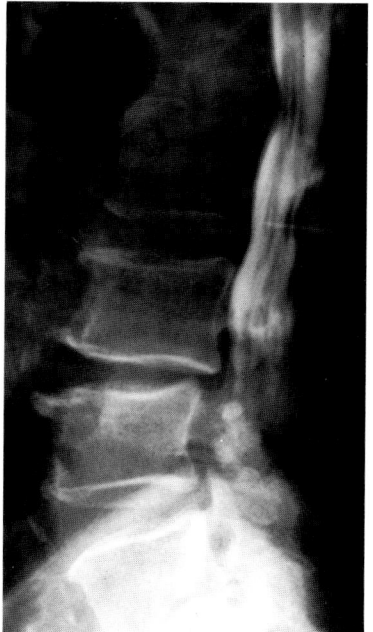
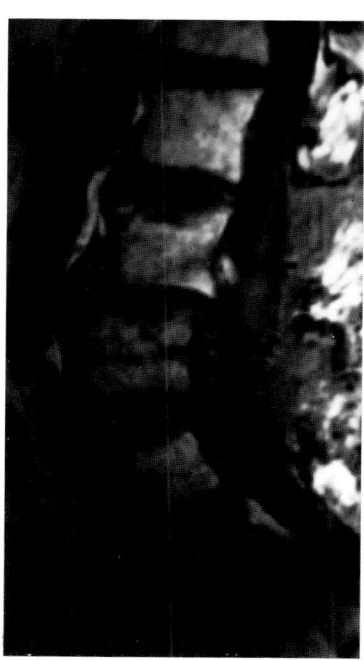
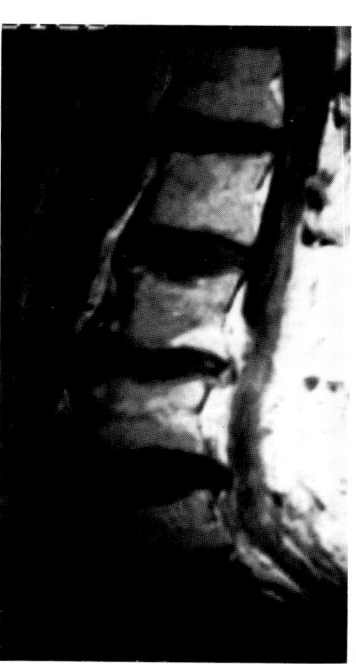

FIG SP24-3. Arachnoiditis. (A) Lateral view of a lumbar myelogram shows irregular collection of contrast within the most distally filled aspect of the thecal sac, thickened nerve roots, and a block at L3-L4. Sagittal precontrast (B) and postcontrast (C) T_1-weighted images were performed. After contrast infusion there is inhomogeneous, amorphous enhancement of the contents of the thecal sac. Note also the marked enhancement of the postoperative scar posterior to the thecal sac at the site of previous laminectomy, and enhancement of the epidural venous plexus or postoperative scar (or both) posterior to the L3 and L4 vertebral bodies.[15]

DEMYELINATING AND INFLAMMATORY DISEASE OF THE SPINAL CORD ON MAGNETIC RESONANCE IMAGING

Condition	Imaging Findings	Comments
Multiple sclerosis (Fig SP25-1)	Areas of increased signal on T_2-weighted images. In acute stage, there may be associated swelling of the spinal cord, which can mimic an intramedullary neoplasm. In late disease, the cord may become atrophic.	Enhancement of spinal cord lesions appears to correlate with active disease. In about one third of patients with multiple sclerosis who present clinically with myelopathy, no associated periventricular lesions can be detected on MR scans of the brain.
Transverse myelitis (Fig SP25-2)	Increased intramedullary signal on T_2-weighted images in a cord that may be of normal or slightly expanded caliber. The abnormal signal may extend above the level of clinical deficit. Mild contrast enhancement may occur.	Rapidly progressing myelopathy that occurs in the absence of any known neurologic disease. It has been associated with viral illness, vasculitides (such as lupus), vaccinations, and multiple sclerosis. In patients who recover, follow-up MR scans may demonstrate resolution of the abnormal signal and return of the cord to a normal caliber.
Acquired immunodeficiency syndrome (AIDS)–related myelopathy (Fig SP25-3)	Various patterns may occur. The study may be normal or show areas of increased signal intensity on T_2-weighted images that are indistinguishable from transverse myelitis due to other causes. Some contrast enhancement may occur.	In addition to other cerebral neurologic complications, persons with AIDS may experience a vacuolar myelopathy that is probably related to direct injury to the neurons by the HIV virus. Demyelination of the posterior and lateral columns resembling subacute combined degeneration also occurs.

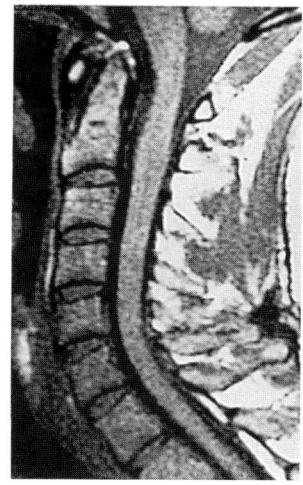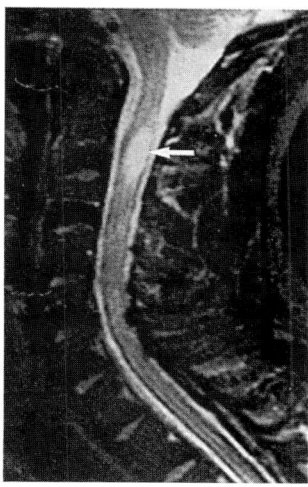

A   B

FIG SP25-1. Multiple sclerosis. (A) T_1-weighted and (B) T_2-weighted sagittal images show focal enlargement of the cord at the C2 level that demonstrates high signal intensity (arrow, B).[16]

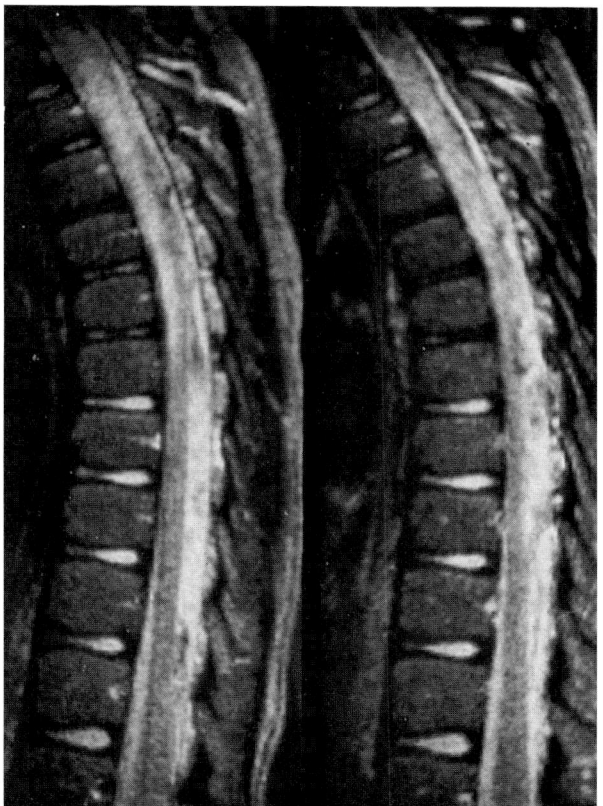

FIG SP25-2. Transverse myelitis. T_2-weighted sagittal images in a young boy with rapid onset of back pain and paraplegia 3 weeks after a viral illness show diffuse increased signal intensity in the cord, consistent with edema.[16]

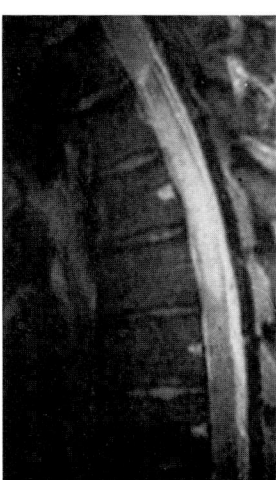

FIG SP25-3. AIDS-related myelopathy. T_2-weighted sagittal image demonstrates high intramedullary signal in a somewhat swollen area of the thoracic cord.[16]

Condition	Imaging Findings	Comments
Postradiation myelitis	Depending on the time elapsed since radiation, the cord may appear normal, atrophic, or enlarged. Lesions may have increased signal intensity on T_2-weighted images and may show contrast enhancement.	The effects of radiation for the treatment of an intramedullary neoplasm may be difficult to differentiate from tumor. Radiation also produces fatty replacement of vertebral body marrow that results in a characteristic high signal intensity on T_1-weighted images.
Sarcoidosis (Figs SP25-4 and SP25-5)	Enhancing intramedullary or pial lesion that is usually not evident on standard spin echo scans.	Although clinical involvement of the CNS occurs in 5% of patients with sarcoidosis, primary involvement is very rare. The involvement may be intramedullary or extramedullary (or both). Pial enhancement is not pathognomonic because it can be seen with tuberculous, toxoplasmic, or HIV-related meningitis; leptomeningeal metastases; and postshunting meningeal fibrosis.

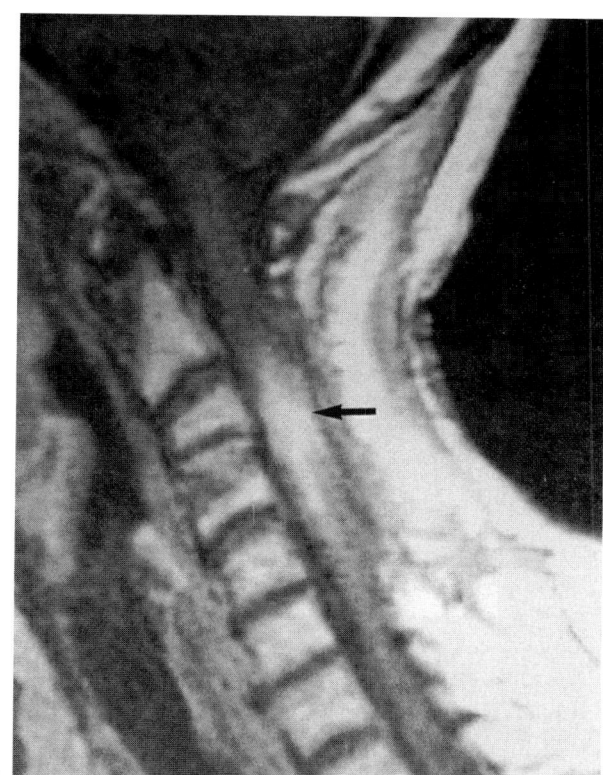

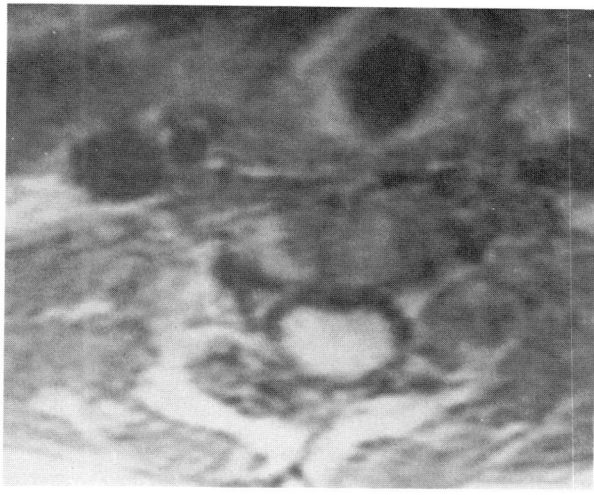

FIG SP25-4. Intramedullary sarcoidosis. (A) Sagittal and (B) axial T_1-weighted images after injection of contrast material show an enhancing intramedullary mass (arrow, A) indistinguishable from a glioma.[16]

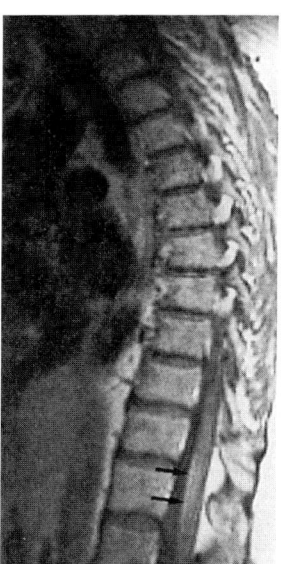

FIG SP25-5. Pial sarcoidosis. T_1-weighted axial image of the thoracic region of the spine after injection of contrast material demonstrates pial enhancement along the conus (arrows). The patient's bilateral lower extremity numbness resolved following steroid therapy.[16]

CONGENITAL ANOMALIES OF THE SPINE ON MAGNETIC RESONANCE IMAGING

Condition	Imaging Findings	Comments
Tethered cord syndrome (Fig SP26-1)	Caudal displacement of the conus below the L2-L3 level in neonates and young children or below the middle of L2 after age 12.	Clinically presents with motor and sensory dysfunction of the lower extremities (unrelated to myotomal or dermatomal pattern), muscle atrophy, decreased or hyperactive reflexes, urinary incontinence, spastic gait, scoliosis, or foot deformities. Causes include lipomatous lesions (intramedullary lipomas, lipomyelomeningoceles, lipoma of the filum terminale); myelomeningocele; diastematomyelia; and a short, thickened filum terminale (>2 m).
Syringomyelia/hydromyelia (Fig SP26-2)	Fusiform widening of the spinal cord, which contains a dilated central cavity filled with CSF-intensity material.	Usually associated with the Chiari I malformation. In adults without this malformation, syringomyelia/hydromyelia suggests the presence of a spinal cord tumor.
Failure of fusion of posterior elements (Fig SP26-3)	Various patterns of posterior protrusion of meninges, neural elements, and fat through a midline bony defect.	Meningocele; myelomeningocele (usually with Chiari II malformation); lipomyelomeningocele.
Diastematomyelia (Fig SP26-4)	Longitudinal splitting of the spinal cord.	Often occurs in association with a bony or fibrous spur (best seen on plain films or CT) that divides the cord and may cause tethering.
Dorsal dermal sinus	Single or double low-intensity line extending downward and inward from the skin through the subcutaneous tissue. If present, the dermoid/epidermoid lesion can be clearly delineated.	Epithelial tract connecting the spinal canal with the skin of the back (most commonly the sacrococcygeal or lumbar region). About half terminate in an epidermoid or dermoid lesion (about 25% of dermoids are associated with dermal sinuses). Clinically, the sinus most frequently appears as a pinpoint hole or a small atrophic zone in the skin. A tuft of short, small, wiry hairs may emerge from the ostium.

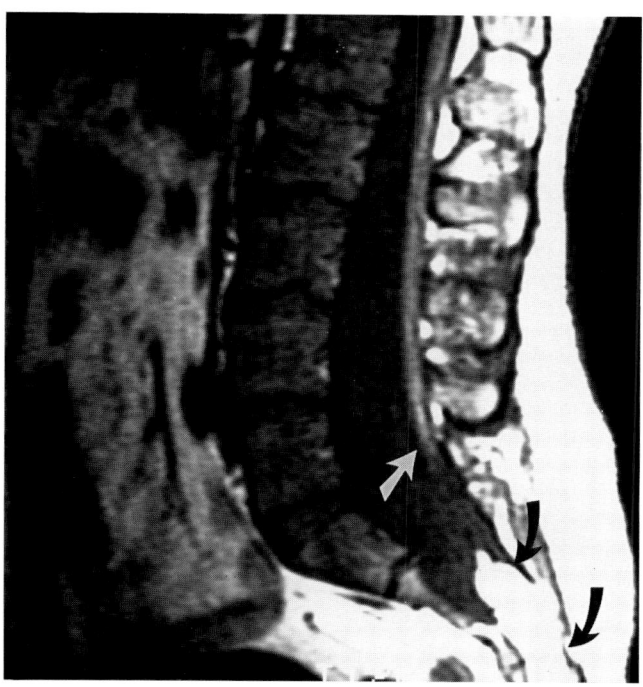

FIG SP26-1. Tethered cord syndrome. Sagittal T_1-weighted image in a patient who had undergone a myelomeningocele repair at birth shows that the cord ends at the L5 level (straight arrow). Note the absence of the posterior elements of the sacrum, as well as the presence of a high-signal-intensity mass (lipoma) within the sacral spinal canal (curved arrows).[12]

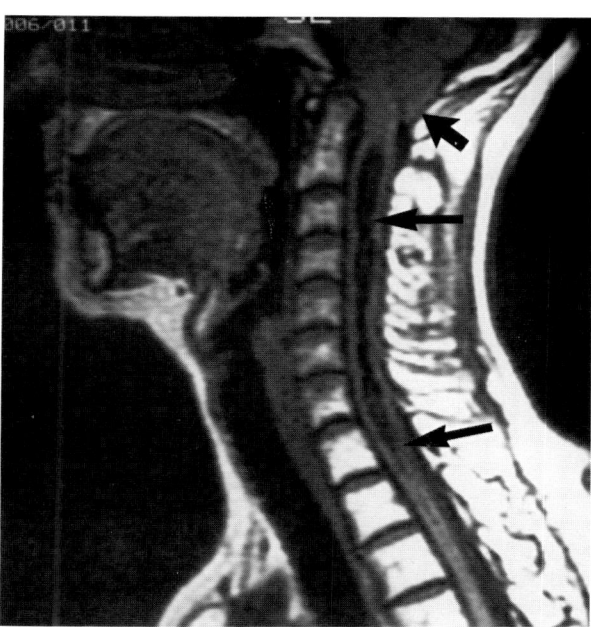

FIG SP26-2. Syringomyelia in Chiari I malformation. Sagittal T_1-weighted image of the cervical region of the spine shows the characteristic low position of the cerebellar tonsils (short arrow). The intramedullary cord syrinx extends from C_2 to T_2 (long arrows).[12]

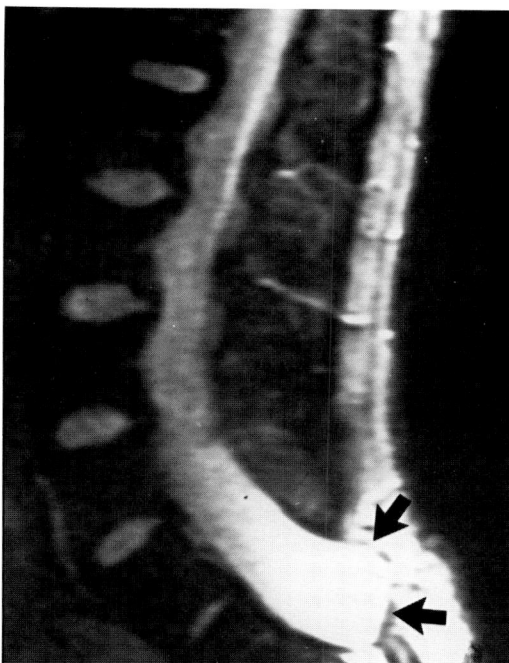

FIG SP26-3. Meningocele. Sagittal T_2-weighted image shows extension of the meninges and subarachnoid space through a bony defect in the upper sacrum (arrows).[12]

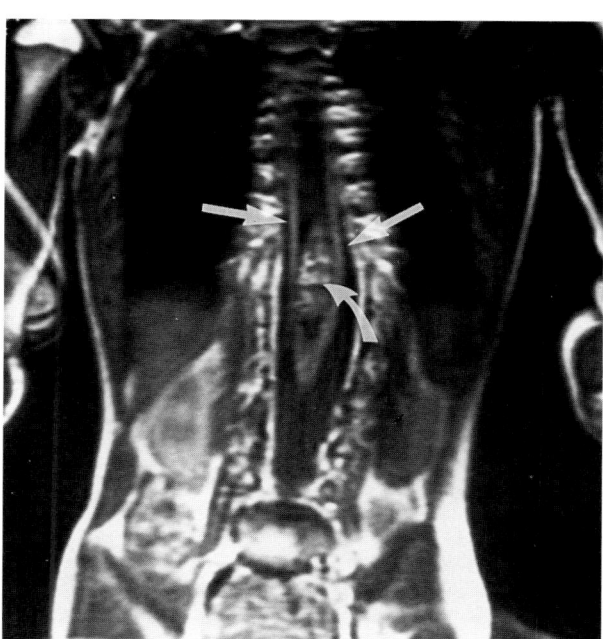

FIG SP26-4. Diastematomyelia. Coronal MR scan shows the two hemicords (arrows) separated by a bony spur that contains marrow (curved arrow). The hemicords unite inferior to the bony spur.[12]

SOURCES

1. Reprinted with permission from ''Radiologic Diagnosis of Metabolic Bone Disease'' by WA Reynolds and JJ Karo, *Orthopedic Clinics of North America* (1972;3:521–532), Copyright © 1972, WB Saunders Company.

2. Reprinted from *Diagnosis of Bone and Joint Disorders*, ed 2, by DL Resnick and G Niwayama, with permission of WB Saunders Company, © 1988.

3. Reprinted with permission from ''Benign Tumors'' by JW Beabout, RA McLeod, and DC Dahlin, *Seminars in Roentgenology* (1979;14:33–43), Copyright © 1979, Grune & Stratton Inc.

4. Reprinted from *Roentgen Diagnosis of Disease of Bone*, ed 3, by J Edeiken with permission of Williams & Wilkins Company, © 1981.

5. Reprinted from *Clinical Radiology in the Tropics* by WP Cockshott and H Middlemiss (Eds) with permission of Churchill Livingstone Inc, © 1979.

6. Reprinted with permission from ''The Radiologic Assessment of Short Stature'' by JP Dorst, CI Scott, and JG Hall, *Radiologic Clinics of North America* (1972;10:393–414), Copyright © 1972, WB Saunders Company.

7. Reprinted from *Radiology of Bone Diseases* by GB Greenfield, JB Lippincott Company, with permission of the author, © 1986.

8. Reprinted from *Caffey's Pediatric X-Ray Diagnosis*, ed 8, by FN Silverman with permission of Year Book Medical Publishers Inc., © 1985.

9. Reprinted with permission from ''Ghost Infantile Vertebrae and Hemipelves within Adult Skeletons from Thorotrast Administration in Childhood'' by JG Teplick et al, *Radiology* (1978;129:657–660), Copyright © 1978, Radiological Society of North America Inc.

10. Reprinted from *Introduction to Neuroradiology* by HO Peterson and SA Kieffer with permission of JB Lippincott Company, © 1972.

11. Reprinted with permission from ''Gd-DTPA–Enhanced MR Imaging of Spinal Tumors'' by BD Parizel et al, *AJR* (1989;152:1087–2020), Copyright © 1989, Williams & Wilkins Company.

12. Reprinted from *MRI of the Musculoskeletal System*, ed 2, by TH Berquist (Ed) with permission of Mayo Foundation, © 1990.

13. Reprinted with permission from ''Non-neoplastic Lesions of Vertebral Bodies: Findings in Magnetic Resonance Imaging'' by CW Hayes, ME Jensen, and WF Conway, *Radiographics* (1989;9:883–903), Copyright © 1989, Radiological Society of North America Inc.

14. Reprinted with permission from ''MR Imaging of the Postoperative Lumbar Spine: Assessment with Gadopentetate Dimeglumine'' by JS Ross, TJ Masaryk, M Schrader et al, *American Journal of Roentgenology* (1990;155:867–872), Copyright © 1990, American Roentgen Ray Society.

15. Reprinted with permission from ''Benign Lumbar Arachnoiditis: MR Imaging with Gadopentetate Dimeglumine'' by CE Johnson and G Sze, *American Journal of Roentgenology* (1990;155:873–880), Copyright © 1990, American Roentgen Ray Society.

16. Reprinted with permission from ''MRI of Infectious and Inflammatory Diseases of the Spine'' by AS Mark, *MRI Decisions* (1991;5:12–26), Copyright © 1991, PW Communications, International. All rights reserved.

17. Reprinted with permission from *Clinical Magnetic Resonance Imaging*, RR Edelman, JR Hesselink (Eds) Copyright © 1990, WB Saunders Company.

18. Reprinted with permission from ''Tumors of the osseous spine: staging with MR imaging versus CT'' by J Beltran, AM Noto, DW Chakeres, et al, *Radiology* (1987;162:565–569).

19. Reprinted with permission from ''MR Imaging of Sacral and Presacral Lesions'' by LH Wetzel, E Levine, *AJR* (1990;154:771–775).

Subject Index

**Library and Learning
Resources Center
Bergen Community College**
400 Paramus Road
Paramus, N.J. 07652-1595

Return Postage Guaranteed